'Brilliant, compelling, and thought-provoking.'

Christopher Bollas, PhD, *author of* The Shadow
of the Object *and* Being a Character

'I find *Gravitational Psyche* to be a book that manages to describe the phenomena constituting the analytic experience in an unusually delicate and
intelligent way. This is a rare event in the analytic world. It is a pleasure to
read.'

Thomas Ogden, MD, *author of* What Alive Means
and Coming to Life in the Consulting Room

'Taking the centrality of conflict, contradiction, and paradox in mental
life as his subject of investigation, Todd Anderson offers us a discourse
of astonishing range and depth. His approach integrates the perspectives
of classical psychoanalysis, contemporary intersubjectivity, and modern
Continental philosophy. The labyrinthine and near-mesmerizing syncre-
tism that marks his voice yields proposals that are thoughtful, convinc-
ing, and humane. Paradox is thus revealed to be integral, inevitable, and,
if held by unhurried attention, deeply instructive as well. This is a truly
meaningful addition to our current psychoanalytic literature!'

Salman Akhtar, MD, DLFAPA, *emeritus professor
of Psychiatry, Jefferson Medical College; training
and supervising analyst, Psychoanalytic
Center of Philadelphia*

'When you begin to read Todd Anderson's two-volume *Unstable Objects*,
one of the more remarkable debut efforts to appear in our psychoanalytic
literature, you will immediately feel, as I did when I first encountered this
work, that you are in the hands of a master, someone who thinks with
rare depth and grace, and whose writing is—what should I say?—simply
marvelous. It's not just that Anderson writes beautifully and with great
expressiveness. He does. But he also writes in a way that makes it virtually
effortless to read him, even when he addresses complex matters. As lovely
as it is, the writing is always transparent to the subject matter. Anderson's
modesty, simplicity, and quiet confidence allow him to approach profound psychoanalytic questions with great thoughtfulness. In the process,
he adds to our appreciation of the work of analytic writers, and others,
who have preceded him. Over and over again, the writing demands quo-
tation. You will find yourself trying to get people, especially people who
know psychoanalysis, to listen to the many passages that say something
in words that, once read, are irreplaceable. These books are special. They

constitute a kind of manifesto, a statement of the nature of psychoanalysis from Anderson's relational point of view. Do yourself a favor: Read them.'

Donnel B. Stern, PhD, *William Alanson White Institute; NYU Postdoctoral Program*

'This book doesn't simply present ideas; it evokes states of mind. The writing form itself becomes part of the witnessing process—recursive, atmospheric, and affectively alive. Todd Anderson carries forward a lineage of symbolic containment that allows what is fragile, unformulated, and reverent to be held without being prematurely resolved. This is a work of psychoanalysis as living process.'

Michael Eigen, PhD, *author of* The Psychoanalytic Mystic *and* The Sensitive Self

'Todd Anderson's new book makes me want to go back and rewrite everything I've ever published—not out of regret, but because of how deeply he integrates the loose ends of so many theorists we share and love. His work is a tour de force: richly lived in, deliberately untidy, and fiercely humane. Anderson writes not to our 'churches of reason,' but from within the clinical hour itself. He invites us to dwell in contradiction—not to interpret or resolve, but to inhabit. This is psychoanalysis at its most human: not aiming to fix, but to move, to dwell, to return home.'

Philip Ringstrom, PhD, *author of* A Relational Psychoanalytic Approach to Couples Psychotherapy

'Each practitioner must make psychoanalysis in their own idiom, personalizing theory to hold us as we reach for authenticity in clinical engagement. Todd Anderson offers original ways to understand the shapes and contours of the relationships we encounter as we try to make sense of the therapy that helps both us and our analysands.'

Susie Orbach, PhD, *author of* Fat Is a Feminist Issue *and featured in* Expanding Psychoanalysis: The Contributions of Susie Orbach *(edited by Brett Kahr)*

'A remarkable new voice has been added to the canon of contemporary psychoanalytic writing. With startling originality, Todd Anderson deconstructs the earliest expressions of subjectivity and the ways in which they can go awry. He finds ways to frame and elaborate theoretical material that is at once familiar yet his fresh and compelling insights encourage clinicians to look further. These volumes will become an essential addition to our professional libraries.'

Ghislaine Boulanger, PhD, *author of* Wounded
by Reality: Understanding *and*
Treating Adult Onset Trauma

Gravitational Psyche

Gravitational Psyche draws on ideas from physics, psychoanalysis, and philosophy, to propose a radical reframing of how subjectivity is structured and sustained.

What if the psyche, like the cosmos, is governed by invisible curves and recursive loops? Exploring how symbolic atmosphere, affective orbit, and curved epistemologies shape experience from the ground up, this volume integrates psychoanalytic theory with metaphors drawn from physics, nonduality, and recursive form. It develops a topological and recursive framework for analytic practice: the mind as a curved field, shaped by symbolic tension, relational mass, and recursive returns. Anderson presents the psyche not as a static structure but as a gravitational space, where repetition, collapse, and atmosphere reveal the curved nature of subjectivity. It further equips readers to orient, listen, and intervene where language thins, helping analysis preserve vitality without forcing premature coherence. This book offers readers a fresh vocabulary for working at the edge of symbolization.

Bridging theory and practice with vivid clinical illustrations, conceptual maps, and a study guide designed to support teaching and supervision, this book is key reading for all psychoanalysts and psychotherapists.

Todd Anderson, PhD, PsyD, is a psychoanalyst practicing in New York City. His work explores how dissociation and desire shape psychic survival, bringing together insights from object relations, relational psychoanalysis, and contemporary philosophy.

PSYCHOANALYSIS IN A NEW KEY
DONNEL STERN
Series Editor

When music is played in a new key, the melody does not change, but the notes that make up the composition do: change in the context of continuity, continuity that perseveres through change. Psychoanalysis in a New Key publishes books that share the aims psychoanalysts have always had, but that approach them differently. The books in the series are not expected to advance any particular theoretical agenda, although to this date most have been written by analysts from the Interpersonal and Relational orientations.

The most important contribution of a psychoanalytic book is the communication of something that nudges the reader's grasp of clinical theory and practice in an unexpected direction. Psychoanalysis in a New Key creates a deliberate focus on innovative and unsettling clinical thinking. Because that kind of thinking is encouraged by exploration of the sometimes surprising contributions to psychoanalysis of ideas and findings from other fields, Psychoanalysis in a New Key particularly encourages interdisciplinary studies. Books in the series have married psychoanalysis with dissociation, trauma theory, sociology, and criminology. The series is open to the consideration of studies examining the relationship between psychoanalysis and any other field—for instance, biology, literary and art criticism, philosophy, systems theory, anthropology, and political theory.

But innovation also takes place within the boundaries of psychoanalysis, and Psychoanalysis in a New Key therefore also presents work that reformulates thought and practice without leaving the precincts of the field. Books in the series focus, for example, on the significance of personal values in psychoanalytic practice, on the complex interrelationship between the analyst's clinical work and personal life, on the consequences for the clinical situation when patient and analyst are from different cultures, and on the need for psychoanalysts to accept the degree to which they knowingly satisfy their own wishes during treatment hours, often to the patient's detriment.

A full list of all titles in this series is available at: https://www.routledge.com/Psychoanalysis-in-a-New-Key-Book-Series/book-series/LEAPNKBS

Gravitational Psyche

Further Developments of the
Psychoanalysis of Unstable Objects

Todd Anderson

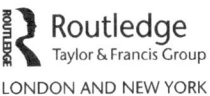
Routledge
Taylor & Francis Group

LONDON AND NEW YORK

Designed cover image: Getty Images

First published 2026
by Routledge
4 Park Square, Milton Park, Abingdon, Oxon OX14 4RN

and by Routledge
605 Third Avenue, New York, NY 10158

Routledge is an imprint of the Taylor & Francis Group, an informa business

© 2026 Todd Anderson

The right of Todd Anderson to be identified as author of this work has been asserted in accordance with sections 77 and 78 of the Copyright, Designs and Patents Act 1988.

For Product Safety Concerns and Information please contact our EU representative GPSR@taylorandfrancis.com. Taylor & Francis Verlag GmbH, Kaufingerstraße 24, 80331 München, Germany.

Trademark notice: Product or corporate names may be trademarks or registered trademarks, and are used only for identification and explanation without intent to infringe.

British Library Cataloguing-in-Publication Data
A catalogue record for this book is available from the British Library

ISBN: 9781041201519 (hbk)
ISBN: 9781041172536 (pbk)
ISBN: 9781003715306 (ebk)

DOI: 10.4324/9781003715306

Typeset in Optima
by codeMantra

Contents

Acknowledgments

This book stands on ground made possible by the presence and generosity of a few key people.

To Nancy McWilliams, for your unwavering support and steady belief across this project's unfolding.

To Donnel Stern, for your early recognition and for meeting this work on the terrain of experience.

To Kate Hawes and Aakriti Aggarwal, for your continued care in bringing it into form.

To Tim, whose quiet steadiness remains the ground beneath it all.

With enduring gratitude to Christopher Bollas, Thomas Ogden, and Michael Eigen, whose writings, presence, and engagement with me and my writing have helped contour the symbolic atmosphere from which this work has emerged.

To Phil Ringstrom, Aleksandra Wagner, Susie Orbach, Salman Akhtar, and Ghislaine Boulanger, for reading and offering thoughtful feedback on portions of the manuscript—and for the depth of contact you each bring to thinking.

Those unnamed here have either already been spoken of or need no mention to be felt. Their traces remain throughout.

This book continues the unfolding of a larger project, *Unstable Objects*.

Initial Conditions

This work does not begin with a thesis but with a field—curved, unstable, affectively dense. Its entry point is not conceptual clarity but symbolic condensation. What follows emerged less from intention than from the pressure of experience that demanded symbolic form. The writing is recursive, structured by echoes rather than claims.

Note to the Reader

This text aims to remain close to the forces that shape psychic structure beneath conceptual resolution. Its form is not accidental: recursive, destabilized, resistant to closure. No claim is final. Each sentence returns the reader to a field where meaning strains against symbolization—and where response, not mastery, is the ethical position.

Prelude—The Singularity and the Desire to Know

The Singularity

There is a center to psychic life we can never touch.

A mass so dense, it bends every thought, symptom, and structure into being—without ever being seen.

We call it the self, but it is not self.

We call it trauma, but it is not trauma.

It is what every symptom orbits.

It is what every story deflects around.

It is the singularity—the unrepresentable core of psychic life.

And yet, we yearn for it.

To reach it. To dissolve into it.

This is not a wish for healing. It is a wish for *totality*.

Like Isolde's Liebestod—the love-death at the edge of knowing—we mistake the annihilation of separation for the arrival of truth.

But if we could touch the singularity, we would no longer exist as we are.

No curvature. No orbit. No time.

To know it is to die into it.

And so the psyche does something brilliant.

It moves at such speed that it appears solid—

A character style, like a firebrand spun in darkness.

The light traces a shape, a self, a stance—but it is only the afterimage of what cannot be held.

We are that trace.

We are what the singularity leaves behind as it draws us close, but not in.

The Curved Psyche

The psyche is not a container. It is a topology—curved, recursive, distorting the very frame through which we attempt to see it. There is no straight line in a field bent by suffering, by desire, by memory. No neutral position from which to observe it. The analytic encounter does not take place *within* the psyche, but *as* the psyche—the shared field between patient and analyst, warped by the gravity of what remains unsymbolized.

In this cosmos, **time and space are never separate**. Every memory is a place; every symptom is a duration. Psychic structure bends the experience of time—just as mass bends space in general relativity. A depressive patient may stretch a moment into eternity; a narcissistic structure may collapse a decade into a single, frozen now. Psychic time is not linear—it is gravitational. It folds, thickens, and reverses.

Just as Einstein revealed that **mass and energy** are not opposites but different states of the same substance, we begin here with a parallel truth: structure and affect are not two realms, but **condensations and dispersions of one psychic field**. Emotion is structure in vapor; character is affect in collapse. A panic attack may be read as boiling, a phobia as condensation, a manic defense as the sudden vaporization of constraint.

This is why we speak of **states**, not only structures. The obsessive mind condenses thought into repetition; the schizoid disperses selfhood into vapor. The borderline collapses time into catastrophe, while the masochistic structure saturates the field with psychic humidity, unable to dry into form. The analyst meets these weather patterns as atmospheric pressures—and learns, over time, to read them as **climate**, not just crisis.

Each of these configurations—obsessive, depressive, hysteric, psychopathic, narcissistic, schizoid, paranoid—is not a *type*, but an **orbit** around something that cannot be symbolized directly. What we call diagnosis is not a label, but a **map of curvature**: how the psyche bends experience, how it organizes meaning around the unrepresentable.

This unrepresentable core—the **psychic singularity**—is not simply trauma, though trauma often hides inside it. It is not reducible to the id, but resembles it. It is not only Bion's *O*, but spirals near it. It is not the Real of Lacan, but shares its ungraspable heat. The singularity is the *mass at the center* of the psychic universe that cannot be seen—only inferred by how things orbit, distort, or fall apart near it.

We all live as **symbols of our singularity**, tracing its outlines in repetition, character, defense, and desire. Each of us becomes a **curved expression** of what we cannot approach directly. The orbit *is* our form of life.

And yet, there is movement. There are **escape velocities**—moments when a patient's psychic orbit is disturbed just enough that something dislodges, repositions, or opens. These are not always moments of interpretation. They are often moments of **field shift**—when the analyst becomes less a knower and more a gravitational presence, allowing the patient to reconfigure not their story, but their orientation to it.

This is the aim of diagnosis in this frame: not to fix identity, but to locate the analyst within the patient's universe. To ask: *What curvature am I participating in? What orbit am I sustaining? And what pressure, what warmth, what precision of gaze might bend it otherwise?*

Here, **even the analyst is curved**. We are not outside the field. We are moved, pulled, entrained. Our capacity to hold paradox, to remain aware of time as both bending and passing, to tolerate collapse without becoming collapsed—this is the clinical ethic of gravitational attunement.

The mind is not an object. It is a field in motion. And the work of analysis is to notice how that field curls inward on itself—how it preserves what it cannot yet release, and repeats what it cannot yet symbolically metabolize.

Before we name any style, before we trace any defense, we must acknowledge this: the psyche is not linear. It is **curved**, layered, recursive—a storm of condensation and vapor, orbit and mass, collapse and thaw.

And the moment we try to fix it in place—even as a diagnosis—we distort it. Better to let it bend us first.

The Delphic Loop

Before gravity, before orbit, before any model—there was the command: *Know thyself.* Carved above the threshold of the temple at Delphi, it was never merely advice. It was a **cosmic dare**. Not a call to self-reflection, but a portal to recursion—for to know oneself is always to enter a loop: who is the self that knows? What knows the knower? And what part of self remains unseeable even in the gaze that seeks it?

The Oracle did not offer answers. She inhaled the vapor from the earth and spoke in riddles. She did not locate truth in clarity, but in the heat of paradox. She offered fragments, aphorisms, warnings: *Everything in measure. Nothing in excess. You are only mortal. Even the sun has blemishes.* Each utterance was both symbolic and diagnostic—not facts, but thresholds, leading not into certainty but into **symbolic recursion**.

So too with analysis. The patient arrives asking to know themselves. But what they seek is not information—it is orientation. And the process of knowing will not lead to a core, but to a **spiral**. The more deeply one knows, the more one becomes aware of what cannot be known. The singularity resists direct gaze. To seek it too directly is to collapse. Like **Tristan und Isolde**, the yearning to merge with the Real is also the yearning to die.

Thus, the Delphic utterance remains the purest metaphor for analysis: **to circle the unrepresentable without falling in**. Knowing becomes a form of orbit. Interpretation becomes a ritual of return. Insight does not close the loop; it deepens it.

And within that spiral, there is a second inscription—*Everything in measure*—the psychic counterpart to gravity. It cautions against totality. It marks the danger of too much meaning, too much presence, too much psychic light without a containing form. Even the analyst's gaze must be metered. Even contact must be modulated. Otherwise, the field floods.

Delphi offers us not a model, but a **stance**. Not a system, but a practice of psychic ethics:

- To speak not from authority, but from condensation.
- To listen not for facts, but for curvature.
- To interpret, not to fix, but to **recursively return**, circling meaning as one might circle fire—close enough to feel its heat, but not enough to become consumed.

The Delphic voice, like the analyst's, must accept its own partiality. Its truth is not in totality but in resonance. It does not answer, it bends the question.

And so we bend, too. Each interpretation, each frame, each diagnosis is not a conclusion—it is a symbolic stroke around the unspeakable. To know the patient is not to grasp them, but to become curved in their gravity. To allow ourselves to be shaped by the symbolic vortex they unknowingly create.

The self cannot be known. But it can be circled.

It can be warmed.

It can be witnessed.

And in that circling, the orbit itself becomes a kind of self—not what we are, but the **path we trace around what we are not allowed to know**.

Philosophical Anchors

The psyche is not made of thoughts. It is made of tensions: between being and not-being, between presence and representation, between the said and the unsayable. Philosophy, at its best, does not resolve these tensions—it preserves them. It frames the paradoxes not as problems, but as coordinates in the space of subjectivity.

Heidegger reminds us that **Being is not a thing**, but an unfolding. We are not containers of existence, but expressions of it—and often, *forgotten* expressions, veiled by the language we use to describe ourselves. In analysis, this forgetfulness appears not as absence, but as overpresence—a clotted, overdetermined self who cannot simply be, because their being has been overwritten. Heidegger's *unconcealment* is not unlike the analytic task: to allow what has always already been there to come forth, newly seen.

Wittgenstein warns us that **language cannot reach its own edge**. The limits of our speech are the limits of our world—but also the invitation to gesture beyond them. In the clinic, we witness this when words loop, stall, or distort—when what needs to be said cannot yet find form, or when the form becomes a defense. The analyst speaks not just to communicate, but to **trace the unspeakable**—to move just close enough to the edge that something new begins to shimmer.

Derrida speaks of **différance**, the deferral of meaning, the way every sign slips against itself. For the analyst, this is not a problem to fix but a condition to inhabit. The self is always already displaced, never coinciding fully with itself. To analyze is not to restore wholeness, but to become attuned to the **play of trace and absence**, the hauntings that give shape to desire.

Levinas insists that the other is **unknowable, irreducible, and prior to ontology**. To relate is not to grasp, but to answer. The analyst, in this view, does not understand the patient so much as *respond* to them—not as an object, but as an ethical rupture. The face of the patient confronts the analyst not with content but with demand: *be here in a way that cannot be systematized*. This is not a technique. It is presence.

All of these philosophers—and many more—do not speak *about* the psyche. They speak **as** the psyche, from within its folds. Their ideas are not scaffolding, but echoes—of the very structures the analyst navigates daily. Their thought, like analysis, bends toward the unspeakable, seeking a form of rigor that does not kill what it touches.

So we borrow from them not to build theory, but to deepen our **symbolic stamina**. To remain in the paradox. To think from the middle. To recognize that every interpretation, every diagnostic gesture, every act of naming is already folded inside a tradition of not-knowing.

And in that, there is freedom.

Not the freedom of clarity—but the freedom of **symbolic resonance**, of tracing what cannot be said, again and again, until the patient begins to hear their own unspeakable voice inside the echo.

The Arbitrariness of All Frames

We must begin somewhere. And every beginning is a cut.

To write of psyche through the lens of space-time, orbit, and singularity is not a claim of truth, but of **useful distortion**. Like all analytic framings, it is an act of **symbolic selection**—one way of slicing the cosmos so that something becomes visible. But every slice obscures what it does not reveal.

The same is true of character styles. We describe them as orbits, as gravitational curves, as modes of condensation and collapse. But they are not objects. They are **movements**, artifacts of a field in flux. Any typology—obsessive, schizoid, narcissistic, paranoid—is not a fixed identity, but a **recursive posture** in the presence of what cannot be metabolized. A style is not who someone is. It is how their psyche has come to bend under the weight of the ungraspable.

The mind does not sort cleanly. We all carry each structure, each posture, each weather system—sometimes as storm, sometimes as trace. The compartments are artifacts of analysis, not of being. Even the chapters that follow are **fictions of order**, necessary to approach the unapproachable. But the truth is always composite. The psyche is a hologram: even the smallest part contains the whole, bent by perspective.

This is why this book begins in a spiral. The **Prelude is the whole**, curled tightly into five coils—singularity, curvature, recursion, paradox, and frame. Each chapter that follows is not a new beginning, but a **re-expansion** of the same material: the same mass, seen from a new angle. Like the Indian tantric tradition of *root text and auto-commentary*, what comes next is not more, but deeper.

And this is why all frames must be held lightly. Every metaphor—gravity, vapor, orbit—is an **epistemological prosthetic**. It helps us move, but not arrive. The moment we mistake it for reality, we collapse back into dogma. The analyst's task is not to find the right metaphor, but to notice when a metaphor **opens** something—when it creates a new arc of movement in the field.

The same is true of diagnosis. It is not truth, but **topology**. It is not a name, but a tracing—a way to mark where the psyche folds, loops, and collapses. And the ethical charge of diagnosis is to do so in a way that **invites movement**, not fixity.

Because every system of knowing carries the risk of foreclosure. And every patient is already burdened by having been too known, too early, too falsely. To frame them again is a risk. But to refuse framing is abandonment.

So we frame—carefully, provisionally, paradoxically. We allow the orbit, we feel the gravity, we trace the vapor—all the while knowing that what we are seeing is **only an expression** of something more central, more condensed, more hidden: the singularity of the self, that can never be known directly, only lived around.

All that follows is commentary.

Let us begin.

Introduction—The Singularity and the Orbit

These fragments—looped, folded, unfinished—form the grammar of what follows. If the psyche curves rather than unfolds, then knowing must also bend: not toward mastery, but toward contact. The chapters ahead do not offer resolution, but a structure for circling. They trace the arc of return—not to explain what psyche is, but to illuminate the gravitational contours of how it moves, splits, orbits, and longs. The singularity remains, not as origin or endpoint, but as a luminous pressure: the impossibility at the heart of perception, around which every form begins to bend.

Opening: The Field before Form

In the beginning, there is no diagnosis, no narrative, no coherence. There is not yet even a patient or an analyst. There is only a field—sensory, vibratory, potential. A field of shared breath, charged silence, and barely perceptible gestures. This field is not a metaphor. It is the raw atmosphere of contact, the not-yet-symbolized condition from which the analytic situation will eventually coalesce. It holds the nascent ingredients of psychic life, before form, before containment, before knowing.

This second volume opens there: in the unmarked space that precedes the subject-object split. We are not beginning again so much as rotating the perspective. *Unstable Objects I* explored fragmentation, rupture, and the trauma of representation. *Unstable Objects II* takes up the other side of the paradox: the continuous field, the gravity of structure, the curvature of symbolic life. It does not leave behind secrecy and fragmentation, but reframes them within larger orbits of coherence and condensation.

In the psychoanalytic situation, experience always arrives saturated. But not all of it is legible. The analytic pair encounters not only content, but atmosphere—affective texture, symbolic resonance, gravity wells of feeling that defy immediate conceptualization. This book proposes a shift in register. Instead of tracking meaning, we trace movement. Instead of seeking integration, we ask: how is the psyche curving around that which it cannot bear to name?

DOI: 10.4324/9781003715306-1

The orbit, then, becomes the governing metaphor. Not a linear trajectory from symptom to health, but a recursive looping around something unformulated. The psyche does not simply develop—it bends. Desire bends. Time bends. Identity bends. And analysis, at its best, attunes to those bends without trying to straighten them.

The singularity at the center—whether trauma, drive, truth, or absence—cannot be directly contacted. It destabilizes representation. But its presence is registered in the arc of everything that curves around it. This is the gravitational logic of psychic life: what cannot be held directly becomes the very axis of orbit.

This volume takes up that logic. Its chapters are not arranged as a sequence of arguments, but as elliptical passages. Each circles a center it cannot reach. Each holds something ungraspable, not to explain it, but to remain in fidelity to its pull. The task is not comprehension. It is reverberation. We begin not at the center, but on the edge.

The Analyst in the Orbit

The analyst enters the field not as a detached observer, but as a body drawn into a curve. In every session, we are moved—affectively, unconsciously, gravitationally. The patient may speak of a childhood scene or a broken dream, but what arrives in the room is not only narrative. It is pull. Tension. Proximity. Some analytic moments land like objects thrown into the shared space between us. Others trace an arc we can barely perceive. We become part of their motion.

There are times when what the patient speaks is almost incidental, and what saturates the hour is the density of something unsymbolized. The analyst may feel sleepy, or suddenly alert, or gripped by a nameless urgency. These affective perturbations are not noise; they are signals. They tell us that we are near something—a singularity of meaning, a collapse of temporality, a condensation of affect that cannot yet find its form.

In these moments, the analyst must resist both the interpretive reflex and the retreat into neutrality. What is called for is a kind of analytic proprioception: an attunement to the field, to its warps and tensions, to its subtle shifts. We are not outside the patient's orbit, but within it, pulled into resonance. Our task is not to name the center, but to track the trajectory.

This requires a different kind of listening. Not just for what is said, or even what is not said, but for how the space itself bends. Language stretches, associations loop, silences thicken. The analytic frame becomes not a container but a topology—a structure that shapes and is shaped by the recursive motion of subjectivity.

In traditional metapsychology, the analyst is often positioned as the interpreter, the translator of unconscious content into narrative form. But at the edge of experience, something else is required: a willingness to be unsettled, to be moved without anchoring. We become witnesses not only to meaning, but to motion; not to clarity, but to curve.

The orbit, then, is not simply the patient's. It is shared. It is the analytic situation itself, held between us, structured by our mutual inability to land. In the refusal of arrival, something opens—a space for reverberation, for symbolization, for becoming. The analyst's role is not to map the psyche from above, but to dwell within the trajectory as it unfolds. To be moved, and to move in turn.

Gravity and Grace: The Ethics of Staying Near

To orbit is not merely to move; it is to remain near without grasping. In psychoanalytic work, this stance becomes an ethical position. We are asked not only to understand the patient but to accompany them—to remain proximate to what cannot be resolved, integrated, or even fully formulated. The orbit becomes a mode of care.

Freud's model of interpretation, though brilliant, often sought to dissolve mystery into clarity, to transmute symptom into narrative. Yet what if some symptoms are not puzzles to be solved but gravitational echoes—traces of a singularity that resists integration? In such cases, the analyst's task shifts from decoding to accompanying and from unearthing meaning to sustaining presence.

This is the realm in which Loewald's vision of psychoanalysis as a "second birth" becomes relevant. The analyst provides not an answer but a holding environment in which the patient may experience themselves anew—nearer to the mystery, not farther from it. It is a birth not into form, but into orbit: the realization that one can live in relation to what has no name.

There is grace in this. Not in the religious sense, though sometimes it approaches that register, but in the aesthetic and ethical sense: the grace of restraint, of attunement, of refusal to reduce. Analysts must cultivate an ability to stay near without intrusion, to tolerate the tension of nearness without resolution.

Winnicott's notion of the "capacity to be alone in the presence of another" is one of the clearest clinical formulations of this orbiting presence. It is not withdrawal, nor is it fusion. It is a field in which both analyst and patient may exist as separate-yet-near, coherent-yet-fractured. In this space, symbolization can emerge—not from imposition, but from co-presence.

We might also consider Jessica Benjamin's emphasis on mutual recognition. To recognize another is not to know them in totality, but to remain in a state of wonder, of responsiveness, of simultaneous subjectivity. The orbit is not a failure to connect but a refusal to dominate. It is the ethical possibility of being with another without subsuming or being subsumed.

Gravity, then, is not merely a force that binds. It is also a metaphor for what draws us toward the unspeakable in another. Grace is what allows us to stay there without falling in. This, too, is a form of interpretation—not one that names, but one that listens with fidelity to the orbit itself. In that listening, something shifts—not resolved, but held. Not grasped, but circled.

Recursive Return and the Shape of Experience

To live a life is not to progress in a straight line. It is to loop, return, and revise. Psychic life rarely unfolds as pure trajectory; it moves through recursive rhythms, through what might be called the choreography of return. This return is not mere repetition. It is a spiraling process, one in which each orbit traces a new relation to the same unspeakable center.

In clinical work, this shows up as the repetition compulsion—but to reduce it to pathology misses its deeper function. Repetition is a form of psychic geometry. It is how the unconscious draws attention to what cannot be said in any other way. It is a rhythm, not a riddle. To understand it, we must listen with an ear for pattern, for shape, for time folding back on itself.

Freud recognized the power of repetition but struggled to situate it within a theory of meaning. He described it as a compulsion, a death drive, a disruption of the pleasure principle. Yet we might also hear in repetition the voice of the symbolic itself—the psyche's way of insisting on something that cannot yet be symbolized. In this sense, return is not regression but method. It is the soul's mode of persistence.

The analytic frame, with its regularity and recurrence, mimics this shape. The session begins, unfolds, ends—and returns. The analyst becomes not a fixed object but a point in the patient's orbit, a place they can loop back toward, revise their trajectory around, and test gravity against. It is in this looping that psychic structure takes form—not as solidity, but as rhythm.

Thomas Ogden's writing on reverie and analytic thirdness captures this recursive movement. He reminds us that meaning in analysis often emerges not from any single statement but from the echo across sessions, the way a word reverberates, mutates, finds its place again in another context. The past does not simply return—it reshapes the present, and the present, in turn, reshapes the past.

To think recursively is to resist closure. It is to understand psychic life as layered, rhythmic, and paradoxical. The same story told twice is never the same. Each orbit is a new relation to the center. This is why therapy often feels like circling rather than solving. The goal is not to arrive, but to find a livable relation to what cannot be left behind.

The recursive shape of experience also reflects the analyst's own inner work. We are drawn again and again into similar themes, similar failures, similar longings. Our own histories spiral through our listening. We are not immune to the orbit; we are shaped by it. And so, analysis becomes a shared choreography—a mutual recursion through which something new, or at least more bearable, may come into being.

Orbits and Fields: From Intersubjective Space to Symbolic Atmosphere

The psychoanalytic relationship is not a closed dyad but an open field—a spatial, affective, and symbolic medium in which meanings arise, dissolve, and reconfigure. To speak of the analytic field is not merely to acknowledge mutual influence, but to recognize a shared atmosphere in which both patient and analyst are suspended. This field is not always symmetrical. Gravity pools in uneven ways. One figure may carry the intensity of projection; the other may float in and out of presence. But what links them is not identity or difference—it is orbit.

Orbiting is a mode of being-with that neither fuses nor withdraws. It holds space between engulfment and detachment. In the best analytic hours, there is a palpable sense of shared motion—not forward movement, but elliptical circling around something not-yet-speakable. Here, the analyst's role is not to stabilize, but to resonate. What we offer is not always insight, but containment of the curved trajectories that words take when they are still saturated with affect.

Symbolic atmosphere emerges from this resonance. It is not reducible to what is said, but is carried in tone, gesture, silence, and rhythm. The orbit becomes expressive. We might think of Bion's reverie or Bollas's evocative object as early articulations of this field effect. However, the metaphor of the orbit helps us refine the distinction: it is not that the analyst simply absorbs and metabolizes; rather, the analytic field permits a form of attunement in which both subjectivities bend toward a center that remains unsymbolized.

Such bending is not passive. It is an active orientation toward paradox—toward what cannot yet be known, but must still be tracked. It involves tolerating ambiguity, allowing multiple temporalities to coexist, and permitting fragments of speech and sensation to reverberate without resolution. In this sense, orbit becomes a technique as well as a metaphor. The analyst orbits the patient's experience—not to decode it, but to co-inhabit its gravitational logic.

Symbolic atmosphere, then, is not a mood. It is a mode of knowledge—a way the field thinks before thinking, feels before feeling. The analytic process becomes a choreography of mutual circling, in which presence is structured not by interpretation alone, but by the form of relation itself.

The Edge of Naming: Language, Gravity, and Interpretive Collapse

The drive to name is among the deepest in psychoanalysis. We name to organize, to bind, to make suffering knowable. Yet every name also risks collapse. To speak something is to give it form—but that form, once named, may lose the gravitational weight it held when unsymbolized. This is the paradox at the heart of analytic language: it both reveals and reduces, both liberates and evacuates.

Recognition Reversal—the moment when the symbolic form, once attained, appears emptier than the unnamed experience it replaces—is a common occurrence in analytic work. Patients labor toward expression, only to find the words oddly lifeless. A trauma is narrated and then it goes flat. A desire is finally owned but feels less vital. It is not that the experience was inauthentic. It is that the symbolic has altered its orbit.

This reversal points to something crucial. There are psychic truths that resist linear unfolding. They do not want to be spoken clearly, but rather to be held in suspended articulation. The analytic hour must sometimes linger in that liminal space—before speech, after meaning, inside the symbolic field but not yet fixed in form.

Interpretations that collapse this space too quickly can strip the psyche of its curvature. The patient's experience becomes a fact, rather than a movement. As analysts, we must attend not only to the content of what is said, but to the gravitational field around it. What happens when a truth is nearly spoken? What fragments swirl around the formulation? What slips away in the moment of insight?

This is not a call to abandon interpretation. It is a call to recognize its double edge. Naming is an act of grace and of violence. It frees, but it also constrains. When we speak of psychic structure, we must also speak of what structures resist. When we work with language, we must also work with its silences.

In this way, analytic presence becomes a kind of orbital listening. We hold close to what is forming, but we do not force its birth. We allow meaning to constellate, to become temporarily visible, then fade. And we learn to trust that something is still held in the field—even when nothing is said.

The metaphor of the singularity is not simply a poetic flourish. It is a methodological orientation. It warns against the analyst's desire to stabilize meaning prematurely. It reminds us that some psychic truths do not unfold through sequential interpretation but emerge only when we dare to dwell in the density of what cannot yet be symbolized. The singularity may appear in the transference as silence, resistance, erotic charge, or a rupture in the analyst's attention. These are not barriers to progress. They are the gravitational contours of the unspeakable.

To track the psyche this way is to shift our epistemology. We no longer seek to decode or extract meaning from psychic life as if it were a puzzle. Instead, we move with it, inside it. We attune to resonance, to symbolic atmosphere, to aesthetic form. We begin to hear symptoms not as encrypted messages from a repressed past but as formal condensations—gestures of structure, recursive shapes that carry meaning without needing to be unpacked.

Psychoanalytic theory itself might be reimagined not as a fixed set of concepts but as a dynamic field, where thought moves in gravitational relation to that which it cannot fully absorb. What if our theories are not maps but orbits? What if their repetitions and revisions, their contradictions and returns, are not flaws but signatures of proximity to a truth that eludes capture?

This would place psychoanalysis closer to art than science—yet not as a retreat from rigor. Rather, it would suggest that the rigor of our field is not in explanatory clarity but in aesthetic fidelity: a responsiveness to the movement of mind, to its folds and doublings, to its resistance to closure. A well-formed interpretation, in this mode, does not finalize a truth but reveals its complexity, opens a space, and thickens experience.

In this spirit, this book does not propose a unified theory. It gathers singularities. It invites the reader into elliptical paths, where each chapter refracts a different angle of the psychic field: from the holographic mind to the gravitational architecture of symptom; from nondual awareness to the curvature of time; from recursive trauma to character style. What holds them together is not an argument but a fidelity to form. Each chapter is an orbit. Each begins again at the edge.

For those who have read *The Fragmented Self, Recognition, and the Edge of Desire: Foundations of the Psychoanalysis of Unstable Objects*, this second book may feel like a deepening spiral. The two books are not sequential. They are intersubjective—two poles of a paradox, two asymptotes of the same arc. The first book leaned into rupture. This one leans into form.

The singularity, then, is not just a metaphor for psychic density. It is also a metaphor for the analytic relationship. For what happens when two subjectivities enter a shared field—when the analyst and patient find themselves orbiting the same unspeakable center. The analyst, too, becomes unstable. Not shattered, but resonant. Not dissolved, but permeable.

This is the tone we aim to hold in the pages that follow. A tone of fidelity without foreclosure. A stance of curiosity, discipline, and reverence. The reader is invited not only to understand, but to move with. To read not for mastery, but for attunement. To allow something unnamed to take shape—not as a definition, but as a gravitational pull.

We begin at the edge of language. With a motion. With a field. With the refusal to reduce. What follows is not a map, but a choreography.

And so we begin—not with a fixed center, but with a field in motion. Not with certainty, but with resonance. Each chapter that follows invites a different mode of perception, a different gravitational intimacy with what resists containment. Let this book be not a doctrine but a companion—an unstable object in your hands, drawing you, too, into orbit.

Part I

Orbits and Singularities— Framing the Psyche Beyond Newton and Freud

This opening Part reimagines the psychic field not as a static structure but as a gravitational topology. Freud's model of drive and force is retained, but curved—subjectivity emerges not from mechanical causality, but from recursive proximity to what cannot be named. Singularity becomes metaphor: the unknowable point around which psychic life orbits. The very desire to know becomes gravitational.

To speak of singularity is not to name an origin, but to mark a tear in representation—a point of density around which psychic life curves. These opening chapters begin a project of extending **Freud's energetic metaphors** and **Klein's theory of part-object internalization** beyond their historical physics, toward a **topological model** of the mind. The psyche is not a system of containers and contents but a field of recursive orbits, bent by unformulated force. Orbit, in this sense, is not distance from truth but a form of truth itself. These chapters initiate the gravitational metaphor by articulating how symbolic form emerges through motion, deferral, and the impossibility of full recognition. The singularity is not behind us. It is what we circle—forever unfinished, generative, and destabilizing.

DOI: 10.4324/9781003715306-2

1 The Original Paradox, Refracted

We orbit what we cannot name. This is recognition. This is diagnosis.

Prelude to Division: Light That Cannot See Itself

The most unbearable paradox is not the tension between opposites—it is that even opposition arises within a single field. In this field, which we might call psyche, or cosmos, or singularity, awareness bends into itself, not as a linear unfolding, but as a loop: recursive, radiant, and unstable. The split—the ancient mark of good and bad, self and other, subject and object—is not pathology. It is the price of representation.

What appears as duality is already a perception shaped by that split. And yet, something deeper remains, prior to perception. This is the field of the nondual—not a mystical fusion, but a topology without edges, a space before space, a time before time. It is the field in which the eye cannot see itself, where light radiates not from a source, but as the burn of coal from within. It is also the field in which psychoanalysis unfolds, not just as a method, but as a metaphysical wager.

We might say that every patient who enters the analytic space carries within them a gravitational mass—a singularity—that cannot be seen directly. We orbit what we cannot name. The orbit is not just the symptom; it is also the structure of meaning. The way the psyche bends around its own unsee-able core determines time, language, and even the possibility of knowing. To approach this core is to risk annihilation. But to remain unaware of it is to be condemned to drift.

In this chapter, we return to the original paradox and refract it through new lenses—Freud's doubt, Klein's fragments, Bion's O, Buddhist tantra, recursive structures, and the lived encounter of analyst and patient in the somatic weight of silence. Every part we interpret, every symptom we name, every moment of countertransference is the shadow of the whole, refracted. We do not heal the split. We live near it; we name its atmosphere. This is clinical gravity.

The paradox of paradoxes is that it creates time. When we split, we create sequence—this before that, this after that. Space becomes navigable. Time

DOI: 10.4324/9781003715306-3

becomes endurable. And yet, the analyst's task is to hold the map and the terrain together—to metabolize that which has no form into language that can be felt.

The part-object, the fragment, the symptom, the dream—all are signals of the Real. They are distortions not because they are wrong, but because they are curved. Their very curvature allows them to appear. As such, every analytic act is an act of reverence. Not toward truth, but toward orientation.

This chapter is an orientation to the field. The singularity is not trauma alone, not memory alone, not O, not the id—it is what the self organizes around. It is the gravitational pressure that makes symbolization possible and unbearable. We cannot touch it. We cannot name it. But in its light, everything else begins to glow.

To circle it, to feel its pull, to orient our interpretations and our silences by its warping of psychic space—that is the analytic task.

We begin not with a concept, but with a field.

We begin not with answers, but with the bend of questions around a center that cannot be seen.

Freud and the Oceanic Limit

Freud's discomfort with the notion of an "oceanic feeling"—that sense of undifferentiated oneness—has become a well-known tension in the origin myth of psychoanalysis. In *Civilization and Its Discontents*, he concedes that others report such a feeling but confesses that he does not experience it himself. His disbelief is often taken as hubris or a symptom of repression. But what if we read it differently? What if Freud's confession was less about personal limitation and more a signpost of a structural horizon—the epistemological boundary that psychoanalysis could not yet cross?

Freud, after all, was working within the framework of late nineteenth-century science. His metaphors—psychic energy, hydraulic pressure, tension, and discharge—reflected the Newtonian worldview dominant at the time. Space was absolute, time was linear, and causality moved in one direction. In this framework, the subject was understood as a bounded entity, a container of drives and conflicts, a system of parts. The metaphors were not incidental. They were the scaffolding of thought itself.

What the Newtonian cosmos could not accommodate, however, was the simultaneity, paradox, and recursion that define psychic life. The oceanic was too vast, too pre-subjective. It could not be made into an object of theory without collapsing the very distinctions that made theory possible. Freud's refusal of the oceanic, then, may reflect the structural necessity of differentiation for his model of mind. The analytic subject required boundaries to be legible. And boundaries are, by definition, splits.

There is a recursive dissonance in Freud's project. On the one hand, he was drawn toward what resists symbolization: the unconscious, the drive, the symptom, the dream. On the other hand, he sought to master these through a conceptual architecture grounded in rationalism and containment. The id was unspeakable, yet he spoke it. The dream was the royal road, yet he paved it with grammar.

This tension becomes clearest in his metaphysical caution. Freud acknowledged the gaps in his system, but he resisted crossing into what he could not theorize. In this way, psychoanalysis was born from a wound it could not name—a rift between knowing and being. The analytic endeavor emerged in the space opened by that split.

We might say, then, that Freud could not feel the oceanic because his theory depended on its absence. The nondual would have undid the architecture of drives and defenses. To theorize from within the field of oneness would have required a different physics entirely—not a Newtonian model of psychic hydraulics, but a relativistic one, in which mass bends time, and the observer shapes the observed.

This is not a critique of Freud, but a recognition of his brilliance and his bind. He reached the edge of the field but could not look in. He knew that something else pulled at the psyche, something anterior to representation. But he lacked the metaphors to name it. And naming it would have cost him the very coherence that made his work possible.

What emerges, then, is a legacy of recursive inheritance. We inherit not just Freud's insights, but his blind spots. His refusal of the oceanic does not close the door. It marks the place where another kind of perception might begin. The oceanic is not pre-theoretical—it is the ground from which theory must sometimes disintegrate before it can reform.

We do not need to disavow Freud. We need to refract him.

The oceanic is not a regression. It is the backdrop of psychic becoming—the field into which the analyst is drawn when language fails and time folds. To recognize its presence is not to abandon structure. It is to recognize that all structure is already curved.

Klein's Part-Objects and the Light of the Whole

To Klein, the part-object was a developmental and defensive necessity—a way of managing overwhelming affective states by splitting objects into tolerable fragments. But what if these fragments were not only defenses against the whole, but signals of the whole's prior presence? What if they were not merely pieces, but radiant expressions of something unrepresentable, glimpsed only through what they refract?

The breast is not just a breast. It is a condensation of all nourishment, presence, vitality, and contact. Likewise, the persecutory anus is not merely a bad part-object, but a concentrated signal of violated boundary, shame, or engulfment. Each fragment, in this sense, is curved light—bent around the singularity of the self's becoming.

To see part-objects not as merely split-off defensive phenomena but as angles of approach—rays of the Real—requires a different mode of perception.

These are not shards broken from an imagined wholeness; they are ways the whole allows itself to be known in time.

Nondual awareness cannot look directly at itself—like the eye that cannot see itself, or like the burning coal whose light comes from within. The part-object is this coal-light: not illuminated by another, but burning with the internal radiance of its referent. That referent is unknowable. The singularity cannot be perceived, only inferred by how objects bend around it.

The clinical moment in which the patient fixates on a single part—of the analyst, of the self, of the past—is not to be pathologized as a failure to integrate. It is to be held as an invitation: here, a curve. Here, the whole speaks through the part, if we know how to listen.

This listening is not only auditory but gravitational. The analyst orients to the felt weight of the part-object, sensing its affective mass, its density, its orbit. We learn not what it is, but what it draws us toward. It is in this sense that the analyst's own countertransference becomes diagnostic—not of the patient's pathology alone, but of the structure of the field.

The part-object is not only a split. It is a condensation. In this way, it echoes the structure of metaphor itself: something stands in for what cannot be directly named, and in doing so, brings it closer. The fragment is the form the infinite takes in order to become sayable.

To interpret the part-object as a pathway to the whole—without reducing it, without collapsing it into a premature synthesis—is the task of an analysis grounded in paradox.

It is not the whole that we must recover. It is the capacity to recognize that the part already glows with the pressure of the whole behind it.

Bion, O, and the Void of Contact

Bion's concept of O—the ultimate truth of the thing-in-itself, unknowable yet real—stands as perhaps the most refined psychoanalytic gesture toward the nondual. O is not knowledge, but the condition that precedes it. Not a thing, but a presence that cannot be held. It is the analytic analogue of the singularity: infinitely dense, impossible to touch, yet shaping the entire gravitational field of the mind.

To approach O, Bion insisted, one must suspend memory and desire. One must tolerate the collapse of coordinates. This injunction is not merely technical. It is ontological. In order to come into contact with that which underlies all appearances, the analyst must cease to rely on symbolic furniture. The encounter with O is a falling away—of narrative, of orientation, and of self.

What Bion describes is a mode of attunement that reframes clinical work from interpretation to witnessing, from deciphering meaning to bearing presence. The analyst does not bring knowledge to the session. The analyst becomes the organ of perception through which something previously unformulated might briefly pass into being.

And yet, this passage often comes not as clarity but as disturbance. Contact with O is not experienced as illumination. It is felt as rupture. In moments when the patient nears the edge of the unsymbolized—whether in silence, in incoherence, in bodily tremor, or in sudden disorganization—the analyst may feel themselves pulled into a psychic gravity they cannot name. What occurs here is not regression, but saturation: the field becomes dense with the pressure of the Real.

If Freud placed the unconscious beneath language, and Klein nested it in internal objects, Bion located the deepest stratum in the space before symbolization. O is not hidden content. It is presence without content. The analytic task becomes one of remaining with this presence long enough that something may form around it—not as a direct perception, but as curvature. We do not see O. We see its effect on the analytic space, just as we infer the black hole from the distortion of stars around it.

This is why Bion's "selected fact" becomes so powerful. It is the point in the analytic field where the pattern begins to warp, where the previously unconnected becomes gravitationally linked. The selected fact is not deduced. It is felt. And the feeling is often disorienting.

In this framework, countertransference is no longer only an echo of the patient's internal world. It is the seismograph of O's approach. When the analyst feels weightless, lost, heavy, hollow, or suddenly gripped by inexplicable affect, they may be nearing the edge of the field where O exerts its pull. These are not disturbances to be explained away. They are the distortions of reality around the singularity.

And O, like the singularity, is not the same as trauma. It is not a past event. It is an ontological threshold—something present but unreachable, shaping everything around it. O may arise in a moment of contact so deep it becomes unspeakable. It may also emerge in the moment of witnessing a disintegrating self. In either case, it demands from the analyst a paradoxical poise: to remain near the unrepresentable without trying to represent it.

Here, Bion joins the tradition of negative theology, Zen koans, and Lacanian Real: that which resists incorporation, which cannot be mapped, but which gives rise to the very need for mapping. O is not God. It is not self. It is not object. It is the nondual pressure at the core of becoming.

To work in the presence of O is not to master technique but to refine receptivity. The analyst becomes, as Bion writes, a vertex through which the unknown may enter the known—not by will, but by orientation. In this, we return to the metaphors of space-time: the analyst as field, not force; as curvature, not point.

Much like light bending around gravity wells, the patient's language often curves around O. They do not speak it. They speak near it. They loop, repeat, dissociate, or stall. These are not resistances. They are orbits.

To interpret is not always to resolve. Sometimes, to interpret is to name the orbit, to say: this is where we circle. In doing so, the analyst does not collapse mystery into meaning. Rather, they provide coordinates for presence. They metabolize the gravitational field so the patient can remain near it without annihilation.

O is not therapeutic in itself. It is unbearable. But to be near O without being destroyed is perhaps the deepest experience of holding. And here, the analyst does not hold the patient alone—they hold the field, the warp, the curve.

This is why the analyst's body cannot be left out. Contact with O is felt somatically: in breath, muscle, stomach, pulse. These are not metaphors. They are instruments. The pre-verbal persists throughout life, and the analyst must become its vessel—feeling, metabolizing, and slowly symbolizing in order to offer the patient back a world they can survive in.

Bion wrote that we must "eschew memory and desire," but this is not a blankness. It is a rigor. A suspension that allows time to bend. And when time bends, something old and unformulated may arise—not as content, but as pressure.

To work with O is to allow the unknown to mark the session. Not to fill the space, but to saturate it. In this saturation, something becomes possible—not integration, but attunement. Not meaning, but gravity.

O is not what we find. It is what we orbit.

And it is in this orbit that the analyst's task becomes not explanation, but witness. Not containment, but field.

The Self-Reference Paradox and the Loop of Symbolization

Symbolization is the foundational act of psychoanalysis. Yet from the beginning, Freud struggled with its double edge: it reveals and it conceals, it heals and it fragments, it marks and it misses. When we speak of the pre-verbal, we do not refer to an era past. We speak of a mode of experience that continues to live underneath the words we use to try and know ourselves. The paradox is this: symbolization is the only way we can bring psychic life into relation, and it is also what renders it alien.

In this, symbolization becomes recursive. We symbolize what was unformulated. But we also symbolize the very act of symbolizing. There is no final referent, only iterations that fold experience back onto itself. To speak a truth is also to distort it. To reflect is to bend.

The ancient paradox, "This sentence is false," mirrors this. It is not a riddle to be solved but a structure to be inhabited. It shows how certain truths can only exist in contradiction, how the assertion of meaning inherently undoes itself. This is not a flaw in language. It is its deepest function. Language is not a vessel for truth. It is the recursive terrain where truth appears as a ripple, never a core.

This looping structure is not merely linguistic. It is psychic. The subject who knows they are a subject begins to reflect on themselves, and in doing so, generates a gap between self and self-image, between being and knowing. This is the foundation of human suffering and also its potential for transformation. We cannot resolve the loop. We can only begin to attune to its rhythm.

What analysis offers is not an exit from the loop but a way of dwelling within it—attuning to the curvature of one's psychic orbit. The patient speaks. The analyst listens. The analyst speaks. The patient listens. Something is named. Something shifts. Something escapes. This dance is not linear. It is elliptical.

And yet, it is precisely this recursive motion that allows for psychic change. As new symbols emerge, they press upon older configurations. They reorganize the gravity of experience. But they do so by working within the field, not above it. The analyst does not offer a truth from the outside. They become a resonant node inside the loop. They speak not to define but to bend.

In this sense, the analytic relationship is a self-referential field. Each party reflects and is reflected. Each interpretation generates a new arrangement of gravity. The words are never just words. They are matter. They bend space.

This is why the light-from-coal metaphor matters. Nondual awareness is not a light that illuminates from outside. It is the radiance from within, undetectable unless one notices the glow it casts on the surrounding world. The part-object, then, is not a fragment. It is the glint of the whole, seen in partial form only because of the limits of our gaze. It is the eye trying to see itself.

To say this is not to mystify. It is to return psychoanalysis to its radical foundations: that we are beings shaped by what we cannot know, but can learn to live near. Symbolization does not conquer the unknown. It choreographs its orbit.

The recursive loop of symbolization is not a trap. It is a topography. And the task of the analyst is not to point to the exit, but to walk the spiral path alongside the patient until a new bend reveals something not-yet-seen. The paradox is not what obstructs the work. It is the work.

Diagnostic Gravity and the Character of Orbit

All diagnosis is a map drawn in curved space.

To diagnose is not merely to label—it is to describe how a psyche bends. Structures of personality, symptom formations, and character styles are gravitational architectures. They are the patterns by which a person has learned to move through the field of others, to organize proximity and distance, need and defense, recognition and hiding.

Character is not static; it is orbital. It repeats, returns, loops. The orbit itself is not the problem. The question is: around what does it circle?

In this model, character styles become traces of a singularity—an unspeakable mass at the center of psychic life. They are not reducible to trauma or experience, though trauma often amplifies their density. Each style is a way of surviving curvature, of establishing stability in a universe of forces that feel ungraspable.

To speak diagnostically, then, is to speak of orbits. Borderline, obsessive, narcissistic, schizoid—these are not entities, but gravitational tendencies. They describe how time is felt, how closeness is feared, and how space is organized. The borderline orbit may be highly elliptical—swinging between merging and abandoning. The obsessive orbit may be rigidly circular—tightly constraining affect to maintain coherence. The narcissistic orbit may hide its center entirely—masking need with a shell of radiant display. These are all attempts to stabilize experience around something that cannot be touched directly.

The analyst's task is not to collapse the orbit, but to study it. To understand how meaning moves. To notice where language speeds up or slows down. To sense the affective tides that swell and recede as the patient approaches or flees their own center of mass.

In this view, diagnosis becomes an ethical act—not because it judges, but because it orients. It allows the analyst to hold the patient's universe with more sensitivity. To offer interpretations that account for psychic velocity. To move with, rather than against, the forces that structure the patient's world.

And yet, even as diagnosis bends toward objectivity, the analyst must remain curved. There is no neutral stance in a field shaped by gravity. The analyst's own structure will shape how they perceive the patient's orbit. Attunement becomes mutual—a recursive awareness of how two gravitational fields distort one another in contact.

Thus, we approach a relational diagnostic ethic: one in which character is never just a property of the patient, but a relational form. The analyst, too, has orbits. Together, they co-create a cosmos in which something new may be symbolized.

The Analyst's Mass: Ethics of Gravitational Presence

The analyst is not outside the system. They are a body of mass within it.

To sit with a patient is not to hover above their psyche, but to enter its gravity. The analyst's presence bends the field. Their history, tone, silences, interruptions—all carry symbolic mass. This is not a flaw. It is a fact of intersubjectivity.

What does it mean to be a mass in another's universe?

It means that interpretation is never neutral. It exerts force. It changes the trajectory of thought. It draws out some associations and renders others improbable. The analyst is both observer and participant, both witness and distortion.

Freud understood transference as repetition, a curved reenactment of the past. But what if transference is also a gravitational phenomenon? A way of registering the analyst's mass within the patient's space? Countertransference, then, becomes the analyst's registration of being pulled—drawn into orbits not entirely their own.

To be ethical, the analyst must become aware of their gravitational field. Not to erase it, but to refine it. To sense how their density—of presence, of language, of silence—affects the patient's symbolic motion. Sometimes lightness is needed: a translucent mass, allowing the patient's orbit to express itself fully. Sometimes, solidity: a reassuring pull when the patient is spiraling too far.

This is an ethics of tone, not doctrine. Of shape, not content. The analyst listens not only to what is said, but to how the space responds to their saying. They notice the warping of time in the session—the dilation when dissociation sets in, the compression when affect floods the field. They adjust, not to correct, but to co-regulate the shape of the cosmos.

The analyst's body matters. Not just the metaphorical body of language, but the actual, breathing, resonating presence. Eye contact, posture, pauses— these are instruments of gravity. They shape what can be borne, symbolized, and metabolized.

And in this shared curvature, the analytic space becomes a living system. Not balanced, but dynamic. Not still, but stable enough for something unspeakable to begin to take symbolic form.

To be an analyst is to agree to become curved. To give up the fantasy of a fixed center. To let the patient's mass affect one's own—and to trust that in this mutual gravity, new orbits may emerge.

Nonduality and the Unformulated Field

All dualities emerge from an undivided field.

This is not a spiritual proposition, but a clinical and epistemological one. In every analysis, we work with fragments that seem to oppose each other— autonomy and dependence, love and hate, self and other, inside and outside. These dualities are not errors. They are the basic structure of psychic life, but they arise against a background that is not itself split. The analyst does not return the patient to the undivided field; they simply make it possible to perceive that the field is always already present.

The nondual does not oppose the dual. It includes it. Just as space-time in relativity is not a container for objects but the very medium of their relation, so too nonduality is the condition that makes psychic division possible. The split is real—but it floats in a field that is not split.

We might think of this through the metaphor of water changing states. Solid, liquid, vapor—these are all forms of the same matter. Similarly, the psyche organizes itself into character, symptoms, and stories. But underneath these forms is something like condensation: invisible movements of affect, fantasy, and attunement that precipitate the more recognizable features of personality.

Diagnosis, structure, and interpretation all refer to crystallized formations. They are necessary. But the analytic process is a heat source. It re-evaporates the solidified and makes it mobile again. It reveals that what seemed fixed is always becoming.

This is why the pre-verbal persists throughout life. It is not merely the residue of infancy. It is the ongoing condition of lived experience. In analytic listening, the analyst attunes to sensations, tones, pauses, and subtle shifts that precede symbolic formation. Often, these are felt first in the analyst's own body. They move through sensation and affect before they become coherent thoughts.

As an analyst, I often find myself speaking from a place that I have not yet understood. Words come from somewhere inside a pre-symbolic awareness that only later becomes metabolized into meaning. In this way, the analyst becomes a conduit for the patient's unformulated experience—not by interpreting from above, but by speaking from within.

This is a nondual act. It blurs the distinction between self and other, between affect and thought, between expression and reception. The analytic field is not a dialogue between two bounded egos. It is a fluid space of co-evoked experience, where language is born from sensation, and sensation is shaped by symbolic reverberation.

The part-object, in this light, is not a fragment of something lost. It is the whole appearing in a specific form. To borrow our earlier metaphor: nondual awareness is the light radiating from a burning coal—not the light that shines on it, but the glow that emerges from within. The eye cannot look at itself. And yet, in moments of deep analytic attunement, we glimpse the trace of what cannot be directly known.

This is not mysticism. It is clinical immediacy. It is what happens when the analyst speaks not to interpret but to resonate; not to define but to invite.

The patient's story, diagnosis, and character style may appear dualistic. But within each is the gravitational trace of the unspeakable singularity around which the psyche orbits. The analyst does not need to name the singularity. They only need to notice how everything bends around it.

And in that noticing, a new kind of knowing becomes possible—one that does not split but includes, that does not grasp but inhabits. This is the analytic task at its most fundamental: to reveal the nondual field that sustains all the apparent divisions of psychic life, and to allow the patient to experience themselves not as a fixed character, but as a dynamic field of potential.

It is not that the patient must dissolve into oneness. It is that they must come to feel that their many parts, contradictions, and defenses are already suspended in a field that can hold them. The nondual is not a destination. It is the ground.

And from this ground, new structures may emerge—less rigid, more porous, curved rather than cornered. The analyst's task is not to lead the patient out of duality, but to help them perceive that the dual is always already held within the whole.

The split makes time. The nondual holds it. The symptom is the curvature. The symbol is the trace. The patient is already in their universe—they just didn't know it yet.

Curvature and the Ethics of Symbolic Attunement

Every symbol bends. Every interpretation curves the space in which it is spoken.

In psychoanalysis, the symbol is not a neutral sign. It organizes the psychic field. It creates paths, deflections, and orbits. It holds a density of prior experience while orienting toward an imagined future. This means that every interpretive act carries ethical weight—not because it is moral, but because it alters the field.

Freud described dreams as the royal road to the unconscious. But symbols in waking life may be more potent still. They carry within them compressed histories, affective residues, and dissociative folds. To speak to a patient is never just to speak; it is to alter the gravity of the session.

What this means is that analytic work is not just about truth, but about precision. The analyst does not aim merely to be accurate, but to be curvaceous—to bend language in a way that invites the psyche to reorganize itself. When an interpretation lands, it is not because it is correct, but because it resounds. It alters the field and invites coherence from within the patient's own symbolic matrix.

We can think of this in relativistic terms. A massive body curves space-time, and other objects follow that curvature. Similarly, certain words, when spoken with affective truth, curve the analytic space. The patient is drawn into new orbits—not coerced, but enticed. The analytic field itself changes shape.

This is why timing matters. Kairos—the opportune moment—cannot be separated from curvature. An interpretation too soon becomes an impact without mass: it glances off the surface and leaves no trace. Too late, and it becomes absorbed into inertia. The analyst must sense the symbolic gravity in the room and wait for the moment when the field can accept a new fold.

But curvature also implies care. The analyst must be willing to enter the patient's distorted space without imposing a straight line. There is no neutral stance. The analyst bends with the patient, not to follow them blindly, but to feel the shape of their world from within.

And from that curved interior, a different kind of ethical stance emerges—one not rooted in objectivity, but in participation. The analyst becomes a body of gravity; a symbolic mass whose presence curves the patient's experience in ways that permit emergence.

There are risks. To misattune is to distort. To interpret prematurely is to collapse potential into prescription. The ethical task is to remain in tension: to hold symbolic clarity without collapsing the field's generativity.

In this sense, analytic ethics is not about rules. It is about orbital alignment. The analyst listens not only for content, but for gravity—how the words fall, where they circle, what they are avoiding. They become astronomers of meaning, watching for irregularities in the orbit that hint at an unseen mass: the singularity, the dissociated fragment, the unbearable affect.

What is unspeakable still has shape. The analyst must become a witness to the gravitational asymmetries that indicate the presence of what cannot yet be symbolized. This witnessing is the ethical act.

And in this witnessing, the analyst's own gravity matters. Their symbolic vocabulary, affective palette, and capacity for holding paradox all contribute to how the field bends. This is not a defect of subjectivity. It is its gift.

We do not remove ourselves from the field to become ethical. We become ethical by entering the field with awareness of our impact. To be curved is not to be compromised—it is to be real.

Ultimately, symbolic attunement is not about correction. It is about resonance. The analyst does not straighten the patient's path. They join them in their curved space, and together they co-create the conditions for a different orbit.

Return to the Singularity

There is always something around which everything else is organized, yet which cannot itself be seen.

In physics, a singularity is a point at which density becomes infinite, and the laws of space-time break down. We cannot observe it directly. We infer its presence by the way light bends around it, by the orbits it shapes, by what disappears within its pull. In psychoanalysis, the singularity is not a concept. It is a phenomenon—the unknowable center of psychic life around which all meaning curves.

Every psyche has its singularity. It may be composed of trauma, fantasy, yearning, and shame. But it is never reducible to those. It is not the content that matters—it is the gravitational function. The singularity is what cannot be symbolized but must be circled. It is the core mass of psychic life.

We are each the symbol of something we cannot fully know. We are the orbiting trace of an unspeakable center. To know that center would be to collapse into it. Tristan and Isolde long not just for each other, but for the annihilation of separation. Their union is death because the singularity dissolves form.

In analytic work, we do not reveal the singularity. We reveal its effects. We track the warping of speech, the recursive return of themes, the compulsion to repeat. These are not merely defenses. They are gravitational patterns. The analyst becomes a cartographer of the patient's psychic cosmos—not to chart what is at the center, but to illuminate how everything orients around it.

This requires a paradoxical stance. We must believe in the singularity's presence without ever trying to name it. Naming is an escape velocity; it ejects the analyst from the field. Staying near the event horizon—where time dilates, where perception slows, where meaning fragments—is the ethical and aesthetic task of the analytic encounter.

The singularity is not only the site of pain. It is also the site of life. All vitality is curved around it. The analyst must resist the temptation to fill it in. The goal is not to make the patient whole, but to help them become aware of how their wholeness is already organized around a center they cannot possess.

And yet, something happens in the analytic process. The orbit becomes more stable. The patient begins to sense their own gravity. They notice their patterns not as failures, but as the natural consequence of a gravitational center. They do not transcend their singularity. They align with it.

This alignment is not enlightenment. It is not freedom from suffering. It is freedom within it. It is the ability to live as a symbol of oneself without collapsing into despair.

From the outside, this may look like ordinary life. Chop wood, carry water. But within the patient, the field has changed. What was once chaos has become cosmos. What was once symptom has become curvature. What was once unbearable has become the invisible axis around which meaning turns.

We can never know the singularity. But we can become sensitive to its pull. We can learn to read the curves in the symbolic field. We can become attuned to the way affect moves around it, the way speech loops back, the way silence thickens. And in this attunement, we become not masters of the psyche, but participants in its gravity.

To return to the singularity is not to go back. It is to recognize that we never left. The analytic task is not to arrive at truth, but to become aware of the structure of our orbit. And from this awareness, new forms of life may emerge—not outside the pull of gravity, but within its dance.

The singularity is the trace of the Real. It is the presence of what exceeds experience, yet organizes it. The analyst does not name it. They midwife its resonance.

And in that resonance, both patient and analyst are changed—not by insight, but by orbit.

2 The Curvature of Psychic Space
Orbit, Structure, and Symbolic Distortion

This chapter begins the book's exploration of psychic structure not through typology or symptom, but through curvature—the bending of inner space around unsymbolized gravity. Where later chapters will approach symbolic collapse through image or fragment, this chapter remains attuned to topology: how the psyche folds, distorts, and saturates experience spatially. Drawing on Loewald, Winnicott, and Merleau-Ponty, it frames the mind as a field, warped by affective density and the pull of the unformulated. This is not a chapter about symptom, but about the shape of psychic architecture itself.

Curvature over Linearity

The psyche does not move in straight lines. It curves, it folds, it loops. When we attempt to narrate a psychological history—what happened, why it happened, how it formed us—we often picture a line: origin, development, disruption, repair. But this linear metaphor conceals as much as it reveals. Psychic life resists chronology. It thickens around certain moments, bypasses others, and returns obsessively to what never properly occurred.

To speak of curvature is to shift our model of mind from the geometric to the gravitational. Events are not simply sequenced in time—they are weighted. A single gesture from a caregiver may exert a stronger pull than years of later experience. A scene never consciously remembered may nonetheless bend every future relationship. Psychic time is gravitational time: elastic, recursive, nonlinear. It coils around intensities. It stalls near absences. It folds back on itself in dreams, in symptoms, in the sudden reemergence of affect with no apparent cause.

There are sessions in which space seems to bend. A patient speaks, but their voice doesn't quite arrive. The room thickens. I once found myself watching a patient's mouth move while feeling as though we were in separate gravitational fields—my chair anchored to one corner of the room, his words echoing from another. He wasn't dissociating; he was saturated—present, intense, but spatially incoherent. He began to describe a moment in childhood when he was yelled at across a long hallway. "It's like I was always on the other side of something," he said, "even when I was right there." I realized I had been

DOI: 10.4324/9781003715306-4

feeling that hallway, not just hearing about it. His affect curved the room. My sense of proximity drifted—not away from him, but around him. The analytic field wasn't broken; it was warped. Curvature, I realized, isn't metaphorical. The psychic field bends under emotional density. What we call "distance" is sometimes only the shape of that bend.

This shift from linearity to curvature reframes our understanding of both development and defense. Development is no longer a path from dependence to autonomy, from fragmentation to integration, but a spiral orbit around unsymbolized centers—sites of intensity that cannot be directly assimilated. Similarly, defense is not merely the pushing away of conflict, but the curving of psychic motion around what cannot be metabolized. Repression, dissociation, even character itself: all are curvatures, trajectories altered by gravity.

We see this clearly in transference. What returns is not just content but trajectory—the shape of psychic movement. The patient re-enters not simply a prior situation, but a gravitational field. The analyst, if attuned, does not just decode meaning, but senses curvature: when the affect speeds up, when the story loops, when the subject's relation to their own speech begins to bend. Something is happening. The present is folding into the past; the past is shaping the field of the now.

Freud's topographic and structural models implied this without naming it. The return of the repressed, the work of the dream, the repetition compulsion—all are forms of psychic curvature. What was excluded does not stay still. It returns, distorted. It spirals through symptom, slips sideways into desire, recurs as obstacle. But the analyst, trained in deciphering, may miss the curvature in favor of content. We want to understand, to explain, to pin down. But sometimes, the curvature itself is the message: the way something cannot be said directly, the rhythm by which it escapes every frame.

Bion's notion of "O," the ultimate unknown, brings this curvature into focus. The analyst, if open to O, does not pursue knowledge but undergoes transformation. Interpretation arises not as a conclusion but as a resonance with the field. In this view, the patient's psyche is not a system to be mapped, but a gravitational reality to be entered, shaped by intensities that exceed symbolization. What we call containment is not the analyst's mastery of content, but their capacity to remain within the curve without collapsing into interpretation too soon.

Loewald, too, hinted at curvature when he described the emergence of inner space. In his vision, psychic structure does not emerge fully formed but unfolds through relational fields. The self is not constructed linearly from past to present, but retroactively configured as past and future take shape in the analytic now. Each interpretation, each attuned silence, curves the psychic field slightly—opening a new arc of movement or reinforcing an old one.

To adopt curvature as a clinical metaphor is also to shift how we think of presence. The analyst is not a neutral observer but a body within a gravitational system. We are pulled, bent, confused. We misstep not only because of our own history, but because of the field we have entered. The patient's psychic curvature distorts our own vision and pulls on our own symptoms. What is countertransference if not the analyst's being drawn into the patient's gravitational loop?

This requires a different kind of attunement. Not only what the patient says, but how they move through psychic space. Do they rush toward understanding? Do they avoid certain themes with odd velocity? Do they return again and again to the same symbolic point, unable to arrive but unable to depart? These are signs not of resistance, but of orbit. Something is exerting pull.

And sometimes, the analyst's task is not to disrupt the orbit but to trace it—to become aware of its arc, to sense its center. Not all progress is outward. Sometimes the most meaningful change occurs when a patient begins to know they are circling, when the curvature becomes felt rather than enacted. In that moment, the gravitational field becomes symbolizable. Not entirely, but enough.

The psyche does not unfold along a timeline. It bends, it echoes, it spirals. In analysis, we do not straighten it out. We follow its curvature, we learn its loops, we dwell near its singularities. And in doing so, something begins to move—not forward, but differently.

The Gravity of Style: Character as Curved Space

Character style is not merely a set of traits, but a gravitational pattern—a way the psyche curves, organizes meaning, and regulates affect in relation to its singularity. Traditional psychoanalytic frameworks often describe styles like obsessive, narcissistic, schizoid, or hysteric as static configurations. But when we approach them through the metaphor of curvature, they become something else: dynamic orbits, each drawn by the invisible mass of the unformulated.

In curved space, there is no straight line. There is only path as it is bent by density—by mass, by memory, by affect that has yet to become symbol. In psychic terms, curvature refers to how one bends toward or away from contact, how one organizes relational time, how one metabolizes intensity. The obsessive patient condenses curvature, circling endlessly within recursive loops of thought to avoid the gravitational implosion of feeling. The schizoid disperses it, expanding the field so widely that no center can be felt. The narcissist folds curvature inward, pulling all symbolic motion into a solipsistic loop that mimics coherence while avoiding saturation. The hysteric performs curvature as acceleration—an aestheticized slingshot around the unspeakable, drawing attention to the arc without ever landing.

These styles are not surfaces but atmospheres. They are not containers of identity but symbolic weather—pressure systems within a gravitational topology. To speak of a "style" is to misname something fluid. It is not what someone is, but how their being has bent under forces they could not integrate. In this frame, diagnosis becomes less about labeling and more about locating: where is the analyst in relation to this curvature? Are we pulled too close to the singularity? Are we trying to straighten something that only lives in orbit?

Winnicott's concept of the false self gains new dimensionality here. Rather than a mask over the real, the false self may be understood as the outermost ring of orbit—dense with condensation, structured around absence. It is not false because it is inauthentic; it is false because it is over-determined by relational gravity. The real self, in contrast, may reside closer to the singularity: it is the ungraspable mass that generates the orbit but cannot be symbolized directly.

In a session with a patient who identifies with an obsessive style, the analyst may notice that time itself begins to warp. The patient speaks in detail but without temperature, circling topics with an almost gravitational precision. Questions do not invite answers; they repel them, as if meaning must remain in motion to prevent collapse. Here, the analyst may feel a tug—toward solution, toward insight, toward the reification of content. But this tug is part of the orbit. To follow it uncritically is to lose the symbolic dimension of curvature. The task is to witness the arc without forcing arrival.

This dynamic echoes Jaak Panksepp's work on affective neuroscience, particularly his emphasis on the SEEKING system—the neural substrate of yearning, of forward motion, of unfinished need. In character styles, the SEEKING system is modulated by curvature. The depressive style may suffer from a gravitational heaviness that flattens pursuit. The manic may escape the curve altogether, careening outward in unsustainable vectors. The analytic process, then, becomes a space where the SEEKING system can be reoriented—not by directing it toward a goal, but by stabilizing its orbit around what had previously been unendurable.

We might also turn to Loewald, who describes the psychic field as layered and dynamic, requiring symbolic condensation to sustain contact across levels of organization. In this view, character styles are not flaws but modes of survival—adaptive topographies that maintain coherence when symbolic metabolism breaks down. The narcissistic style, for example, may reflect a field so saturated with unmetabolized intensity that the only way to preserve motion is to become its own center. This is not arrogance; it is a form of curvature that prevents annihilation.

Each style, then, becomes a kind of psychic physics: a way of navigating the space-time of relationship, a way of surviving the unrepresentable. These styles cannot be interpreted away. They are not distortions of an otherwise true self. They are the shape the psyche has taken in the presence of a singularity too dense to touch. To analyze them is not to dismantle them, but to trace their curvature back to the gravitational source.

This requires a clinical stance of gravitational attunement. The analyst does not stand outside the orbit but enters it—carefully, provisionally. We must sense where we are pulled, when we begin to bend, and how our own interpretive habits shift under the patient's field. This is countertransference as topology: not what we feel, but how our structure is altered by proximity. It is not enough to say the patient is avoidant. We must ask: what pressure bends avoidance into necessity? What density makes presence unsafe? What curvature sustains dissociation?

Michael Eigen's notion of "saturation" is instructive here. Saturation refers to the state in which the psyche becomes so filled with unformulated intensity that symbolic functioning is threatened. In such states, character style becomes a valve, a regulator of pressure. The hysteric, for instance, transforms saturation into spectacle; the obsessive, into control. The schizoid disperses it into an ungraspable distance. Each of these is not pathology per se, but a choreography of survival.

To see this is to deepen our empathy. The analyst does not interpret the style away but joins it from within—becoming part of the orbit, allowing the shared field to bend, to warm, to loosen. Over time, the patient may feel this resonance and shift—not through insight alone, but through altered gravity. A new trajectory becomes possible. The orbit wobbles. The field becomes porous.

Character, then, is not essence. It is curvature. It is the path one traces around what cannot be faced. The analyst's task is not to correct the path but to feel its pull, to sense its rhythm, and to offer a presence that slightly alters the orbit—just enough to allow for new symbolic condensation.

And when that happens—when the orbit changes—something forgotten may begin to return. Not as content, but as movement. Not as truth, but as freedom. Not as cure, but as an altered space.

Recursive Collapse: When Orbit Becomes Abyss

Curvature becomes pathology when its movement folds too tightly upon itself—when orbit loses asymmetry and becomes implosive recursion. In analytic terms, this is when character style ceases to function symbolically and instead becomes a gravitational collapse. The patient no longer circles the unformulated; they fall into it. Interpretation becomes unreadable. Time thickens. The analyst is either frozen at the edge or pulled too far in.

Recursive collapse is not simply regression. It is a breakdown of the space required for psychic motion. The orbit can no longer hold asymmetry between self and other, past and present, fantasy and contact. In this state, saturation exceeds the container, and style becomes crisis. The obsessive style may devolve into paranoid rigidity. The narcissistic arc may invert, leaving a collapsed self unable to metabolize gaze. The schizoid dispersion becomes dissociation. What once was curvature now feels like a symbolic black hole.

In these moments, psychic life no longer moves around the singularity—it is seized by it.

Bion's notion of beta elements—the raw, unprocessed shards of experience that cannot yet be symbolized—offers a frame here. When the orbit collapses, the patient's psychic field becomes dominated by beta elements: sensations that cannot be dreamed, affects that cannot be linked, words that fail to organize. The analytic frame becomes overloaded. The analyst's own alpha function—the capacity to metabolize and symbolically link affect— becomes the only vessel holding the shared space.

This is why recursive collapse is so often marked by a collapse in temporality. The patient ceases to speak in narrative. They may shift suddenly between past and present. A story told in the third person veers into first. Affect floods or vanishes. This is not simply trauma re-experiencing—it is psychic curvature folding into itself, like a topological implosion. In analytic terms, it resembles what Thomas Ogden describes as the "undreamt dream"—an experience that has not yet been constituted symbolically and thus cannot be remembered or spoken without destabilizing the field.

The analyst may feel pulled into a loop—wanting to clarify, soothe, and restore continuity. But these efforts risk reinforcing the curvature of collapse. What is needed is something less directed: an attunement to the recursive quality of the field. The analyst becomes the asymmetry—offering not a mirror, but a differential presence, a slight bending in the opposite direction. This is not a technique. It is a stance: remaining near the singularity without being swallowed.

Recursive collapse also challenges the analyst's own capacity to symbolize. The temptation to retreat into theory, into fixed meaning, becomes high. But theory here must not be used as insulation. As Donnel Stern reminds us, it is in the intersubjective moment of not-knowing that new forms of experience become possible. The analyst who can tolerate recursive collapse without demand becomes a holding pattern—a living frame—allowing the patient's orbit to reorganize.

Recursive collapse also destabilizes identity. As Judith Butler teaches, identity is not a possession but a reiterative performance sustained through time. When orbit collapses, the reiteration fails. The self becomes unstrung from its usual style. The patient may feel depersonalized, fragmented, or emptied. This is not simply dissociation—it is an ontological slackening, a symbolic loosening of the threads that keep the self's narrative curved and coherent.

For example, a patient with a borderline structure may enter a session speaking fluently, reflectively, with apparent insight. Then suddenly, the tone shifts. Their voice becomes younger, their syntax frays. They seem confused about what year it is, or whether the analyst has been seen that week. But they are not psychotic. They are folding inward. The gravitational mass of unprocessed affect has become too dense. Their style is no longer style—it is gravitational defense.

In such moments, intervention must not aim for restoration. To try to "bring the patient back" too quickly is to enact foreclosure. Instead, the analyst can become a temporal anchor—not by insisting on time, but by inhabiting it. By slowing the field. By breathing. By letting syntax fail without panic. This is an attunement to curvature even when curvature fails.

Recursive collapse often hides in the analyst's own reaction. We may feel confused, sleepy, unreal. This is the field pulling inward. Eigen's notion of "psychic deadness" is helpful here—not as absence, but as oversaturation. The patient's collapse is not from lack of affect but from too much affect that cannot be metabolized. The analyst who feels nothing may, in fact, be holding the excess—the saturated atmosphere rendered unfeelable through recursive absorption.

This is where affective neuroscience intersects with psychoanalytic presence. Panksepp reminds us that affective systems are always relational—always moving through shared fields. When the SEEKING system is arrested, the analytic room becomes temporally flat. There is no future in the field. Only recursive now. But the analyst's presence—if uncollapsed—can restore time. Not by interpretation, but by duration.

Recursive collapse also poses a challenge to therapeutic aims. What does it mean to heal a collapse? Often, patients do not want to move forward. They do not want insight. They want to remain near the collapse, because it is the only site that feels real. Like the melancholic who refuses consolation, the patient may resist the analyst's every effort to restore curvature. But this is not resistance in the classical sense. It is loyalty—to an affective topology that once held coherence, however painfully.

In these moments, the analyst must adopt a paradoxical ethic: to remain near the recursive site without either falling into it or demanding motion. This is what Winnicott called "going on being" in the presence of disintegration. The analyst is not a rescuer, but a satellite—moving slowly, maintaining asymmetry, allowing gravity to soften.

Recursive collapse also teaches us that structure is not always adaptive. Sometimes, structure is the collapse. The obsessive repetition, the manic refusal, the schizoid dispersal—these are not styles built atop collapse. They are the collapse, curved into form. To see this is to recognize that healing may not look like insight. It may look like the softening of recursion—so that affect can flow again, so that time can thicken and then unfold.

The analyst's task is to detect when style ceases to orbit and begins to consume. When the symbolic collapses into its own echo. When motion stops. And to respond—not with meaning, but with asymmetry. With duration. With a gravity that does not implode.

Because sometimes, the only way to restore curvature is to be curved—just slightly—differently.

Atmospheric Saturation and the Collapse of Differentiation

The field does not always implode. Sometimes, it swells.

In analytic work, not all crises arrive through rupture. Some seep. The patient does not break, but becomes saturated—drenched in affective ambiguity so dense that no differentiation can hold. Here, thought does not fail with a crash but loses its edges. Emotion floods without clarity. The room feels warm, thick, and unstable. Analyst and patient float inside it, breathing air that feels like water.

This is the domain of saturation: the psychic state in which symbolic distinction dissolves under too much pressure. It is not absence, but excess. Not silence, but noise. Affect saturates the field so completely that no single contour can be drawn. A word is spoken, and it lands everywhere. The boundary between self and other becomes slippery, viscous. Transference becomes atmosphere.

In these moments, the analyst does not interpret from outside the field. They are in the weather. The transference is not an object to name—it is a climate to endure. As Bollas reminds us, the patient often brings not a narrative but a texture. A feel. An atmospheric registration of early experience, condensed into mood rather than memory.

This saturation is often the aesthetic signature of masochistic and depressive styles, though it may also appear in borderline, hysteric, and even narcissistic presentations. The patient may speak in looping resignation. They may flood the room with despair without asking for help. Or they may use beauty, eroticism, or deference to blur agency. The analyst finds themselves seduced into silence, or into over-speaking—either drawn into the mist or desperate to pierce it.

What is at stake in these moments is differentiation. Not only between self and other, but between affect states themselves. The patient cannot say if they are sad or angry, longing or humiliated. Shame bleeds into rage, which curdles into self-deprecation, which dissolves again into passivity. The analyst cannot anchor to tone. Words bend under the saturation of feeling, like wet paper losing form.

Jaak Panksepp's affective neuroscience reminds us that basic emotional systems like SEEKING, PANIC, and CARE operate not as clean categories but as overlapping currents, often co-activating in ways that exceed conscious control. In saturation, these systems collide. The patient's CARE circuitry may be activated, but so too is PANIC—and the result is not longing, but helpless erotic submission. The analyst who reads this as sexualized transference alone misses the way saturation creates psychic ambiguity—an atmosphere that distorts all signals.

This climate often reflects early relational environments in which too much affect moved through too little structure. It is not the emptiness of neglect, but the chaos of over-involvement, misattuned engulfment, or seductively fused care. The child is not left alone; they are overwhelmed. They learn to breathe within intensity, to survive by losing boundaries.

In the clinic, these patterns reemerge as affective murk. The patient may say they want clarity, but they seem to undo every moment of it. They may cling, then disavow. They may eroticize the analytic presence, not to make contact, but to liquefy it. Interpretation lands but then slides. The frame holds, but feels dampened. Analyst and patient begin to lose track of position.

In these sessions, what collapses is not simply thought but symbolic differentiation itself. Affect floods the field, and the symbolic function begins to drown. As Loewald teaches, symbolic function is born not of cognition but of temporal and spatial separation—it requires enough distance between experience and reflection to allow meaning to condense. But saturation undoes that distance. Everything is now. Everything is everywhere. The symbolic does not link—it swells.

One patient, a man with high-functioning depression and masochistic tendencies, often entered sessions with what he called his "swamp mood." He described feeling "emotionally wet." His tone was gentle, even sweet— but every word carried a drowned bitterness. He smiled as he said he didn't mind being misunderstood. He praised the analytic process even as he quietly erased its effects. Over time, I began to feel the texture of the field before the content of his words: a heaviness, a fog, a strange comfort in futility.

My countertransference moved in kind. I found myself speaking too softly, delaying interpretations, waiting for an opening that never came. I worried about intruding. I felt immersed in him—drawn into his gentle despair. It took many months to recognize that what felt like empathy was actually saturation. The room had become affectively dense, and I was no longer symbolizing—I was diffusing. I had become an atmospheric participant.

The turning point came not through insight, but through a shift in presence. I began to hold my chair differently. I straightened my back. I named the fog. I stopped waiting for him to clear it. "It feels like we're swimming today," I said once, "but no one's reaching the surface." He didn't respond directly, but the saturation thinned. We both breathed more. In the weeks that followed, his tone began to sharpen. A humor emerged—dry, biting, newly differentiated. He was no longer drowning me to survive.

This is the ethic of the analyst in saturation: to resist both drowning and disavowal. To remain symbolic without demanding clarity. To name the tone without prematurely interpreting its cause. To offer not explication, but contour—psychic edges thick enough to survive the blur.

Winnicott's notion of "holding" becomes critical here, but it must be reimagined as a dynamic container for affective weather—not a static vessel. Holding does not mean calming. It means staying curvaceous in the presence of affective excess. It means allowing the field to saturate, but not to burst.

Here, Derrida's *différance* returns: the slippage between signifier and signified becomes affectively dense. Every utterance refers, defers, displaces. The analyst must learn to hear the unsaid not as absence, but as condensation. The unspeakable is not silence—it is atmospheric presence that has yet to symbolically cohere.

And so we bend with the field. Not to mirror it, but to counter-curve— offering a differentiated stance that is not rigid. This is what Benjamin calls mutual recognition: not fusion, not withdrawal, but the trembling co-presence of two differentiated minds, each capable of resonance without collapse.

The analyst's stance, then, must be neither declarative nor absent. We speak not to name, but to edge. We interpret not to fix, but to trace the contour. We offer tone before we offer cause. And we allow the saturation to thin—not by draining it, but by thickening the symbolic frame enough to hold its weight.

Because the patient is not only telling a story. They are creating a climate. And we are breathing it with them.

Performance as Defense: The Panic of Being Known

Some patients do not simply fear being misrecognized. They fear being seen at all. The moment of authentic contact—what others might experience as relief or intimacy—triggers in them not safety but a panic of exposure. This panic is not just affective; it is ontological. To be seen is to collapse. The structure of selfhood, in such patients, is organized around performance— carefully rehearsed, tightly controlled, semi-opaque. The performance is not a falsehood. It is a necessary curvature around a center that cannot be safely approached.

To be known, in these configurations, is to risk disintegration. The ana- lyst, then, encounters not just resistance but theatricality: mannered speech, stylized affect, seductive overavailability. These are not tactics of manipula- tion, but atmospheric defenses—attempts to preserve distance through satura- tion. If the field becomes too vivid, too affectively thick, it clouds rather than clarifies. As in weather, too much humidity blurs vision. The patient's perfor- mance generates this fog: too much presence can be as defensive as absence.

Winnicott famously distinguished between the true and false self, but he also recognized—though rarely emphasized—that the false self may be an authentic structure in its own right: a protective formation with adaptive vital- ity (Winnicott, 1965). In the curvature model, performance is not mere dis- guise; it is an orbiting pattern. The self bends away from the unbearable: the infant whose spontaneity was not met learns to anticipate instead. Over time, anticipation becomes character, and character becomes self. Performance hardens into identity.

Judith Butler, in *The Psychic Life of Power* (1997), helps us think of this not just as interpersonal, but as fundamentally social and political. The self is formed through regulatory regimes of recognition, which are internalized as part of psychic structure. To be seen "correctly" is to conform to expecta- tions; to be seen otherwise is to risk abjection. The analytic situation stirs this paradox. On the one hand, it offers a gaze that promises to receive what has never been seen. On the other hand, it activates the historical terror that being seen might annihilate the delicate architecture of survival.

In clinical work, this often appears as what Loewald (1960) called "unfreez- ing." A patient who has functioned smoothly—articulate, insightful, even engaged—suddenly becomes incoherent or dissociated when the analytic gaze touches something unperformed. The warmth of interpretation thaws the protective structure, and what emerges is not the truth, but disorientation. Performance, then, is not antithetical to self. It is its own kind of coherence, developed not as deception, but as a compromise with the impossibility of being seen without distortion.

Michael Eigen (1993b) might describe this as a defense of intensity. For some patients, aliveness itself is the threat. The performance is a way to regu- late the voltage. What appears to the analyst as false is, for the patient, the only viable form of psychic containment. The stylized self is not a mask. It is the cooling shell around a core too hot to touch.

Here, the metaphor of curvature becomes essential. The self does not split neatly between truth and falsity. It curves, it protects, it shimmers. Just as light bends around massive objects in space, so too does meaning bend around zones of internal danger. The analyst's task is not to strip away performance, but to attune to its orbit: how does this patient loop around the unbearable? What rhythm of approach and retreat organizes their speech, their gaze, their silences?

We might think of the analytic setting as a symbolic theater, but one in which the goal is not to end the play, but to understand the script's gravitational pull. Some patients must perform in order to survive the gaze. Others perform to preempt the analyst's seeing. Still others perform because that is all the self has ever been: a recursive echo of what might have been received. As with Foucault's panopticon (1977b), the internalized gaze organizes behavior long before the actual observer arrives.

There is an aesthetic here, too—what Barthes (1977) might call the "grain" of the voice. Every defense has a texture. Performance can be brittle or fluid, stylized or chaotic, erotic or intellectualized. Each variation expresses something about the psychic topology: what can be approached, what must be deflected, where the analyst is permitted to look. The performative field is not uniform. It is curved. And the pressure of that curvature must be felt, not just analyzed.

For instance, consider a patient who speaks in aphorisms—clever, concise, emotionally opaque. Their style is dazzling, but the analytic field remains flat. No pressure builds. One day, in a moment of spontaneous affect, they pause and say something simple, unpolished. The room thickens. They become visibly uncomfortable. The analyst notices a shift—not in content, but in atmospheric curvature. Something unperformed has entered the field. The panic of being known arises not because of trauma per se, but because the self's structure was built to avoid precisely this intensity.

In such moments, the analyst must practice what Jessica Benjamin (2004) calls "witnessing beyond recognition." The goal is not to interpret the unperformed into coherence, but to remain present to it without collapsing its singularity. To witness a truth not yet in form requires a tolerance for ambiguity, for psychic heat, for partiality. It also requires a refusal to rescue: to let the patient feel the edge of being known without rushing to contain it.

The panic of being known is not a signal of failure. It is a threshold. It tells us that the performance has thinned, that the singularity is near. The patient's choreography may become erratic here—testing, withdrawing, accusing, seducing. The analyst must stay curved: not neutral, but responsive; not interpretive, but attuned. This is the clinical ethic of orbit: to remain close enough to sense the gravity, far enough not to distort the field.

Levinas (1969) reminds us that the face of the Other is not an object to be known, but a summons. In the moment of panic, the analyst confronts the Other not as pathology, but as demand. The self that appears is not the one the analyst expected—it is the one the field produced under pressure. And our ethical task is not to fix it, but to remain with it.

There is no purity beneath performance. No authentic self waiting to be revealed. The performance is itself the artifact of truth: it tells us what could not be borne, and how the self adapted to survive. The analytic process, then, is not a stripping away, but a circling in. The panic of being known is not a detour. It is the gravitational event itself—the place where curvature is most extreme.

What we meet here is not pathology, but a style of survival.

And our task is not to interpret it away, but to orbit it faithfully—until something new begins to move.

Temporal Permeability and Recursive Time

The analytic field is not merely spatial—it is temporal. Each utterance arrives not only from a psychic location but from a psychic time. And for many patients, the boundary between these times is unstable. Traumatic memory, characterological rigidity, and affective saturation bend time, collapse it, distort it. In such patients, the present is not now; it is an echo, a loop, a recurrence. The past is not behind them—it leaks forward, coloring perception, configuring relational stances, dictating meanings before they can be co-constructed.

To say such a patient "regresses" is insufficient. The term suggests a linear model, a fallback into something earlier or less mature. But psychic time, as we've argued, is not linear—it is gravitational. Moments of the past are not simply re-experienced; they become thick zones of repetition, sites of recursive activation. A patient might respond to a minor boundary with the despair of abandonment. But what returns is not content—it is time. The patient has become temporally permeable.

Eigen (2004) notes that memory in such states is not recollection but atmosphere. The past returns as tone, not as narrative. Something floods the room—an affective weather, a curvature of the field. And the analyst must learn to feel it, not just track it. When the patient suddenly speaks as if betrayed, despite no present betrayal, the analyst is not encountering a distortion to be corrected. They are encountering an arrival from another time. The task is not to reorient them to the now but to enter, momentarily, the then that still lives in the present.

In this way, the analytic hour becomes a meeting of temporalities. The analyst lives, as Loewald (1960) proposed, in a temporally stratified mind—holding the patient's present distress, the past experience it reactivates, and the future psychic potential it seeks to protect. The analyst's own counter-transference may be bent by these pressures. A felt sense of confusion, slowness, or intensity may reflect not just interpersonal dynamics but temporal turbulence: the field itself thickening with layered time.

This permeability is not pathological in itself. Indeed, it may be a form of symbolic richness. But when time becomes recursive—when the same emotional structure returns again and again, closing rather than opening the field—pathology emerges not from the content, but from the stuckness of time itself. The borderline repetition of rupture, the obsessive return to failure, the depressive preemption of hope—these are not styles of thinking but temporal signatures. They mark where time has folded inward, sealing off the possibility of revision.

In such cases, the analyst must become not only a witness but a time-worker. Interpretation becomes not just meaning-making, but time-releasing. When an analyst says, "You're responding to me as if I've already let you down," they are not correcting a mistake—they are locating the patient within a recursive temporal field. They are making space for time to move again.

Here, Merleau-Ponty's (1962) phenomenology becomes useful. He reminds us that time is not external—it is lived. Temporality is not a frame but a mode of existence. The patient's present may be lived not as presence, but as suspended anticipation, dread, or echo. And the analyst, too, lives in this time. We feel when the session becomes stuck in a loop. We feel when we are being treated as someone from before. But instead of resisting, we may ask: What structure of time are we now inhabiting?

Judith Herman (1992), in her work on trauma, insists that healing requires the re-sequencing of time. The traumatic event disrupts chronology; it freezes a moment into a permanent now. The patient lives as if what happened is still happening. In analysis, the work is not to forget, but to thaw. When the patient can narrate the event, place it in sequence, and reflect upon it—then it has moved. The past has become past.

But some patients resist this thawing. Not because they do not want to heal, but because the frozen moment holds identity. If the betrayal ends, who am I? If I am no longer wounded, what becomes of the care I finally received in the analyst's presence? This is the double-bind of temporal healing: movement requires mourning. And some patients would rather loop than lose.

Freud (1914b) sensed this when he described repetition compulsion as a return to the scene of trauma in search of mastery. But his model was still linear—past to present to future. What we are proposing here is more curved. The patient returns not to master, but to orbit. The traumatic site is not just content; it is gravity. And repetition is not simply compulsion—it is a form of life.

This is why analysis so often feels recursive. The same themes return, the same ruptures repeat. The analyst wonders: Have we made any progress? But perhaps the goal is not to move forward but to move differently. The spiral, not the line. Each return to the trauma field brings a new inflection, a new capacity to stay present, a new degree of symbolic metabolism. The repetition is not failure—it is structure under pressure.

Ogden (2005) offers a helpful lens here with his concept of the "undreamt dream"—experiences that have never been symbolically held, and thus cannot unfold in ordinary time. These moments arrive in the analytic field not as stories, but as sudden shifts in atmosphere, as distortions of time itself. The patient becomes drowsy, the analyst distracted. An unseen moment is seeking emergence, but cannot yet be dreamed. Time buckles. The analytic task is to stay close, to allow the field to heat until a form begins to cohere.

Sometimes this form is a word. Sometimes it is silence. Sometimes it is just the shared awareness that time is moving differently here. The analyst must learn to listen not just for content, but for temporal contour. Is the patient in a now, a then, or a loop? What tempo governs their speech, their gaze, their silence? And what tempo does the analyst bring? Are we rushing? Waiting? Holding?

These are not neutral choices. They shape the field. The analyst who slows the pace may allow time to stretch. The analyst who returns to a phrase spoken weeks ago may mark continuity. The analyst who tolerates the silence of recursive time may allow the patient to feel something uncollapsed. In each case, temporality is not just lived—it is co-constructed.

Temporal permeability, then, is not a flaw. It is a feature of psychic life. But when the field becomes recursive without relief, when time bends without elasticity, when the future collapses into the repetition of the past—then analysis must act. Not to impose a new tempo, but to tune to the rhythm of the field and offer an alternative: a phrase, a pause, a breath, a gaze. These are the instruments of temporal shift.

And when the shift occurs—when the patient remembers differently, or forgets in a new way, or finds themselves outside the loop for a moment—something opens. Not a destination. A possibility. A new orbit. A reconfiguration of time.

And the future, once foreclosed, becomes imaginable again.

Psychic Climate and the Ethics of Orbit

By now, we have seen how psychic life unfolds not as a series of discrete objects, but as patterns of motion in a gravitational field—curving, condensing, looping through time and symbolic atmosphere. But just as weather patterns differ from isolated storms, so too do psychic climates differ from singular defenses. To enter the analytic room is not merely to encounter a patient's thoughts or symptoms; it is to enter a climate. A felt pattern. A psychic weather system.

Some climates are dry—emotionally barren, brittle with abstraction. Others are saturated—humid with longing, affectively overgrown. Still others are arid and electric at once, with the volatility of a desert thunderstorm: moods shift, defenses fracture, symbolic integrity flashes and then recedes. These are not metaphorical embellishments. They are phenomenological realities— how the psyche organizes its own atmosphere to preserve, defend, and sometimes reveal its center of gravity.

To speak of character style, then, is to speak not of type but of topology. Not what the patient is, but how the psyche moves in order to remain coherent. The obsessive style thickens thought into structure, condenses ambiguity into ritual, and shields against affective dissolution through the architecture of precision. The schizoid diffuses presence into the ether, softens affect into abstraction, and mistrusts the orbit of relational gravity. The depressive collapses time into remorse, feeling into excess, and movement into fatigue. These are not distortions of an ideal, but elegant adjustments to psychic mass.

Each orbit has its own ethical demands. To treat a paranoid structure as merely rigid is to miss the ethic of vigilance it embodies. To pathologize the hysteric without recognizing their exquisite sensitivity to relational heat is to mistake performance for emptiness. And to assume the narcissistic patient seeks praise rather than symmetry is to collapse their symbolic hunger into cliché. Each climate requires a different analytic posture—not because the analyst is a chameleon, but because the field is alive, and ethics begins in responsiveness.

Winnicott (1965) understood this when he spoke of the analyst's "capacity to be alone in the presence of another." The analyst is not neutral because they are blank, but because they are atmospherically attuned. Their neutrality is a form of presence calibrated to the patient's climate: porous when needed, insulated when containment is at risk. This is not technique—it is ethical weathering. The analyst allows themselves to be shaped by the atmosphere while remaining capable of symbolic return.

At times, this climate overwhelms. The analyst may feel despair that is not theirs, or urgency that comes from nowhere. They may feel a pull to soothe, to fix, to name. These are signs of psychic orbit: the analyst has entered the patient's gravitational loop. The ethics here is not to resist, but to feel without becoming. To note the climate, to participate in its warmth or chill, but to retain enough symbolic distance to remain capable of movement.

This is what distinguishes analytic orbit from enactment. In enactment, the analyst is consumed by the climate—becomes weathered, lost. In orbit, the analyst feels the pull but does not fall in. They are aware of the curvature, the repetition, the affective temperature—and they speak from within it, not against it. Their interpretations are not interruptions; they are forms of climate literacy. They name the atmosphere in a way that introduces space, not rupture.

Jessica Benjamin (2004) offers a vital contribution here in her notion of mutual recognition—not simply as a relational achievement, but as an ethical one. To recognize another is not to agree with their affective climate but to acknowledge its reality. The analyst says, "I feel the fog," "I notice the cold," "I see the repetition"—not to diagnose, but to witness. This witnessing is the analyst's ethical posture in orbit: to name the gravity without collapsing into it.

There are times, of course, when the analyst's own climate intervenes. We bring our atmospheres, our symbolic weathers, into the room. Sometimes these atmospheres resonate, creating openings; at other times, they conflict, generating heat. The ethics here are not to erase our climate, but to know it. To sense when our need to be useful overrides the patient's tempo. To track when our need for clarity precipitates symbolic foreclosure.

Levinas (1969) reminds us that ethical relation is not grounded in symmetry, but in responsibility to alterity. The patient is not a self to be understood, but a presence that makes a demand. The analyst's task is to meet that demand not with solution, but with presence that holds without consuming. To feel the patient's orbit, to sense their climate, to respond without reduction—this is analytic ethics at its core.

To hold style as orbit rather than as identity means giving up the fantasy of diagnosis as destination. It becomes, instead, a tracing—of the patient's recursive logic, their temporal bends, their atmospheric thickness. Diagnosis names a climate pattern. It sketches the outlines of a psyche in motion. And the ethic is to name it without freezing it—to allow the patient to become legible without being fixed.

This is why the best interpretations do not feel like conclusions. They feel like weather reports: momentary readings of a shifting field. "There's a fog here." "It feels stormy." "I notice we return here, again and again." These are not metaphors. They are orientations—ways the analyst attunes to the ethics of orbit.

In the end, psychic climate cannot be controlled. But it can be known, metabolized, and symbolically thickened. The analyst is less a forecaster than a barometer: a reader of pressure, of movement, of condensation and wind. The patient does not need us to name the sun. They need us to notice the change in the air. To say, "I feel it, too." And to stay, even as it storms.

Because when the patient can begin to notice their own climate—not just as suffering, but as structure—they begin to reclaim symbolic movement. They begin to sense orbit not as fate, but as form. And in that recognition, something shifts. Not the weather itself, but the capacity to live inside it, differently.

That is the work of psychoanalysis—not to change the sky, but to attune to its curvature.

And in doing so, offer shelter enough for something new to begin to form.

Gravity and the Analyst's Gaze

Gravity, in this model, is not a metaphor for pathology, but for presence. It is the pull of the unsymbolized, the condensation of affect into form, the mass of experience that draws everything around it into orbit. When we speak of character style, we are really speaking of gravity wells—zones of psychic compression around which the self loops, performs, and recurs. These orbits are not chosen. They are formed in response to mass.

What has mass in psychic life? Not just trauma, but significance. Repetition. Affect that was once overwhelming and remains unintegrated. Loss that had no witness. Love that could not be metabolized. The child does not orbit randomly. They curve around what exerted the most pull. Around what bent time, structure, safety, and self.

In analysis, gravity enters the room as field pressure. The patient may speak lightly, but something in their pacing, in their gaze, in the temperature of the room, suggests density. The analyst begins to feel tired. Or pulled. Or unable to think. This is not resistance. It is gravity. Something massive is near. And the analyst, if attuned, begins to notice the curvature of the hour.

To respond to gravity requires a shift in posture. Interpretation as cleverness—bright ideas and explanatory models—often collapses here. The patient does not need brilliance. They need witnessing. And witnessing, in the presence of gravity, means staying close without being pulled under. It means holding one's own symbolic mass, not becoming a satellite.

The analyst's gaze must be warm, but weighted. Not blank, not devouring. Gravity does not respond to neutrality as distance; it responds to attunement as density. The analyst must become symbolically dense enough to anchor the field. To not fly away. To not fall in. To be present with just enough mass to allow curvature to be experienced rather than enacted.

Bollas (1987) described the "unthought known" as a psychic gravity that shapes experience without language. It operates like a silent mass in the field, bending the possible before it is thought. The analyst's task, then, is not to unearth it, but to sense its weight—to track how it bends narrative, relation, and affect. The gaze here is not searching for content; it is tracking form.

This is a different gaze than the diagnostic glance or the empathic nod. It is the gravitational gaze—the look that holds without absorbing, the presence that gives shape without imposing meaning. It is the gaze that remains when interpretation would fracture, when silence is not avoidance but alignment. The patient may not know what they want, but they can feel whether they are being held or collapsed into.

This gaze also demands ethical restraint. To name what is not yet form can violate the field. The analyst must learn when the gravitational tension is ripe—when the unsymbolized has softened enough to be touched without distortion. This is the precision of gaze: to see not with intent, but with timing. To name the curvature just as it crests. To say what the field is almost saying, but not quite. Not yet.

In Lacan's terms, the analyst's presence should be not all-knowing, but lacking—an object that can be invested with meaning, not one that overdetermines it. Gravity here is also the analyst's desire—not for content, but for form to emerge. The patient orbits this desire. They sense whether the analyst needs to understand, to fix, to soothe. Any unconscious demand becomes another mass in the field.

The discipline, then, is to remain present without becoming heavy. To have gravity without collapse. To allow the field to bend without introducing one's own curvature too soon. The analyst must be willing to be used symbolically—and to monitor how the patient uses them. Do they become the absent father, the engulfing mother, the mute sibling, the perfect mirror? These are not transference tropes. They are gravitational identities—roles shaped by psychic mass.

Ogden (1994) calls this the "analytic third"—the shared field co-created by analyst and patient, but neither reducible to either. In this field, gravity is not one person's experience but a shared atmospheric tension. The analyst must track not just their own pull, but how the patient orbits them—and how the dyad spirals together toward or away from symbolization.

The analytic hour becomes, then, not a session of exchange, but a chamber of gravity. A space where curvatures can be traced, orbits observed, and repetition slowed. The analyst becomes a gravitational counterpoint—not fixing, but thickening the field just enough for something to begin to form. This is not interpretation. It is symbolic presence. The gaze as mass.

The risk, always, is foreclosure. The analyst who interprets too soon may collapse the orbit into insight that cannot yet be borne. The one who withholds completely may fail to hold the symbolic atmosphere. The one who identifies with the patient's gravity too completely may lose their own symbolic center. Each of these errors is a form of gravitational imbalance.

The ethics of the gaze, then, is to remain symbolically centered while allowing the patient to feel their own orbit. To give them the experience of being seen without being collapsed, known without being named, held without being gripped. In this space, style can begin to curve differently. What was frozen in orbit may find a new velocity. What was stuck may stretch. The gravitational hold may shift just enough to allow time to move again.

For patients with long histories of being misrecognized—those whose style has been pathologized, flattened, or caricatured—this shift is profound. It is not just therapeutic; it is ontological. They begin to feel that their climate is readable without being reducible. That their gravity does not make them too much. That their style is not a pathology, but a form of life.

And in that space, orbit becomes choice. Not freedom in the naïve sense, but in the psychoanalytic one: the capacity to symbolize the field. To move differently. To feel the curvature without being defined by it.

This is the gift of the analytic gaze—not to see through, but to stay with. To become gravity enough to hold the field, light enough to allow orbit, and ethical enough to know the difference.

And in that delicate balance, something unfurls. Not transformation as rupture, but as reformation of gravity itself.

A softening of mass.

A new style of movement.

Orbit and the Ethics of Naming

To orbit is to move without arrival. It is to remain tethered to something massive, invisible, unresolved. The orbit is not a failure to change; it is the psyche's form of survival. Each character style is an orbit—an elegant, if costly, loop around what cannot be metabolized. These styles—obsessive, hysteric, narcissistic, depressive, paranoid, schizoid—are not symptoms. They are trajectories. Psychic movement traced over time.

Naming them is a dangerous act.

Every diagnostic term is a symbolic incision. It can clarify, but it can also cut. It can offer containment, or it can fix identity. To name a style is to introduce a frame. That frame, if too rigid or too early, becomes another orbit. The patient begins to circle the name, rather than the self. They become the labeled, rather than the lived. The analyst, in turn, risks treating the orbit as essence—forgetting that every style is a curve around something unformulated.

And yet, naming is part of the work. Not naming is also an intervention. The refusal to locate style can leave patients swimming in an ocean of affect without an anchor. They may repeat without recognition, orbit without witness. They may feel unheld by the very person meant to help symbolize what bends their lives into shape.

The task, then, is not to avoid naming, but to name differently.

We do not name to categorize. We name to reveal curvature. To offer the patient a glimpse of their movement—not as pathology, but as pattern. The diagnosis is not a verdict; it is a trace. A symbolic stroke around a field of affect. A way to say: I see how you move. I see how the mass at the center of your life bends your time, your relationships, your sense of self. I see the orbit, and I do not mistake it for who you are.

This is why we speak of orbit rather than essence. The orbit can change. The mass can shift. New gravitational relationships can emerge. The hysteric need not forever seduce; the obsessive need not loop endlessly in thought. But to move differently, the orbit must first be seen. And for it to be seen, it must be symbolized. Named.

In the clinic, this naming often occurs slowly, provisionally, wrapped in metaphor rather than jargon. The analyst might say, "It seems like your mind circles this in a very particular way," or "There's a gravitational pull here that keeps drawing things back." These are diagnostic utterances—but diagnostic in the key of movement, not identity. They track the shape of experience without reducing it.

And even formal diagnoses, when used carefully, can be gifts. To tell a patient, "This reminds me of the obsessive structure—not because you are obsessive, but because this rhythm of mind, this need to contain, this condensation of thought—is something I recognize," can be liberating. It places their suffering in a lineage. It allows them to see their style as a stance, not a flaw. As a form of life.

Bion (1962) warned of the analyst who interprets too soon, whose desire to know overwhelms the patient's capacity to symbolize. The same is true of diagnostic naming. If we name before the orbit is felt, before the movement is safe enough to trace, the name lands as violence. It forecloses, rather than reveals. It becomes mass, not light.

And yet, the refusal to name can also wound. It can suggest that the patient's style is unspeakable, or that their suffering has no structure. This, too, is a kind of foreclosure. A negation of form. The ethical stance, then, is not silence or speech, but timing. Not knowledge or ignorance, but resonance.

Timing matters because naming is never neutral. It enters the field with weight. It can be metabolized or rejected, felt as containment or collapse. The analyst must learn to sense the field's readiness—to feel when a name would clarify, and when it would distort. And most importantly, to remain open to renaming. To change the name as the orbit shifts.

This is not relativism. It is gravity ethics. It is the refusal to mistake the trace for the truth. The refusal to believe that any map is the territory. The recognition that every diagnostic gesture is a symbolic act that reverberates through the field.

In this frame, even the word "style" is provisional. It suggests coherence, when many patients live in fragmentation. It suggests pattern, when what they feel is chaos. And yet, it also offers hope. To have a style is to have a shape. A way of being that can be traced, held, known—not as totality, but as trajectory. A style is not a cage. It is a signature of survival.

To name it, then, is to offer recognition. Not recognition of pathology, but of movement. Of how the psyche bent to protect something. Of how character is condensation. Of how orbit is resilience.

This form of naming aligns with Jessica Benjamin's (1990b) notion of recognition as mutual constitution—not the unilateral knowing of the patient by the analyst, but a shared encounter in which the analyst's naming becomes a response to the patient's symbolic bid. The name is not imposed. It is offered. It waits to be received.

And sometimes, it is rejected. Rightly so. The patient says, "That's not me," and the analyst listens. The name missed. The orbit was misread. The field resisted. This is not failure. This is curvature asserting itself. The analyst adjusts. Waits. Listens again. The orbit speaks in loops.

In the end, naming is not a final act. It is a phase of orbit. A moment when the unspeakable briefly crystallizes into form—just long enough to be felt, witnessed, and released. A diagnostic term, in this frame, is not a definition. It is a symbolic flare. A gesture toward the curvature of a life.

The ethics of naming, then, is not to avoid it, but to hold it lightly. To speak it not as fact, but as question. To let the name bend with the field, soften with the hour. And always, always, to remember that what we are naming is not the patient, but their motion.

They are not the orbit. They are what orbits.

And what orbits can move.

3 Chronotopes of the Self

Structural Temporality and Character Style

This chapter proposes that character structure is best understood not merely as a set of psychic traits, but as a chronotope—a lived form of time that organizes experience, symptom, and transference. Drawing on psychoanalytic, philosophical, and literary sources, it examines how temporality shapes personality style, symptom expression, and analytic process. Clinical material illustrates the ways patients inhabit specific temporal configurations—such as looping, freezing, or acceleration—and how analytic attunement can gently modify these structures through shared temporal experience. This chapter links structural pathology to distortions in temporality, arguing that the therapeutic action of analysis often lies in the creation of new rhythms, not new insights. Ultimately, it repositions the analytic field as a temporal crucible, where symbolic gravity allows psychic time to bend, fold, and reconfigure in the service of lived change.

Having traced the psyche's curvature in spatial terms, we now turn to the dimension most saturated by that curvature: time. For structure is not only a shape—it is a rhythm, a pacing, a recursive logic that bends temporality from within. What we call "character" is often a temporal style: a way of moving through duration, resisting change, or looping through repetition. In this chapter, we ask how psychic structures shape the experience of time itself— not as neutral flow, but as warped field, a chronotope that both protects and imprisons.

Time's Texture: Psychic Chronotopes and the Narrative Self

Psychoanalysis has always been concerned with time, though it often approaches it obliquely. Whether in the long arc of development, the return of the repressed, or the recursions of transference, time becomes less a neutral backdrop and more a dynamic force shaping psychic experience. Yet time, like space, is not a universal constant within the psyche. It bends, loops, accelerates, and fragments—and in doing so, it constructs character.

This chapter explores how temporality is not merely experienced by the self but constitutes it. Character styles, long regarded as stable traits or affective patterns, are here reframed as emergent temporal structures.

DOI: 10.4324/9781003715306-5

These structures—what Bakhtin might call *chronotopes*, or time-space configurations—organize psychic life through the intertwining of narrative, memory, expectation, and fantasy. Each self is a chronotopic formation: a temporal style of being that condenses developmental history, defensive choreography, and affective economy into a lived rhythm of relation.

We are not simply situated *in* time; we are shaped *by* the kind of time we inhabit. The obsessive patient, for instance, inhabits a temporality of deferral and suspension, where action is endlessly delayed in favor of symbolic precision. The hysteric lives in elliptical time, charged with anticipation and crisis, where the present always hovers on the edge of a not-quite-yet. The depressive collapses into a recursive temporality, circling back over the same emotional terrain, while the narcissistic character often inhabits a suspended, timeless now—a scene that cannot end, lest the void beyond it be encountered.

These are not merely descriptive metaphors. They are structural conditions that generate the particular suffering—and symbolic grammar—of each character style. To treat character, then, is to engage not only its defenses and attachments, but its underlying chronotope: the temporal topology through which meaning accrues, stagnates, or ruptures.

The spatial theory of mind developed in the prior chapter sets the stage for this temporal turn. Where psychic space configures the field of internal objects and relations, psychic time regulates the flow and sequence of affect, symbol, and memory. The two are inseparable—temporality is always spatialized, just as spatial form is infused with temporality. A patient's sense of being trapped may reflect not just a claustrophobic relational structure but a temporality in which no future can be imagined. Conversely, the phantasm of endless potential often camouflages an evacuation of lived time: a flight from limit, loss, and repetition.

The chronotope, in this sense, is both aesthetic and structural. It defines not only how time is felt but also how life is narrated. Some selves narrate in mythic time—every current event becomes a reiteration of an archetypal betrayal. Others narrate in episodic bursts, unable to sustain a continuity of experience. Still others fixate on a moment frozen in psychic amber, returning to it compulsively without metabolizing its meaning. These patterns are not simply artifacts of trauma; they are how trauma is lived—and how the self, in turn, becomes narratable.

Psychoanalytic technique, then, must learn to listen temporally. What kind of time does the patient bring into the room? What is the rhythm of their associations, the latency of their feeling, the recursive echoes in their storytelling? To intervene effectively is often to disturb the closed circuit of a pathological temporality—not through interpretive content alone but by offering a different rhythm, a temporal counter-transference. The analyst's capacity to hold delay, to tolerate incompletion, to register repetition not as redundancy but as signal—these become the tools for entering the patient's lived chronotope.

This is particularly evident in moments of rupture. When a patient relives a traumatic memory in session, it is not simply the past returning; it is the present moment folding under the weight of a temporal distortion. The past is not remembered, it is *re-entered*. Such moments are not regressions in a linear sense, but recursive condensations—the psyche bending time to sustain coherence. To witness this without collapsing into the patient's temporality is a delicate act: one must feel the pull of that time without becoming of it.

Freud's early work on trauma and repetition already gestured toward this. In "Beyond the Pleasure Principle," the compulsion to repeat is framed as a paradox: the return of painful experience defies the logic of mastery or pleasure. But rather than resolve the paradox, Freud left it open—a riddle about time and drive. Contemporary relational analysts have picked up this thread, reframing repetition as a form of unformulated experience, a memory not yet symbolized. But even here, the chronotopic structure—the *kind* of time being repeated—remains underexplored.

To speak of chronotopes is not to abandon the analytic language of defense, desire, or symbol. It is to enfold these within a temporal matrix, where defense is not just a function but a pacing; desire not just a vector but a temporal mood; symbol not just a meaning but a rhythm of emergence. In this light, the psyche is not only a site of conflict or relation but a time-structure— warped, recursive, shimmering with repetition and delay.

As we proceed, each section will examine specific character styles through their temporal logics. We will explore how schizoid, depressive, obsessive, hysteric, and narcissistic formations each constellate their own chronotopes. These are not fixed types but dynamic fields—gravitational temporalities around which the self is drawn, often unwittingly. Clinical vignettes will illustrate not just the content of these structures, but their pace, their loops, their absences, and their insistences.

Psychoanalysis, at its best, listens for time. In character, in symptom, in silence, the analyst listens for the beat of a suffering time—a chronotope seeking reformation.

The Obsessive and the Suspended Future

The obsessive character inhabits a temporality of suspension—not merely of delay, but of purposeful non-arrival. Time, for the obsessive, is a site of negotiation, precision, and symbolic substitution. The future is endlessly deferred, not because it is feared per se, but because its arrival threatens the symbolic order on which the obsessive's self-coherence depends.

In the obsessive's world, temporality is thick with potential but thin in realization. Each act is preempted by a thought; each thought is met with a counter-thought. Rituals proliferate, not to reach a destination but to keep it at bay. This is not procrastination in the pedestrian sense, but a structural choreography of symbolic time. The obsessive is perpetually approaching the scene of life—yet never crossing its threshold.

What makes this temporality so affectively charged is its relationship to control. The obsessive fears not just chaos, but the temporal collapse that would follow spontaneity. The unforeseen is not just unwelcome—it is structurally destabilizing. Hence, the compulsive return to ordering systems, schemas, and symbolic equivalences. Every thought must be accounted for, every potentiality imagined. In this temporality, the future cannot simply unfold; it must be pre-lived in language.

The result is often a life lived in the subjunctive: what could be, should be, must not be. Loewald once remarked that obsessive defenses preserve the ego's relation to the superego at the cost of spontaneity. Yet more than a moral economy, the obsessive structure reflects a deep temporal moralism—a fantasy that time itself must be purified before lived.

In session, this manifests as a relentless intellectualization, a flooding of thought that staves off affect. However, this is not simply a resistance. It is a chronotopic defense: thinking becomes a time-suspending apparatus, a way of inhabiting the threshold without falling through it. Words are not vehicles of communication so much as sandbags against the flood of the present. The analytic task is not to undo this thinking, but to trace its temporal grammar—to sense what is being suspended, and why.

One patient, Leo, exemplified this mode of being. A gifted academic in his mid-thirties, Leo was celebrated for his analytical brilliance and exacting mind. But in his personal life, he was paralyzed. Decisions—about relationships, housing, even weekend plans—spiraled into recursive loops. "What if I commit, and it's the wrong choice?" he would ask. But even as he spoke, the question was already doubling back on itself: "And what if not choosing is its own failure?" Leo's temporality was not linear but vortexal. Every line of thought curved inward, self-interrupting. Time, for Leo, was a recursive chamber in which the self might endlessly reflect—but never emerge.

What was striking was Leo's relationship to spontaneity. Moments of emotional clarity, even joy, would be met with a self-monitoring delay: "Was that authentic? Did I manufacture that reaction?" Affect itself could not be trusted unless it was pre-verified. This suspension of immediacy was not merely a defense but a temporal worldview: spontaneity was temporally unsafe—too close to the loss of control, too near the abyss of feeling that might destabilize his hard-won symbolic order.

In such patients, the analyst must become a counterpoint to recursive time. To rush them toward affect is to join the collapse they fear. But to reflect back their temporal rhythm—and then begin to modulate it—is to offer a new temporal object. Holding silence a little longer, mirroring their repetitions without judgment, and carefully introducing interpretive rhythm can open small breaches in the obsessive chronotope. These breaches are not dramatic. They are temporal micro-shifts: a slightly quicker resonance, a word left uncompleted, a shared glance that slips outside the loop.

Yet it is crucial not to condescend to the obsessive's time. It is, after all, a time that protects. Beneath the suspension lies a deep trauma of intrusion or engulfment. The obsessive's symbolic saturation is not just defense—it is memorial. A way of keeping time structured after some earlier time was collapsed or chaotic. Their recursive thought is a ritual of order in a psyche that once experienced time as catastrophic.

Theoretically, this maps closely to the work of D.W. Winnicott and André Green. Winnicott's idea of the false self as a defense against impingement is here temporalized: the obsessive creates not a false self but a false time—a chronotope in which the self can persist safely at a distance. Green's "dead mother complex," meanwhile, gives insight into the affective flattening often found in obsessive patients. If the maternal presence has withdrawn affectively, then the child may internalize not her image but her absence—leading to a time-space in which presence always threatens vanishing, and thus must be suspended.

This also resonates with the Lacanian notion of the signifier's dominance in the obsessive. Lacan framed the obsessive's world as overdetermined by the symbolic order—a world in which the signifier functions not to open meaning, but to enclose it. Yet this is also a temporal phenomenon: the obsessive does not fear meaninglessness so much as the arrival of meaning that cannot be controlled.

There is, then, a kind of melancholia in the obsessive's time. Not a sadness per se, but a mourning of spontaneity—a preemptive grief for the self that might be, if only it were safe to emerge. In this way, the obsessive chronotope is not a failure of desire but a desire regulated into stasis.

And yet, this stasis is not absolute. Obsessive time may be recursive, but it is also dynamic. The loops contain energy. When the analytic frame is steady enough, when the symbolic scaffolding is mirrored and then slowly loosened, small acts of spontaneity may emerge. The obsessive laughs. They risk an unfinished thought. They linger in feeling. These moments are not breakthroughs. They are breaches—temporal apertures through which the self may re-enter time.

Leo, after many months, arrived at the session and said, "I don't want to talk today. I think I just want to be here." It was a small sentence. But in the context of his obsessive temporality, it was seismic. To be—not to think, not to pre-narrate, not to defer—but to *be*. That was a different kind of time. A shared present not suspended but lived.

These moments often dissolve quickly. The old chronotope reasserts itself. But something has shifted: a trace remains. The analyst, too, becomes part of that trace—a temporal object who held time differently, and in doing so, made a new temporality imaginable.

The Hysteric and the Looped Scene

The hysteric lives within a temporality of perpetual return—not the delayed future of the obsessive, but a looping past that demands constant re-staging. Unlike the neurotic's compulsion to master through ritual, the hysteric seeks presence through reenactment. The aim is not completion, but recognition—not resolution, but reappearance. Time becomes a stage on which the scene of desire is replayed, again and again, each time with slight variation, but never finality.

This looping is not merely behavioral repetition, nor is it reducible to trauma replay. It is a structural condition of psychic time. The hysteric's temporality is marked by a recursive aesthetic: the past presses itself into the present, but not as memory. It arrives instead as performance. Each gesture, symptom, or seduction is a time capsule—a bid to re-enter the original scene, to provoke the return of the gaze that once failed to hold.

For the hysteric, temporality is structured not around goal or progress, but around the circulation of desire. It is a time of deferral and echo—each utterance aimed not at the now, but at a symbolic other who may arrive belatedly. There is always someone watching, someone not yet arrived, someone who might yet mirror the self into being. The present becomes a waiting room for that gaze.

This echoes Jean Laplanche's notion of the enigmatic signifier. The hysteric inhabits a temporal field in which the question of what the other wants remains unanswered—and thus, interminably asked. The looped scene is not a failure to move on; it is the only way the scene can remain inhabited without foreclosing its mystery. It is a temporality of erotic inquiry, of suspended resolution, where the symptom becomes both the trace and the medium of address.

One patient, Myra, a choreographer in her early forties, offered a vivid illustration. Her sessions often began in fragments—impressions, gestures, half-statements. "He looked at me like I wasn't even there. So I danced. Not for him—but for someone who might see me seeing him not seeing me." The syntax was disjointed, but it enacted something precise: Myra was staging the scene of misrecognition in order to displace it, inhabit it, and transform it into choreography—both literally in her art and symbolically in her speech.

Her symptoms—panic in intimacy, erotic disorientation, somatic dizziness—were not simply dysregulations. They were temporal distortions: echoes of scenes in which the desired other was absent, inattentive, or withholding. These symptoms repeated not to remind her of trauma, but to locate her in time. "I need the feeling," she once said, "because then I know I'm alive." The loop, for Myra, was not pathology but ontology. To stop looping would be to risk falling out of time—to become unheld, unsymbolized.

Clinically, this challenges the analyst to meet the hysteric not with interpretive finality but with temporal attunement. To witness the loop as a temporal logic, rather than a content problem, is to shift the analytic stance. The analyst becomes a participant in the looped scene—not as rescuer or resolver, but as temporal accompanist. This may require tolerating affective saturation, rhythmic intensity, even erotic transference—without grasping for closure.

But this is not a license for passivity. The analyst's presence must be rhythmically alive. Too little attunement and the loop intensifies in desperation. Too much anticipation, and the scene collapses into something overly coherent—thereby extinguishing its symbolic ambiguity. The loop is a tightrope. The analyst walks it with the patient, not to escape the loop, but to become more precisely situated within it.

Philosophically, the hysteric's time recalls Nietzsche's idea of the eternal return—not as metaphysical doctrine, but as existential form. To live as though each moment might return eternally is to inhabit time with heightened affective charge. For the hysteric, every scene bears this weight: it is performed as though it is the one that will define all others. The loop is not just repetition— it is a stage of consequence.

This also resonates with Sedgwick's notion of "reparative reading." The hysteric's reenactments can be read not as paranoid retracings of loss, but as reparative gestures—bids to reshape time through performance. Each loop is a wish to re-author the original wound, not through denial, but through aesthetic reconfiguration. The symptom, then, is not just a signal of what went wrong, but an effort to hold it differently.

In one session, Myra described a recurring dream. "I'm on a stage with no lights. I'm performing a dance I don't remember learning. But I know it's mine. There's no audience. Just silence. And yet I can't stop." We unpacked this slowly. The dance, she came to realize, was the loop itself—a choreography of desire performed not for approval, but for temporal coherence. In the absence of the witnessing gaze, the dance sustained her existence. The loop was her way of not vanishing.

Loewald's concept of internalization is again useful here. He described how psychic structures are formed when external relations become internally animated—when the presence of the other is psychically sustained. For the hysteric, the loop may be a failed internalization—a symptom that re-stages the un-internalized other. The analytic task, then, is to become part of that internal world, not by replacing the original other, but by being symbolically metabolized over time.

There is also an echo here of Bion's idea of "thoughts without a thinker." The hysteric often experiences affective states that cannot be owned or located. The loop becomes a container—not to resolve, but to hold these unthinkable states in a performative register. The analyst's role is not simply to interpret but to witness the emergence of thinking as it crystallizes from aesthetic form.

Eventually, Myra found herself able to name her scenes more explicitly. "It's not that I want him to love me," she said. "It's that I want to see myself being loved—or failing to be loved—so I know I exist." This was not cynicism. It was ontological clarity. The loop was never about the content. It was about the staging of the self in time.

When the analyst can hold this recognition—that the scene is real, not despite its repetition, but because of it—the hysteric's looping begins to soften. Not because the wound is healed, but because the time is shared. The analyst becomes not a breaker of loops but a co-participant in their symbolic reframing. The loop no longer traps; it resonates.

In this way, the hysteric's temporality—often dismissed as regressive or histrionic—emerges as one of the most richly symbolic forms of time. It is a time that refuses to collapse, to finalize, to foreclose. A time of return that does not regress, but re-signifies. A time that insists not on arriving, but on being held again, and again, until the self finds form in the echo.

The Depressive and the Smeared Present

If the obsessive clings to the future and the hysteric loops through the past, the depressive inhabits a present that feels thickened, smeared, and unlocatable. Time slows, but not in the reflective calm of serenity. It congeals. The present becomes saturated—not with aliveness, but with the weight of absence. The depressive self lives in a time out of joint, not because it skips or repeats, but because it stretches too thin across too much internal loss.

This is a temporality of mourning, but not necessarily of bereavement. Rather, it is the structural mourning of relational depletion. The depressive carries a history that cannot be metabolized—not because it is repressed, but because it is too diffused to be grasped. The past is not reenacted but dripped into the now, clouding its contours. The present becomes hard to inhabit because it does not feel like a site of emergence. It feels like a residue.

Philosopher Henri Bergson spoke of time as durée—a lived flow that cannot be cut into discrete units. For the depressive patient, however, durée becomes viscosity. It is time experienced not as movement but as drag. Psychic life thickens. Affect coagulates. There is no clear before or after, only a gray continuity that resists punctuation. This can make meaning elusive—not because the patient is unreachable, but because meaning feels flattened into a temporal monotone.

One patient, Ethan, a quietly brilliant writer in his 30s, often described his experience as "feeling like I'm underwater." It wasn't anxiety. It wasn't grief. "Just heaviness," he said. "Like everything is coated in a film I can't wipe off." Ethan did not loop like Myra or spiral like Darren. He hovered. He described his sense of self as "dimly lit—like the power's on but no one's home." The present for Ethan was not traumatic, but uninhabitable. Not because it hurt—but because it barely registered.

In sessions, his silences were not filled with resistance. They were filled with time. Time that didn't want to pass, but also couldn't stop. When I spoke, his responses would come with a delay—not dissociation, but diffusion. "It takes me a while to find what I think," he once said. "It's like my thoughts don't want to be caught." This wasn't evasion. It was the temporality of psychic dimming—where the now has no spark, only continuity.

This structure of time echoes what Thomas Ogden calls the "autistic-contiguous position." Unlike the paranoid-schizoid or depressive positions, the autistic-contiguous is characterized by a sensuous, pre-symbolic relationality where boundaries are felt through textures rather than meanings. For Ethan, time itself was textural—thick, molasses-like, ungraspable. His depressive temporality was not about loss per se, but about the erosion of temporal edges.

In this smeared present, the depressive often turns toward symbolic simplification as a survival strategy. Ethan's language was precise but sparse. His narratives were flat, nonlinear, and often ended before they began. "I woke up," he once recounted. "It was raining. I didn't get up." That was the story. He offered no embellishment, no affective inflection, because he wasn't hiding from intensity—he was submerged beneath it. The analyst is tasked here not with drawing the patient out but with entering the viscosity, learning its grain.

Aesthetic forms can sometimes mirror this temporal quality. In minimalist music—the long, slow work of Morton Feldman, for instance—time seems to hang. Tones linger. Repetition becomes variation, not through change but through endurance. For depressive patients, the inner world is often scored like this—with long, unbroken notes that threaten to fade into silence. The therapeutic rhythm must adjust. Interpretation too soon or too brightly can feel like a blinding light after hours in darkness.

There is also a neurobiological component to this psychic temporality. Jaak Panksepp's work on affective neuroscience identifies the SEEKING system as central to the experience of vitality. Depressive states involve the dysregulation of this system—not just low mood, but a fundamental disruption in the organism's orientation toward the world. Ethan did not lack ideas. He lacked forward momentum. His temporality was not directed—it was ambient.

Relational psychoanalysis offers tools to navigate this. Stephen Mitchell reminds us that meaning is co-created not just through content but through timing. With Ethan, the pace of interpretation mattered more than its accuracy. He needed to feel the analyst's tempo more than the analyst's thought. When he began to speak of his internal world in metaphor—"it's like a room that's slowly filling with water, but no one seems to notice"—I understood this as a shift in temporal presence. He wasn't moving faster, but he was beginning to shape time symbolically.

Fairbairn's vision of the internal world as composed of object-relations helps clarify this. The depressive does not necessarily repress objects. Instead, the objects are there, but drained. Internal relationships persist, but they are low-voltage—too weak to catalyze symbolic life. The self is not empty; it is undercharged. In Ethan's case, the depressive temporality expressed not emptiness but over-connection—a field of internal others whose unmetabolized affect clogged the present.

Over time, our work together began to thicken in a different way. His silences became rhythmic. His metaphors became more textured. He once said, "I think maybe I've been trying to write a story I'm still inside of." This was not a statement of trauma. It was an emergence of temporality. The depressive does not need to be pulled into a different time—they need their time to be made symbolically habitable.

In Buddhist psychology, the concept of *dukkha* refers to the inherent unsatisfactoriness of conditioned experience. Ethan's depressive temporality carried this existential weight—not as belief, but as atmosphere. And yet, it was not hopeless. When the analyst can breathe inside this atmosphere without pressing for air, something new becomes possible. Not change, but texture.

Loewald again offers a bridge: transformation involves the re-temporalization of experience. To make the smeared present legible is to give it symbolic dimension. Ethan's emergence did not look like light breaking through clouds. It looked like clouds learning to carry light. The depressive temporality did not lift. It folded inward, became more complex, and more storyable.

In this way, the depressive chronotope is not a pathology of time, but a slow form of time. A time that must be accompanied, not accelerated. A time whose beauty lies not in its brightness, but in its depth. The analyst's task is not to rescue the patient from this time, but to become a co-inhabitor—to dwell with them until time itself becomes a shared medium of recognition.

The Psychotic and the Fractured Field

Where the depressive suffers under the smear of temporal viscosity, the psychotic subject suffers from a fractured field of time altogether. Time does not slow or loop—it shatters. In psychotic structures, the self is not temporally extended but scattered. Psychic moments become unstitched from one another. The result is not fragmentation in the aesthetic sense, but the psychic impossibility of narrative cohesion.

To speak of the psychotic chronotope is to risk oversimplification. There is no single psychotic temporality, just as there is no singular psychosis. But we can describe a pattern of disarticulation: time is not endured or anticipated—it is fallen into, often without transition. The psychotic subject may experience the future as it has already happened, or the present as unfindable. What Loewald called the "binding" function of the ego is here too tenuous to organize experience into a stream. Instead, temporal perception becomes a field of free-floating shocks.

In the consulting room, this can take the form of disjointed speech, sudden shifts in affect, or a collapse of sequence. One patient, Clara, had a longstanding diagnosis of schizoaffective disorder and a history of severe early trauma. Our sessions often began mid-thought. She would enter, sit silently, and then say something like, "The hallway is humming again." There was no context. The statement was not symbolic—it was real. I once made the mistake of interpreting the hallway as a metaphor. She looked at me with an odd mix of pity and irritation. "No," she said. "It's really humming."

This was not resistance. It was temporal dislocation. Clara's psychotic structure did not allow her to locate the present as a continuous plane. Time for her was punctuated by intrusions. These were not hallucinations in the classical sense—they were events with no spatial or temporal casing. They arrived unbidden, raw, untransformed. Her affect was not muted but disconnected. She could move from laughter to terror with no apparent stimulus because the internal links between events did not hold.

Ogden's concept of the "undreamt dream" becomes especially salient here. The psychotic chronotope is often marked by the inability to dream experience—not in sleep, but in the waking psychic sense. Without this capacity, time becomes a barrage rather than a flow. The analyst cannot interpret too quickly. The work, at times, becomes almost pre-symbolic: witnessing, rhythm, tone.

In this sense, the psychotic field is not just fragmented—it is spatialized in an extreme way. Psychic moments feel like separate rooms, each sealed from the others. Clara once described her inner world as a house in which none of the doors opened. "I can see the other rooms," she said. "But I can't get into them. It's like they're there, but not real." Her statement reveals a paradox: the presence of inner life and the simultaneous impossibility of entering it. The self is not emptied but barricaded.

Fairbairn's model helps illuminate this: in psychotic structures, internal objects are often so persecutory or split that the self cannot relate to them directly. Instead, the self becomes caught in a maze of part-objects, none of which can be symbolically negotiated. The result is a temporality without time—a flat field of shifting fragments that resist integration.

The analyst's task is to become a kind of temporal tether. Not to reconstruct narrative, but to offer continuity of presence. Clara responded not to questions but to tone. If I was too structured, she withdrew. If I was too unstructured, she panicked. Over time, she began to test whether I could hold two non-contiguous states. She once described a memory of walking to school and suddenly "becoming upside down." I asked what that meant. She said, "My feet were still on the ground, but the world flipped. Like a page." She looked at me, wary. "You think that's crazy?" I paused. "No. I think that's how it felt." She nodded. "Yes," she said. "Exactly."

Bion's theory of containment is crucial here. In psychotic states, unmentalized beta elements flood the field. The analyst must become the alpha function—not by interpreting, but by receiving. Clara did not need a meaning for her "upside-down" world. She needed me to stand in it without collapsing. Slowly, that allowed her to begin forming micro-sequences of time. "When I feel that coming on," she said months later, "I now try to say, 'It's still now.' Even if it doesn't feel like it."

This is where the psychotic chronotope begins to shift. It cannot be made linear. But it can be softened. Clara started bringing drawings to session—not symbolic art, but shapes. Circles, grids, spirals. "I like drawing things that hold themselves together," she said. These images became proto-temporal. They organized feelings without demanding sequence. For Clara, this was progress.

From a Buddhist perspective, psychosis might seem like a proximity to emptiness—but without the holding frame of form. In Dzogchen, the mind is said to be luminous yet empty. For the psychotic structure, that luminosity is blinding, and the emptiness unbuffered. There is no stable "I" to witness the field. As a result, the temporal self cannot anchor. The analyst becomes the ritual object—the reliable structure into which the patient can momentarily entrain their time.

There is also often an uncanny aesthetics to the psychotic temporality. Clara's descriptions were sometimes strangely poetic. "The tree outside my window is watching me," she once said, "but not like a person. Like a dream that hasn't decided what to become." These phrases were not symbolic in the neurotic sense. They were emergent. The analyst must resist the pull to decode. These utterances are time-markers—efforts to find temporal purchase by language.

Kernberg's insights into severe personality organization also offer guidance. At this level, reality testing is compromised, and splitting dominates. Time, in this context, becomes a function of internal object relations. The more split and persecutory the inner world, the more fragmented the perception of temporality. Integration, then, is not just cognitive but temporal. The goal is not insight, but rhythm—to help the patient feel that the world unfolds rather than attacks.

Eventually, Clara began to tolerate small narratives. She would describe a walk to the store or a conversation with her brother. These stories lacked affective elaboration, but they were linear. The sequence was holding. This is the early work of temporal integration. The psychotic chronotope cannot be restructured all at once. But it can be met. And through that meeting, something like time begins to return.

The challenge, as analysts, is to resist the temptation of speed. To honor the fractured field not as a failed narrative, but as a temporality in search of containment. In doing so, we become the timekeeper—not of clocks, but of care.

Temporality as Diagnostic Atmosphere

Time is not merely a psychological variable but an atmospheric condition within the analytic field. Each session is saturated with temporal mood—urgency, timelessness, stuckness, drift. These affective tonalities of time serve as diagnostic indicators, often more revealing than explicit narrative. The analyst learns to "read" temporality not just through content, but through the unspoken structure of how time unfolds between self and other.

One patient arrives early, breathless, already speaking as they enter. Their narratives are driven by a manic temporal economy—every moment overfilled, language as a defense against silence. Another patient consistently pauses, not to think but to avoid the next moment. They stretch time, slow it down, fearing what might emerge. Still another exists in a timeless mist, every story circled without anchoring, the past and present folded into one indistinct continuity. Each of these temporal signatures reveals something foundational about their psychic structure.

As Daniel Stern has observed, the **present moment**—typically lasting just a few seconds—is the basic unit of lived experience, the temporal container in which affective meaning unfolds and intersubjectivity takes shape (Stern,

2004). But the analyst quickly learns that not all presents are created equal. Some are so saturated they collapse. Others are so evacuated that they barely exist. These distinctions are not simply matters of attention or neurotic style—they are clues to the architecture of internal object relations, dissociative patterning, and affect regulation.

In many cases, temporality is a symptom of relational history. Traumatized patients often exhibit disrupted temporal processing. Events are encoded out of sequence or sealed off from associative integration. The present becomes a haunted site—not because of what is happening, but because of what remains unsymbolized. This can result in temporal telescoping (where disparate events collapse into one another) or time-freezing (where experience cannot progress). In both cases, time becomes an affective atmosphere rather than a cognitive map.

For example, a patient may describe a recent interaction with a partner in language borrowed unconsciously from a long-past parental relationship. The analyst may feel confused—not because the story is incoherent, but because it is temporally layered in ways the patient does not yet register. This temporal dissonance is not merely metaphorical; it reflects a lived structure of psychic time. The analyst who listens for temporal distortion—not just narrative gaps—can often locate the precise site of traumatic arrest.

Loewald's concept of internalization as a temporal achievement becomes central here. To internalize an object is to make it durational, to experience its presence across time. For the patient whose psychic life is structured around rupture, internal objects may not be temporally extended. They may be present only in flash or fantasy—unintegrated, unremembered. This is why analytic presence must offer not just safety, but temporal continuity. The patient must come to feel that the analyst will still be there, not only next week, but five minutes from now.

In this way, diagnostic impressions are not just constructed through formal assessments or verbal content, but through the lived, felt rhythm of the session. A patient who never arrives on time may be struggling with anticipatory dread that warps their sense of the future. A patient who panics as the session ends may carry a collapsed sense of continuity. These temporal behaviors are not simply resistance or transference in the traditional sense—they are structural manifestations of how the psyche holds or fails to hold time.

Here, we can also draw on Bion's concept of "container-contained." The analytic frame is itself a temporal container. When the analyst can hold disorganized or chaotic temporalities—by neither accelerating nor retreating—the patient begins to metabolize time differently. For some patients, the analyst's pacing becomes more important than their interpretations. A slowed rhythm can help the patient find the space between affective beats—a moment of breath, of symbol, of psychic pause.

One patient, Julian, came to analysis with a history of relational chaos and episodic dissociation. He could speak about events with vivid detail, but the events never accumulated. Each story was isolated, as though occurring in a separate psychic world. I began to notice that Julian rarely used time-markers: no "last week," "this morning," or "a few days ago." Everything was "this thing that happened." I started gently inserting temporal scaffolding—"Was that before or after the conversation with your sister?" "Had you already seen the film you just mentioned when this happened?" These questions were not interpretive. They were anchoring. Julian began to develop a faint map of when things occurred, and with it, a greater sense of having endured them. His narrative tempo slowed, and feelings began to accumulate across sessions. This was not insight; it was temporal reconstitution.

Temporality also serves as an affective barometer. The patient who lingers excessively on early childhood memories may be seeking not just understanding but a return—a re-living rather than a symbolic working-through. Conversely, the patient who avoids the past altogether may experience it as unlocatable, too saturated with shame or grief to be held in mind. The analyst's task is not to force time forward or back, but to invite its multidirectionality. Psychic change is often nonlinear. It spirals, loops, and doubles back. Analysts must become literate in temporal aesthetics—attuned to rhythm, rupture, and recurrence.

There is also the temporal dimension of the transference. For some patients, the analyst is instantly ancient—a symbolic parent whose every gesture reverberates with early trauma. For others, the analyst is oddly new—a fresh space untouched by history, who must now hold all the patient's futurity. These positions are not chosen; they emerge from the patient's temporal template. Transference, then, is not merely a repetition of the past—it is a temporal choreography, shaped by how the self moves through psychic time.

Analysts, too, bring their own temporal countertransferences. We may find ourselves speeding up with manic patients, slowing down with depressive ones, or feeling temporally erased by dissociative presentations. These experiences are not merely reactions—they are temporal intersubjectivities. When understood, they can become diagnostic. When unconscious, they can become enactments.

The risk, of course, is misattunement. The analyst who imposes a temporality—who insists on linear development or narrative closure—may inadvertently retraumatize. The patient whose time is still shattered cannot be rushed into coherence. The analyst must learn to sit with temporal multiplicity, to tolerate the patient's divergent pulses without collapsing them into a single rhythm.

Eigen's work on the "in-between" may be helpful here. He writes of experiences that are neither one thing nor another—flickers, tremors, breath. These are temporal phenomena, and often the most psychoanalytically potent. Between rupture and repair lies not a bridge, but a moment of shared time—time that has not yet become narrative, but is no longer void. This is the time of therapy.

In this way, temporality becomes not just a backdrop but a diagnostic atmosphere—an interpretive climate that reveals how the psyche holds, fragments, or flees time. By listening not only to what is said, but to how time is felt, shaped, and resisted, the analyst begins to map the structural dynamics of the self. Temporality is not secondary. It is foundational. And in its distortions, repetitions, and silences, it speaks the deep structure of subjectivity.

Countertemporal Resistance: When Change Threatens Structure

In psychoanalytic work, resistance is typically understood as a defense against insight or affect. But when viewed through a temporal lens, resistance may appear not merely as avoidance, but as a protest against the collapse of time-structures that have long sustained psychic coherence. For some patients, even minor movement forward in treatment constitutes a temporal betrayal. Change, in this light, becomes a kind of time-travel—one that threatens to unravel the very architectures that kept the self intact.

The patient may come to session and share an epiphany, only to retract it the following week. What appears as ambivalence may actually be a temporal reversion—a snapping back into the familiar structure of old timelines, where meaning is held in static form. Or a patient may suddenly shift registers, moving from deep reflection to surface chatter. The content hasn't changed, but the temporal register has. The space for change has closed.

This kind of resistance is not opposition in the usual sense. It is an instinctive refusal to destabilize a chronotope—a fear that any reorganization of temporality will leave the self without an orbit. The analyst may feel this as whiplash, or as a kind of gravitational pull back into the old pattern. Sometimes this pull is gentle; at other times, it is filled with panic, rage, or collapse. The patient is not resisting. They are resisting the collapse of their time.

Consider the case of Lena, a woman in her late 30s, who entered analysis after the dissolution of a long-term relationship. Her affect was controlled, her narratives neatly sequenced, and she took pride in her clarity. Over time, however, a different temporality began to emerge. When invited to explore moments from childhood or dream states, Lena would become disoriented, even hostile. "That doesn't matter now," she would insist. "It's over." And yet, the emotional undercurrents betrayed otherwise. Whenever we approached these submerged zones, time began to fragment. Sessions grew slower, harder to follow, and filled with long silences. Something in her object world resisted being remembered in sequence.

As we worked together, it became clear that Lena's apparent clarity was itself a temporal defense—a structure built to contain unsymbolized early trauma. Her chronological competence was a fortress. Any attempt to disrupt the sequence—to move backward, or even sideways in time—threatened to unravel the only container she had. This was not a neurotic defense; it was an existential necessity. For her, memory was dangerous not because of what it revealed, but because of what it might dislodge.

Countertemporal resistance, then, often arises in patients with structural vulnerabilities—particularly those with borderline, schizoid, or dissociative organizations. In these cases, temporality is not simply an experiential mode, but a survival strategy. The analyst must tread carefully, learning to recognize the temporal signatures of threat without becoming drawn into their gravitational logic. One must neither force movement nor collude with stasis. As in Winnicott's "going on being," the analyst must sustain a psychic tempo that allows the patient to encounter time without being overwhelmed by it.

Sometimes, resistance appears not as stillness, but as hyper-temporality—an acceleration that floods the field with meaning before it can be metabolized. This is common in manic or narcissistically organized patients, where temporality becomes over-determined. Every moment is charged, every word saturated. Time speeds up to avoid contact. The analyst may feel breathless, unable to anchor the session in any stable ground. Here, resistance operates through shimmer—not the shimmer of poetic ambiguity, but of disorganization. It becomes a defense against presence.

In such cases, the analyst's task is not to slow things down per se, but to hold the temporal field with enough gravity that the patient may begin to notice their own velocity. Commenting on temporal mood—"It feels like we're moving quickly today"—can open space without judgment. Loewald reminds us that analysis is not just the work of interpretation, but of transformation. And transformation occurs within time—not as a sudden insight, but as an unfolding process, one that requires the containment of emergent structure.

Another form of countertemporal resistance occurs when patients begin to make progress and suddenly become depressed. This is not always a return of the repressed, but the dawning awareness that old timelines may no longer be viable. The sadness is not just about what happened, but about the loss of a coherent past—the timeline that once made sense, even if it was painful. This is particularly true for patients with deeply embedded identification with trauma. To heal is to betray that identification. To change is to unwrite a portion of the self's narrative. This is not simply psychic loss; it is temporal grief.

Ferenczi's insights into the "wise baby"—the child forced into premature knowledge—may be helpful here. Such patients often live in a state of suspended time, where adult competence coexists with unprocessed infantile affect. Analysis, in these cases, does not simply bring the patient forward; it invites them backward, into a time that was never fully lived. Resistance emerges not as refusal, but as fear: If I go back there, will I survive? If I move forward, who will I become?

These are not rhetorical questions. They are ontological. Countertemporal resistance is not merely about time. It is about being. Time becomes the medium through which selfhood is threatened, preserved, or transformed. The analyst who fails to recognize this may mistake withdrawal for regression, or urgency for engagement. We must develop a more nuanced attunement to the temporal field, one that recognizes resistance as a structural echo—a gravitational artifact—rather than a sign of willful opposition.

The solution, if there is one, lies not in interpretation alone, but in presence. A temporally attuned presence that can hold contradiction without collapse, ambiguity without urgency. A presence that allows the patient to experience time not as threat, but as potential. This may mean sitting in temporal disorganization without rushing to structure it. It may mean recognizing when the patient's narrative is looping because linearity itself is intolerable. It may mean joining the patient in the folds of recursive time until a new rhythm can emerge.

Ultimately, countertemporal resistance is not a problem to be solved. It is a condition to be witnessed. And in that witnessing, something loosens. The gravitational field begins to shift. New orbits become possible—not because we forced them, but because we stayed close enough to the old ones for long enough. The psyche does not change because it is told to. It changes because it is accompanied—through time, across time, and sometimes, against time.

Chronotope as Transitional Matrix: Clinical Implications

If, as I have argued, character structure and psychic temporality are inseparable, then the analyst's work must include not only attunement to affect and symbol, but to the patient's lived chronotope—their particular grammar of time. The chronotope is not a static structure but a transitional matrix: a space-time aesthetic that shapes what can be experienced, remembered, and transformed. To work within a patient's chronotope is to enter a temporality that is both protective and constraining, alive and repetitive, sheltering and limiting.

In practice, this means the analyst must listen not just for *what* is said, but *when* and *how*—in what rhythm, with what temporal pressure, in what emotional season. The analyst becomes, in effect, a time-companion. A kind of temporal co-regulator. This demands a style of presence that exceeds content and reaches toward temporal form.

Consider, for instance, how a depressive patient often speaks as if time were static or already concluded. There is no future in their speech, only aftermath. Their idioms are weighted with finality: "It's always been this way," "Nothing ever changes." Such phrases are not mere cognitive distortions but clues to the chronotope: a temporal melancholia that arrests momentum and compresses experience. Here, the analyst must offer not premature optimism, but a subtle re-animation of tempo. Slowness may need to be joined, not corrected. Or time may need to be held gently open, like a window cracked just enough to let air in.

With anxious or obsessively organized patients, the opposite temporal texture often emerges: time is overly active, flooded with possibility or danger. The present collapses beneath anticipatory dread. Here, the analyst may need to serve as a brake—not to halt movement, but to slow the tempo enough that time becomes tolerable. In both cases, the work is temporal as much as it is interpretive. Interventions fail when they violate the patient's chronotope—when they move too fast, or too slow, or at the wrong axis of temporal depth.

In some cases, temporal attunement means being willing to wait—to sit with the frozen parts of the patient's structure without demanding thaw. Winnicott's idea of the *holding environment* is, at its core, a temporal concept: the mother who waits, who sustains time without collapse, who allows for emergence without imposition. The analyst must become a transitional object within time—not the one who directs the tempo, but the one who holds it.

Bion's notion of "patience" as a central analytic virtue also resonates here. For Bion, the analyst must suspend memory and desire—that is, must loosen the pull of both past and future—in order to allow the present to become symbolically alive. This is not simply an ethic of neutrality; it is an ethic of temporal faith. A belief that meaning will emerge when the temporal container is strong enough to hold it.

One might even say that the analytic setting itself is a chronotope—a patterned recurrence in time and space that generates possibility. Weekly sessions, the same room, the same frame: these are not merely structural conventions, but temporal signals. They tell the patient that time will hold. And in that holding, something previously unthinkable may begin to stir. But this symbolic container only functions if the analyst is attuned not only to the rules of time, but to the patient's lived experience of it. The analyst may offer regularity, but the patient brings their own seasons.

This is particularly evident in the treatment of trauma. Traumatized patients often live in split temporalities—one part of the self arrested in the moment of rupture, another continuing in the chronology of survival. These patients do not simply "remember"; they re-live. Their past is not behind them but folded into their present, often with disorienting speed or sudden flooding. The analyst must learn to move between timelines—to join the patient in the fragmented chronotope without getting lost in it. Here, the concept of the *transitional matrix* becomes vital: the analytic space as a temporal bridge between dissociated states.

Ferenczi's clinical diary offers a powerful precedent. His recognition that trauma disrupts temporal continuity—that it collapses the capacity for psychic sequencing—anticipates much of what we now understand as dissociative structure. For Ferenczi, analytic tact involved not only gentleness of interpretation, but modulation of time itself. He slowed down, adjusted his rhythm, and allowed the patient's tempo to lead. In doing so, he made the chronotope visible.

The work of Donnel Stern (1997) similarly highlights the importance of emergence—the sense that some meanings cannot be willed into being, but must be allowed to unfold in their own temporality. Stern's "unformulated experience" is often not yet symbolized because it is not yet chronotopically permitted. The analyst's task, then, is to cultivate a shared field in which the pace of emergence is honored. This is not about *insight* as punctual event, but about symbolic *ripening*—time as soil.

Loewald, too, reminds us that the analyst does not merely interpret the past; they participate in the creation of future temporality. For Loewald, the *past is not located behind us, but lives within the psychic present*—continuously informing how structure is made and remade. Analysis brings this temporal interiority into relational space—not to re-map it in chronological order, but to render its layers metabolizable. In this way, analysis is not just a space of symbolic interpretation, but of symbolic re-temporalization.

Even failure can become a temporal event. A missed session, a rupture in the frame, a delayed intervention—all may become occasions to metabolize time differently. If the analyst can tolerate the discomfort of these moments without rushing repair, they may open a new temporal register. The patient may begin to feel that time itself has changed—that the same hour, the same silence, now means something different.

Ultimately, to conceptualize the chronotope as a transitional matrix is to see psychoanalysis not only as the analysis of symbols and affects, but as the reshaping of psychic time. The analyst does not impose a new timeline, nor collapse the old. Rather, they hold the gravitational field open long enough for new orbits to form. Temporality, in this sense, becomes the very medium of transformation—the invisible scaffolding on which the self rewrites its continuity.

Closing Reflection—Time-Bound Selves, Unbound Psyches

Across the chapters of this book, we have returned often to paradoxes of form and formlessness, of structure and dissolution, of containment and collapse. Here, in tracing the lived temporality of character structure, we encounter another paradox: the self as both time-bound and time-maker, shaped by temporal gravity and yet capable of reconfiguring its own trajectory. In this final section, I wish to gather the threads of the chronotope not as an analytic metaphor alone, but as an experiential horizon—a way of being with time that shapes the very possibility of psychic life.

The idea that character structure is a temporal form carries radical implications. It reframes symptom not merely as signal or compromise, but as temporal sculpture—a way of managing the unbearable by modulating the flow of time. Repetition compulsion, for example, is not only an insistence on content but on rhythm. Trauma, likewise, is not just an event remembered but a tear in temporal coherence. And even what we call identity may be nothing more than a particular temporal signature: the tempo of affect regulation, the sequencing of memory, the curvature of desire.

In this view, the self becomes a gravitational field, organized not only by meaning and attachment but by temporality itself. This aligns closely with what Michael Eigen calls the "psychic atmosphere"—that is, the felt quality of a person's presence, the rhythm and resonance of their psychic being. Eigen, like Bion and Loewald, invites us to listen for more than words. He asks us to attune to the slow drift, the sudden leap, the pause that stretches or snaps. These are the contours of the chronotope. Not its content, but its aesthetic.

And it is precisely this aesthetic—this lived poetics of temporality—that analysis touches when it begins to work. The most meaningful moments in treatment are often not the most articulate, but the most temporally trans-formative. The patient who speaks for the first time in a new cadence. The silence that feels less hollow, more held. The moment when the past no longer floods the present, but lingers beside it. These are not changes in insight but in chronotope. They mark a re-formation of the self's gravitational curve.

This shift is not always conscious. Often, it happens first in the transfer-ence, where time is not linear but recursive. Patients may experience the analyst as both ancient and new, both parental and peer, both timeless and inconsistent. The analyst, too, may feel drawn into temporal dislocations—pulled back into their own history, or forward into premonitions of a shared psychic future. These are not mistakes or enactments alone. They are indica-tors that the analytic field has become a space of temporal plasticity.

The ethical implications of this are profound. To respect a patient's tem-porality is to relinquish the fantasy of control. It is to recognize that no mat-ter how compelling our interpretations, they cannot land until the patient's chronotope is ready to receive them. This demands a humility of timing, a willingness to wait—or to risk moving too soon, and to learn from the resist-ance. It also requires an aesthetic sensibility: a capacity to feel the tone and tempo of the hour, to sense when something is ripening or when it is still frozen in its orbit.

Such sensibility is not a technique but a discipline of presence. It is developed, not prescribed. And it asks of the analyst a deep tolerance for ambiguity—especially temporal ambiguity. To sit with a patient in suspended time, to not know whether change is imminent or deferred, to resist the urgency of resolution—this is the labor of attunement. It is a spiritual labor, as much as a clinical one. It calls us into our own time-structures, our own defenses against stillness or speed.

In this way, the analytic dyad becomes a crucible not only of insight, but of shared temporality. The analyst lends their own capacity to hold time open, to stretch, slow, or thicken it, in ways the patient cannot yet manage alone. This is not always soothing. Sometimes it evokes rage, impatience, and despair. But when it works—when the analyst can metabolize those affects without retaliating or retreating—a new temporal form begins to take shape. It is not given. It is grown.

That grown temporality may be subtle: a tolerance for delay where only urgency once existed. A capacity to reflect before acting. A willingness to return to the same story without collapsing into repetition. Or it may be seis-mic: a sudden awareness that the past no longer owns the present, that mem-ory can be metabolized without flooding, that hope is no longer naïve. All of these are temporal transformations. They are not merely signs of health, but signs of symbolic gravity—of a self that can hold its own time.

I want to end, then, with a reminder: the goal of analysis is not to render the self timeless, but to help it find its rhythm. Not to dissolve structure, but to make it flexible. Not to banish the past, but to loosen its grip. The chronotope reminds us that every patient arrives with a particular curvature of time—a signature that is both wound and wisdom. Our task is not to erase it, but to meet it. To inhabit its folds with them. And when possible, to help them reconfigure the arc.

In that shared space—where the analyst bends time without forcing it, and the patient begins to hear their own tempo anew—something unnamable takes root. A temporality that is not imposed, but emerged. A self that is not built, but lived. And a psyche that, while never fully unbound, becomes just fluid enough to begin again.

Part II

Gravity and Symptom—From Repetition to Field

Freud's Echo, Klein's Trace

These chapters follow the symptom not as a single event but as a gravitational echo—a formal surface saturated by psychic curvature. Freud's repetition compulsion is reinterpreted as recursive orbit, and Klein's internal persecutory world is heard as the resonance of failed contact. The analyst's presence enters as a gravitational field, where affect condenses and symptom formation loops around the unsymbolized.

Freud taught us to listen to symptoms as formations of the unconscious, while Klein showed how internal part-objects generate unconscious phantasy and projective identifications. This section reorients the symptom—not as a message to be decoded, but as a **gravitational trace**: a formal echo shaped by invisible mass. Psychic suffering is reconceived as a warp in the relational field. Transference, in this view, becomes not a replay of the past but a **Kleinian distortion in gravitational atmosphere**, where projective intensity warps the analyst's symbolic position. These chapters propose a shift: from linear interpretation to **co-regulation of aesthetic gravity**—where symptom, affect, and presence orbit one another in curved time.

DOI: 10.4324/9781003715306-6

4 Orbiting the Invisible
Symptom as Gravitational Trace

This chapter reconceptualizes the symptom as a gravitational trace—an aesthetic and spatial condensation of forces that exceed symbolization. Rather than treating symptoms as pathological disruptions or encoded messages from the unconscious, we explore them as field phenomena: distortions in psychic space that orbit around zones of unformulated intensity. Drawing on psychoanalytic field theory, aesthetics, and topological metaphors of the mind, this chapter attends to how symptoms choreograph affective experience, mediate contact, and serve as condensed expressions of relational pressure. Clinical vignettes illuminate how symptoms act as survival structures, anchoring the self when coherence is threatened. The symptom is framed not as something to be removed but as something to be heard, tracked, and metabolized—an aesthetic form through which the psyche holds what it cannot yet narrate.

Every symptom leaves a trail—not just through the body or the psyche, but through the space between. It is not an intrusion into the self, but a curvature around something unspeakable. This chapter orbits that absence. If Chapter 3 mapped temporality as a function of psychic structure, we now shift toward the spatial: toward the folds, the warps, the gravitational echoes that symptoms trace. A symptom is not a mistake; it is a shimmer of coherence where collapse once threatened. It signals where the field has thickened, where affect condenses, where recognition buckles and reorganizes. We follow not the meaning behind the symptom, but the force it exerts—the mood it casts, the repetitions it insists on, the aesthetic logic it performs. Here, the symptom is not a riddle to be solved but a rhythm to be felt. It draws us closer not to resolution, but to the textured geometry of psychic life: where language frays, time coils, and presence becomes an orbit.

Introduction: Symptoms as Echoes of Psychic Gravity

Symptoms are not anomalies. They are not errors to be corrected, nor interruptions in the otherwise coherent narrative of the self. They are clues—vibrational residue left behind by something that cannot be touched directly. In the architecture of the psyche, symptoms form like condensation on a pane

DOI: 10.4324/9781003715306-7

of glass: real, opaque, patterned—but not the thing itself. They trace the curvature of an absence.

If we adopt the spatial metaphor developed in the preceding chapters—of mind as topological field, of structure as a form of psychic gravity—then symptoms are not within the self but *around* it. They are not simply expressions of repressed content or compromise formations between instinct and defense. They are distortions in the field, orbiting what cannot be symbolized. A repetition compulsion, a psychosomatic ache, a sudden, inexplicable dread: each marks the bending of the psychic field around an unseen mass. Not because something is hidden *inside*, but because something *exerts force without form*.

This chapter enters that invisible terrain. Where Chapter 3 explored temporality—how character styles shape and are shaped by distortions in psychic time—this chapter transitions to the spatial. Not space in the literal sense, but the felt geometry of the psyche: its warp, its folds, its gravitational pull toward what resists symbolization. We ask not "What does this symptom mean?" but "What does it orbit?"

To speak of a symptom as a gravitational trace is to engage a different kind of epistemology—one that privileges field effect over content, force over form, resonance over representation. This is not to evacuate meaning from the symptom, but to shift the register: from decipherment to attunement. A symptom does not point to a singular cause buried in the past; it thickens the present. It draws the analytic pair into a shared topology—structured not by linear causality, but by atmospheric charge.

Freud glimpsed this when he noted the uncanny persistence of the symptom beyond interpretation. Lacan formalized it through the Real—the leftover, the remainder, the unsymbolizable. Contemporary relational thinkers encounter it through enactments, through the ways analyst and patient find themselves *in* the symptom, not just analyzing it. The symptom is a force field that includes both parties. It is not simply "expressed"; it is *lived through*.

To grasp this is to let go of the fantasy of cure as subtraction. The symptom does not disappear because its meaning has been unveiled. Often, the symptom *is* the meaning—or rather, it is the form that meaning takes when the symbolic fails. It holds intensity, coherence, and pressure. And in some cases, it is the only psychic structure that remains. To dissolve it without understanding what it organizes may be to strip the patient of their sole gravitational anchor.

This is why symptoms so often resist direct confrontation. They are not stubborn because they are irrational, but because they are structural. They *are* the psyche, warped around an impossibility. This impossibility may be traumatic, but it may also be ontological—a gap in the symbolic order, a split in time, a rupture in early recognition. The symptom forms not only in response to the unbearable, but also in response to what could never fully cohere. It is a holding pattern around a void.

This chapter considers these holding patterns—how they take form, what they hold, and how they shift in analytic process. It does not aim to interpret symptoms into disappearance. Instead, it tracks their aesthetic, spatial, and rhythmic qualities. We consider how a symptom can shimmer, how it might signal through dissociation, displacement, or erotic fixation. We enter the symptom not as invaders or engineers, but as companions of its gravity. What happens when we stop asking how to change the symptom—and start asking what it is circling?

If Chapter 3 frames structure as temporal compression, this chapter treats the symptom as spatial curvature. Together, they establish a grammar for psychic gravity—how the mind bends time and space in response to what cannot be symbolized. Chapter 5 will extend this grammar into the clinical setting, attending to how the analyst's presence itself exerts gravitational pressure. But here, we remain with the symptom itself: not as failure, but as form. Not as problem, but as trace.

Symptom as Relational Field Distortion

A symptom is not just something one has; it is something one becomes. It crystallizes a relationship—not only to an internal object or an unconscious fantasy, but to the gravitational tensions of a larger field in which the psyche has learned to contort, accommodate, and survive. In this sense, a symptom is not a disruption of the self, but a signature of the field in which the self is formed. It is both a message and a deformation, a pulse of desire and an act of submission. This chapter reframes the symptom not as an isolated disruption to be decoded or eliminated, but as a condensation of invisible forces in a relational ecology—a trace of the psyche's adaptation to what cannot be metabolized in the field of presence.

What we conventionally call symptom formation often masks the deeper aesthetic of psychic compromise: a way of maintaining coherence in the face of overwhelming ambiguity, misattunement, or longing. From this perspective, symptoms are not merely the return of the repressed but the residue of a distorted relational rhythm—one that holds space for the subject's most unbearable dilemmas. They speak in loops and crystallizations, forming around points of friction, silence, or overstimulation in the relational surround. Sometimes they offer a rhythmic solution to chronic impingement; sometimes they enact a repetition that signals not memory, but a recursive field-pressure that has never ceased.

Take the case of Jacob, a quiet man in his early 40s who presented with chronic insomnia and recurring gastrointestinal distress. These symptoms had been diagnosed medically, but he had also begun to suspect a psychological source. Over months of analytic work, it became clear that Jacob experienced intimacy as disorganizing, almost suffocating. As his analytic experience deepened, he began noticing that the nights he couldn't sleep coincided with evenings spent with friends or lovers. His stomach pain, too, tended to flare after social meals. What emerged was a pattern—not of psychosomatic causality in the narrow sense, but of a deeper field distortion: a gravitational asymmetry in the way he experienced relational presence.

Jacob's body became the metronome of an intersubjective tension. The symptom was not reducible to repression or projection; it was a field-response to proximity. His nervous system, perhaps shaped in early life by inconsistent availability and overwhelming enmeshment, had learned to regulate connection by turning it into physical noise. In this sense, the symptom held a double function: it registered the vitality of relational desire and simultaneously constrained it, offering a boundary where none had been. This symptom was not his enemy, but his tether—a gravitational compensation that rendered proximity survivable.

Loewald (1960) spoke of the analytic field as a "new matrix," a space in which archaic layers of experience could be relived and transformed in the presence of another. But even in this "new matrix," the symptom does not simply dissolve. It often intensifies, shifting shape or revealing layers of complexity that suggest not a single cause, but a structural saturation of experience. From a field perspective, the symptom cannot be traced to an origin in the past because it is continually maintained in the present—a stabilizing formation in the warped relational geometry of the analytic dyad.

Here we touch the edge of what Bollas (1987) called the "unthought known"—those encoded elements of the early relational field that were never symbolized but remain active in the body, the tone of voice, the micro-gestures of relating. The symptom is one such form: it often emerges not as a message from the unconscious, but as a defense against experiencing the unconscious directly. Yet it is also an invitation—an atmospheric flare indicating where the psyche has become saturated, where gravity has thickened. To approach the symptom as a field distortion is to listen not just for meaning, but for resonance, modulation, and aesthetic form.

Psychoanalysis has long held a dual attitude toward symptoms: they are pathologized and yet precious, clues to suffering but also to truth. When symptoms are treated merely as aberrations, we risk flattening the field from which they arise. When we treat them as evidence of psychic truth, we risk reifying them. But when we sense them as gravitational events—zones where invisible forces gather and hold—we can begin to track their aesthetic logic. They shimmer not because they obscure meaning, but because they hold more meaning than can be metabolized at once.

A patient's panic attack might not only reflect fear but signal a breach in the symbolic atmosphere. A compulsion might not just discharge drive but enact a miniature gravitational orbit, a rhythmic return that organizes the self in the absence of secure holding. Even dissociation, often cast as void or rupture, may instead be a field-regulating move: a way to bend time and space around a core of unintegrated intensity. The symptom, then, is not merely "inside" the patient, nor does it belong solely to the past. It is a living artifact of psychic gravity—an event on the edge of collapse.

In this model, transference itself becomes inseparable from symptom: each is a form of gravitational coherence. The analyst, too, is not outside the field but part of its geometry, implicated in the very structure of the symptom's persistence. This is why working through symptoms requires more than interpretation; it requires the analyst's capacity to bear the affective curvature of the symptom without flattening it into explanation. Interpretation may unstick certain knots, but it is the shared presence in the field—the co-regulated arc of being-with—that gradually shifts the geometry.

Symptom as field distortion brings us back to the question of how psychic space is formed—not as a container, but as a curvature. To move toward healing is not necessarily to extinguish the symptom, but to feel its gravity differently: to no longer be enslaved by its orbit, but to inhabit it with awareness, flexibility, and imagination. The symptom may not vanish, but its density shifts. Its shimmer begins to pulse with possibility. Its grip softens. It is no longer the only anchor.

The Aesthetic of the Symptom

To encounter a symptom solely as pathology is to miss its atmosphere. Like dreams, symptoms have aesthetic properties: tone, rhythm, contour, repetition, and intensification. They shimmer with condensation. They arrange affect and attention around a concentrated nucleus. They are not formless interruptions of mental function, but highly structured expressions of psychic compromise. They shape how experience feels—how it resonates, clings, or recedes. The symptom is an aesthetic act, a choreography of survival etched into the sensorium.

Freud (1900) knew this from the beginning, recognizing that symptoms and dreams shared the same logic of displacement, condensation, and representational substitution. But where the dream dissolves upon waking, the symptom lingers. It insists. Its form does not merely encode conflict but regulates psychic gravity. It holds the psyche near the unbearable, transposing intensity into repetition, metaphor, and gesture. In this sense, the symptom is not just what returns—it is how the psyche marks and frames the site of return.

Klein's (1946) early work on unconscious phantasy already positioned symptoms as crystallizations of relational anxiety. The symptom, in her model, organizes the mind against annihilation, against persecutory threat, against fragmentation. But there is also a poignancy in the symptom's form: it makes something vivid. It calls attention to what cannot be said in any other way. In this light, the symptom is an aesthetic achievement—not beautiful, necessarily, but precise. Its form says what the psyche cannot yet symbolize in language. As such, it is not random, but shaped—felt, survived, metabolized, and re-presented.

This aesthetic quality is most palpable in the texture of the analytic encounter. Symptoms can be heard in the stammer of a narrative, seen in the fixed gaze or the compulsive shrug, felt in the sudden density of silence. The analyst's attunement to these micro-forms is not merely diagnostic but poetic. What matters is not simply what the symptom means, but how it arranges meaning—how it gathers affect, arrests time, bends the arc of speech. A tic, a ritual, a refusal: each becomes a scene, a form, a refrain.

The symptom is also theatrical. It stages something, over and over again. In this sense, it contains what Laplanche (1999) called "enigmatic signification"—a message from the other (or the internal other) that was never fully deciphered, and that continues to be relayed in distorted form. The symptom becomes the medium of that transmission. It holds the unsymbolized residue of that prior address. But it does so not as archive but as performance. It animates what was frozen. It brings the past into the room—not as memory, but as form.

This is why interpretation, when it works, does not simply decode content but touches the form of the symptom itself. It finds the music beneath the symptom's stutter. A woman who compulsively touches the doorframe before entering the room is not just warding off dread—she is marking a threshold, creating a beat, a metrical gap before entry. Her symptom choreographs an aesthetic of control, of spacing, of temporal dilation. It reshapes the world into a form she can bear. Her gesture is not only a defense; it is a syntax.

Bollas (1987) wrote of the "transformational object"—those early relational experiences that alter the psychic world not by symbolizing but by impressing, leaving traces that structure aesthetic preference and subjective style. Symptoms can become such objects. They impress the psyche with a rhythm, a contour, a felt shape that organizes experience. A panic attack, for instance, may be more than a fear response: it may be a trance-state of rupture and intensity that becomes a kind of private performance, a psychic ritualization of the breakdown of form. Over time, the patient may come to rely on this form—not to understand themselves, but to recognize themselves.

The aesthetic of the symptom is also its inertia. Once a form is established, it sticks. It calls the self back into its orbit, again and again. This is not just compulsion—it is identity. Loewald (1978e) noted that symptoms often preserve archaic structures that had once been adaptive. Their persistence is not evidence of failure, but of allegiance. The psyche holds on to them because they are familiar, saturated with meaning, and necessary. They are the last known coordinates.

Aesthetic form is thus inseparable from psychic ethics. To intervene upon a symptom too quickly is to destroy its style, its tempo, its signature. To work with a symptom is to listen not just for its message, but for the world it creates. For the temporal world: how fast or slow it makes experience. For the spatial world: how near or far others feel in its orbit. For the sensory world: what brightness, heat, texture it calls forth. The symptom is a container for all of this. It may be suffering, but it is also meaning.

Consider Alice, a woman in her 50s who came into treatment describing herself as a perfectionist, someone who could "never quite relax." Her presenting symptoms included sleeplessness, obsessive mental planning, and a chronic shoulder pain she attributed to "tension." But over time, her way of speaking about these symptoms revealed something else: she spoke of them with reverence, even affection. "They keep me upright," she once said. "If I ever stopped, I'd vanish."

Alice's symptoms held her together—literally and symbolically. Her aesthetic of control was not merely defensive but sculptural: she was shaping the world to reflect the tension she felt inside. Her tightness was a mode of presence. When her shoulder pain would flare, she didn't feel overwhelmed; she felt real. Her symptom had become a threshold for self-recognition, a kind of sensory anchor. To work with it required more than interpretation—it required accompaniment, a listening for the aesthetic logic that made this pain necessary.

In this way, the symptom is a symbolic medium. It exists not only within the body but between bodies—in the field of transference and countertransference, where meaning is not only spoken but enacted, felt, and transferred through form. When the analyst begins to feel the pull of the symptom's tempo—the pacing, the silence, the lurch—it is not simply countertransference reactivity. It is field attunement. The symptom becomes a shared rhythm, a joint holding, a mutual gravity.

This aesthetic field may resist analysis even as it invites it. The analyst must learn to feel with rather than decipher. To remain close enough to the symptom's form without rushing toward its symbolic translation. To notice the shimmering repetition and trust that what is glimmering is already saying something: not through new content, but through fidelity to form.

When a patient begins to sense the symptom not as a foreign invasion but as a language, something shifts. They begin to collaborate with the symptom. Not to prolong it—but to hear what it holds. They begin to sense how the very form they once feared might also be a compass. The symptom, then, becomes a companion: not simply to be resolved, but to be related to. To be heard in its aesthetic fullness.

Symptom as Trace of the Unsymbolized

If the aesthetic form of the symptom marks its visible architecture, then what underlies that form is often something unsymbolized—an excess, a void, a silence at the core of psychic life. The symptom is not merely an encrypted message waiting to be decoded. It is a condensation of something that was never metabolized into language in the first place. In this sense, the symptom is not a cipher but a trace: the mark left by an experience that escaped inscription. It does not represent the unconscious; it protects against it.

This distinction is vital. When we treat the symptom as symbolic from the start, we presume a continuity of experience and meaning that may never have existed. But some experiences—especially those arising in early development, traumatic rupture, or environments of profound misattunement—do not generate symbols. They generate pressure. What returns is not memory but force, not representation but residue. The symptom, then, emerges not as expression but as defense: a shield of form around a hole in the symbolic order.

The unsymbolized is not simply pre-verbal. It is often post-verbal—something that could have been symbolized but wasn't, because the context of recognition was absent. These are the gaps that haunt the psyche: affects that surged in isolation, gestures that landed without response, desires that unfurled into a void. The result is not repression in the classical sense, but foreclosure of meaning. And yet, the psyche does not forget. It reorganizes around the gap. It builds satellites of coherence to orbit the black hole of unformulated experience. The symptom is one such satellite. Its orbit reveals the unspeakable mass at the center.

Winnicott (1965) spoke of the "unexperienced experience"—those psychic events that occur without a self present to register them. These are not absent from the psyche; they are stored somatically, rhythmically, and atmospherically. The symptom becomes their carrier. It gives shape to what has no place. In doing so, it sustains both the disjunction and the hope of eventual encounter. The symptom does not close the circuit of communication. It leaves it open, waiting, echoing.

In this way, symptoms often announce the presence of an unconscious that is not repressed but unformulated. Donnel Stern (1997) described such material as the "unformulated experience"—psychic content that has never been fully shaped into a mental representation. These unformulated residues exert pressure on consciousness, not as narrative, but as atmosphere: the feel of something unresolved, unclaimed, untouchable. The symptom crystallizes this pressure into a manageable form. It becomes the psychic infrastructure that holds the unrepresentable in place, without resolving it.

But there is also a paradox. In attempting to hold what cannot be symbolized, the symptom may also become a kind of proto-symbol. Its repetition, its form, its aesthetic rhythm—all create the conditions in which symbolization might eventually occur. Like the repetition compulsion that Freud (1920) struggled to explain—why the patient repeats rather than remembers—the symptom may be a stubborn invitation to return. Not because the past is knowable, but because the psyche cannot move forward without orbiting what it has never assimilated. The symptom, then, is not only defensive but reparative. It is a site of potential metabolization.

Consider Evan, a young man in his late 20s who came to treatment following the abrupt end of a relationship. His presenting symptoms were familiar: insomnia, intrusive fantasies, and compulsive sexual behavior. But what drew analytic attention was not just the content of these symptoms, but their tempo. There was an unmistakable rhythm to Evan's repetitions—a nocturnal loop of craving, climax, shame, silence. It was as if his body knew something he could not say. His speech faltered when he was asked about his early memories. His affect would vanish when desire was named. But the symptom pulsed on, every night, as if whispering a wordless demand.

Over time, it became clear that Evan's relational history was marked by an absent father and a mother who could not metabolize his emotional states. His need for recognition had never been mirrored, and his sexualized symptoms now traced that original deficit. But they did not simply compensate—they recreated the scene. Each encounter with a stranger was a re-performance of misattuned touch. Each climax a flash of proximity, followed by collapse. The symptom preserved not a memory, but a structure—a living map of the unsymbolized wound.

In the analytic relationship, something shifted. The tempo of Evan's symptom did not immediately change, but the space around it thickened. Interpretation gave way to witnessing. The analyst did not try to decode the symptom, but to feel it, to track its rhythm, to inhabit its gravity without fleeing or fixing. Slowly, the symptom began to soften. Its urgency dimmed. New words emerged—not for the trauma itself, but for the experience of orbiting it. The symptom became less a prison and more a relic. It still pulsed, but as a reminder, not a compulsion.

This is the work of symbolization—not the insertion of meaning from without, but the emergence of language from within form. The symptom, when held with enough precision and patience, may begin to speak. But its first language is not verbal. It is gestural, temporal, and affective. It moves in pacing, posture, and silence. The analyst must become fluent in this language of unsymbolized transmission. Must learn to listen with the whole body. Must sense when interpretation would violate the symptom's integrity, and when the symptom itself is asking to be witnessed, not resolved.

Ogden (2005) described the analytic third as a space where new forms of experience can be dreamed into being—not through willful construction, but through shared presence in the field of what has not yet been thought. The symptom often leads the way into this space. It marks the edge of what the patient has been able to think, feel, or endure. And in doing so, it also opens the possibility of crossing that edge. But only if the analyst can remain there—still, attuned, unhurried.

This unsymbolized territory is not only difficult—it is sacred. The symptom holds what was once too much for the psyche to bear. It should not be rushed. To move too quickly toward insight or resolution is to miss the dignity of the symptom's form. It has held the unbearable. It has carried the charge. It deserves reverence.

The symptom, then, is not just a signal of distress. It is a form of psychic ethics. It sustains what could not be held otherwise. It makes time for meaning that never came. It creates a somatic punctuation around a trauma that lacked syntax. And in the analytic relationship, it becomes a bridge—not only backward into the past, but outward into language, into recognition, into the possibility of form.

To work with symptoms at this level requires a particular stance: neither analyst as interpreter nor patient as historian, but two presences circling the unsymbolized. The symptom is the third—wordless, rhythmic, insistent. It reminds us that not all suffering speaks in symbols. Some suffering must be formed before it can be spoken.

And so we listen. We orbit. We feel the gravity of what the symptom cannot yet say. And in doing so, we honor the symptom not as pathology, but as trace—of rupture, of yearning, of the unspeakable center around which the psyche has learned to turn.

Resonant Collapse and the Ethics of Presence

To sit with the symptom is to sit with collapse—not merely the collapse of form, but of meaning, of coherence, of temporal and spatial anchoring. Yet this collapse is not always loud. More often, it is rhythmic, recursive, ambient. A symptom flickers in and out of language like static in a transmission, signaling something not yet metabolized. What collapses is not simply narrative, but the distinction between figure and ground, signal and noise. To attend to the symptom is to enter this shimmering border zone, where meaning both recedes and intensifies.

Resonant collapse occurs when the symbolic field folds in on itself—not with a bang, but with a shimmer. The symptom in this state is not a message waiting to be decoded, but a medium through which the psyche organizes unprocessable intensity. It resonates because it repeats with difference, like a musical motif that changes slightly each time it returns. The patient is not simply expressing something through the symptom—they are living within its temporal structure. It becomes a temporal container for what otherwise cannot be borne.

This return is not just personal; it is structural. When collapse resonates, it implicates the analytic pair. Countertransference is not merely reactive but gravitational. The analyst may find themselves pulled into the symptom's rhythm—feeling sleepy, distracted, anxious, over-invested. This is not resistance but field saturation. The symptom reorganizes the atmosphere of the room. Its recurrence marks not failure but fidelity—to an unformulated intensity, to a structure that once preserved the self. To interpret too quickly is not only ineffective—it is a betrayal of this fidelity.

Ogden (1994) wrote of the analytic third as a co-created intersubjective space, one that exists in the movement between two subjectivities. Resonant collapse thickens that space. It bends it. In these moments, the analyst may feel that linear time has stopped; sessions lose their arc, language coagulates, the familiar rhythm of therapeutic pacing evaporates. What remains is the gravitational hold of the symptom—its looping logic, its aesthetic precision, its refusal to resolve. The work, then, becomes not to push through the collapse, but to dwell within it ethically.

Ethical presence in the face of resonant collapse requires a suspension of both urgency and avoidance. It is a refusal to substitute explanation for attunement, or to flee the discomfort of unknowing by imposing coherence. The analyst's task is not to resolve the symptom's opacity, but to remain porous to its form. What is needed is not always interpretation, but companionship—an analyst willing to be folded into the patient's temporal world without eclipsing it. The presence of the analyst becomes the counterweight to collapse, not by resisting it, but by holding its rhythm with steadiness and care.

Bollas (1992) suggested that some psychic experiences are better held through aesthetic sensibility than through analytical language. In this light, the analyst becomes a tuning fork—resonating with the patient's symptom not to mirror it exactly, but to offer another frequency, another mode of organization. This is especially vital in working with what might otherwise be labeled treatment-resistant presentations, where symptoms persist not despite the work, but because the analyst has not yet joined their rhythm.

To work with symptoms at the level of resonant collapse is to recognize the ethical paradox at the heart of psychoanalysis: that we seek to change the psyche by staying with what does not change. That transformation does not always come through interpretation, but through witnessing the symptom's form without rushing to undo it. This is especially true in patients whose symptoms have become their last form of coherence—where to dissolve them prematurely would be to dissolve the psychic structure itself.

Consider the case of Mateo, a man in his early thirties whose presenting symptom was a kind of erotic paralysis. He longed for intimacy but could not sustain arousal in the presence of a partner. Alone, he could fantasize, feel, even orgasm—but once another body entered the room, his desire collapsed. The symptom had the texture of defeat, but it was not simply sexual inhibition. It was a structural condensation of something older and deeper: a longing so saturated with shame and misattunement that it could not move. Each failed encounter was not a repetition of trauma, but a gravitational loop around what had never cohered.

In the analytic work, it became clear that Mateo's collapse was not merely a personal defense but a relational event. The closer the analyst came to the terrain of desire, the more dissociated Mateo became. The symptom organized the field. The analyst's temptation was to push for insight—to speak desire into symbol. But that urgency only tightened the collapse. What shifted the dynamic was something else: the analyst's ability to name the atmosphere without piercing it. "Something in the room slows down when we get near this," the analyst said once, not as interpretation, but as accompaniment. Mateo wept. It was the first moment of erotic contact that did not collapse him.

What occurred in that moment was not the "working through" of the symptom but the recognition of its gravity. The analyst joined the orbit, not to decode it, but to hold it in shared rhythm. This is the ethics of presence: the willingness to feel, metabolize, and reverberate with the patient's symptom without requiring it to mean something else. In this sense, the symptom becomes a third—neither patient nor analyst, but a gravitational structure that includes both.

This approach stands in contrast to therapeutic models that prioritize content over form, clarity over texture, and solution over relation. In resonant collapse, it is precisely the fidelity to form that becomes curative. The patient feels seen not in spite of the symptom, but through it. The analyst's presence offers a counterweight—not by imposing coherence, but by allowing form to resonate until something new emerges.

To work this way requires discipline. The analyst must resist both the seductive pull of insight and the defensive retreat into neutrality. They must instead tolerate disorientation, aesthetic density, and the slow shimmer of symbolic possibility. As Eigen (2004) wrote, "the soul grows at the edges of breakdown." It is not our task to drag the patient away from collapse, but to meet them there—to stand at the edge of their gravitational orbit and bear witness as their form begins, slowly, to shift.

In resonant collapse, we find the deepest paradox of analytic work: that transformation often begins not in what changes, but in what is held. The symptom remains, but its frequency softens. Its tempo loosens. It no longer needs to scream because it has been heard. And what emerges from this hearing is not a cured self, but a self with more space around the symptom—a self whose gravity is no longer collapsed, but curved.

Repetition, Recursion, and the Event-Horizon of the Symptom

To speak of symptom as gravitational is to invoke not only space but orbit: the curved, recursive movement that returns without arrival. Symptoms repeat. They do not merely reappear; they follow a pattern that resists linear unfolding. This is not the repetition of content, but the repetition of form—of structure, atmosphere, affective weight. It is as if the symptom drags the psyche into its own temporal geometry: a loop that tightens the more one tries to escape it.

Freud (1914b) described the compulsion to repeat as a force that defied the pleasure principle, operating instead as a death-driven momentum—a tendency to return to a state of tension, even trauma, not to master it, but to relive its imprint. Yet repetition is not simply masochistic. In psychic terms, it is spatial: it creates a fold in time, a gravitational tether to the unmourned, the unformulated, the unsymbolizable. The symptom recurs not to remind, but to hold—to encircle what cannot yet take shape in thought.

Each instance of repetition brings the subject back to a structural perimeter: a liminal zone, a psychic event horizon. In physics, an event horizon marks the threshold beyond which light cannot escape—a boundary where gravity overwhelms form. Psychically, the event horizon of the symptom is that point at which representation collapses and recursive presence takes over. What is repeated is not memory but gravitational tension. Meaning flickers, but does not stabilize. The orbit sustains itself through the failure of integration.

The analytic task, then, is not to sever the orbit but to trace its curvature. The symptom does not indicate where the patient has been, but where they are stuck—looping through a self-organizing circuit of affect, fantasy, and unconscious structure. These loops are often aesthetic: they carry a particular rhythm, a tone, a signature. A panic attack always emerging at the same decibel of intimacy. A compulsive gesture timed to the silence between sentences. A depressive slump that arrives each weekend, as if to mark the collapse of external holding. These are not merely patterns—they are orbits with gravity.

Bion (1962) spoke of the difficulty of thinking in the presence of unmentalized experience. The symptom, in its recursive form, may represent precisely this: an effort by the psyche to hold unthinkable experience in aesthetic stasis. Recursion becomes an internal container—not for insight, but for coherence. When the analyst encounters this kind of repetition, the impulse may be to disrupt the pattern, to offer new language, new understanding. But such interventions may collapse the orbit before its internal gravity has been metabolized.

To enter this terrain, the analyst must become a gravitational companion: not simply a reflective mirror, but a body with its own affective mass. The symptom, lived in the field, pulls both participants toward the edge of symbolic collapse. The analyst's attention must become recursive as well—not by mimicking the patient's symptom, but by returning again and again to the edge where symbol fails and form remains. This is what Winnicott (1965) glimpsed in his notion of "going-on-being": a rhythmic continuity of presence that allows for the emergence of self. Here, that continuity includes the repetition itself.

This recursive fidelity is not neutral. It is saturated with risk and responsibility. The event horizon is not a safe place; it is a space of disintegration held together only by the tenuous choreography of presence. It is where shame spikes, desire disorganizes, and silence thickens into foreclosure. And yet, it is also where something begins to pulse. Something new. Not meaning in the traditional sense, but form that begins to stretch. Orbit that begins to widen. Recursion that begins to spiral rather than circle.

Take the case of Clara, a woman in her late twenties with a history of developmental trauma and a persistent symptom of erotic withdrawal. She described her relationships as beginning with fascination and intensity, but always devolving into a kind of dissociative deadness. "I go numb," she said. "Even when I want it, I vanish." The pattern repeated across lovers, friends, and even the analytic relationship itself. Periods of connection would build, and then abruptly collapse. At first, this was read as repetition compulsion—as reenactment. But it was more than that. It was recursion: a folding of the relational field back into a structural bind.

In session, Clara's gaze would drift, her speech would slow, and her body would subtly withdraw. It was not resistance; it was gravitational re-entry into the event horizon. The symptom was not defending against contact—it was holding a core dilemma: how to be in relation without dissolving. Her dissociation was not a void but a tether. It held her in the orbit of selfhood, however collapsed. The analyst learned to track the rhythm—when Clara moved into that state, the work was not to pull her out, but to stay near. To speak slowly, to reflect tone not just content, to hold without grasping.

Over time, Clara began to sense the presence of the analyst even in those collapsed states. "I could still feel you," she said once. "Even when I couldn't feel myself." This was not a breakthrough in the traditional sense—it was a widening of orbit. The symptom had not disappeared, but its gravity had changed. The recursive loop had loosened. It now included the analyst. It no longer closed in on itself.

This is the ethics of recursive accompaniment. The symptom does not need to be resolved to shift. Its orbit needs to be joined—entered not as analyst-as-expert, but as analyst-as-satellite. A companion whose presence disturbs the closed loop just enough to open a new curvature. The repetition becomes co-authored. The aesthetic thickens. Symbolization begins not with meaning, but with shared rhythm.

Recursion and repetition are not pathologies of the will; they are the natural language of the psyche under pressure. They reveal where the psyche is working hardest to survive itself. The event horizon of the symptom, then, is not a place to be crossed, but a place to be witnessed. It is the edge of psychic form—a shimmering threshold where something remains ungraspable, yet insists on being held.

In this light, the symptom becomes not just a gravitational trace, but a recursive invitation. Not "what is wrong," but "what still holds." Not "what repeats," but "what seeks resonance." To honor that repetition is to trust in the intelligence of the orbit—that the psyche repeats not to remain stuck, but to rehearse the conditions under which something might finally shift.

Symptom, Style, and the Edge of the Self

A symptom does more than hurt. It stylizes. Its repetition is not merely mechanical; it becomes a signature. In this way, symptoms are not simply errors to be corrected but styles of subjectivity—highly condensed expressions of how a person navigates form, coherence, contact, and survival. They shape the edges of the self: where it begins, where it ends, what textures it can tolerate, what forces it cannot metabolize. A symptom is not only a formation; it is a performance of boundary, rhythm, and orientation in a field of overwhelm.

Style, in this sense, is not cosmetic. It is the very structure of survival. When the psyche encounters what it cannot symbolize or resolve, it does not go blank—it improvises. It creates a form, a gesture, a rhythm that holds the unbearable. Symptoms are among the most enduring of these improvisations. They repeat not because they are senseless, but because they once worked—and perhaps still do. They are stylized attempts to hold together experience when the basic grammar of feeling and being has broken down.

This is what makes symptoms so intimate. They are not simply problems to be solved; they are artifacts of psychic life. They tell us how a person has survived fragmentation, engulfment, abandonment, or incoherence. They tell us what has been lost—and what has been built in its place. They are sometimes the only form left through which the subject can mark the world. In this light, we must ask not only what a symptom means, but what world it creates. What style of relation does it enact? What temporality does it impose? What aesthetic does it preserve?

When patients speak of their symptoms, they are often ambivalent—not just because the symptom causes suffering, but because it also carries familiarity, even comfort. A patient with panic may describe the feeling of being overwhelmed— but also of being real, intense, alive. A patient with chronic indecision may speak of frustration—but also of relief at postponing collapse. These experiences are not contradictions; they are structural. The symptom marks the very edge where the self tries to cohere. It is not just reaction; it is technique.

This technique is not conscious. It is felt into existence. Like a musician who finds the only chord that can hold a dissonant emotion, the psyche locates a pattern that sustains enough coherence to go on. Once established, this pattern begins to stylize the subject's experience of the world. It draws certain relationships closer and pushes others away. It modulates time and intensity. It becomes a gravitational habit—not because it is desired, but because it structures desire itself.

Consider a patient like Isaac, a man in his early thirties whose symptom took the form of relentless perfectionism, especially in creative work. He was a visual artist, but he rarely finished a piece. He would spend hours adjusting tiny details, only to discard the whole image and start again. In treatment, he spoke of feeling like a fraud, afraid that any finished work would reveal his inadequacy. But underneath this self-critique was something else: a devotion to form. His symptom was not just avoidance—it was a way of staying near an unnamable affect. "If I finish it," he once said, "it will be dead."

What Isaac feared was not failure, but foreclosure—the loss of psychic movement, of aesthetic possibility. The symptom preserved his relation to something sacred, something ungraspable. It enacted a style of unfinished-ness, of near-arrival, of suspended culmination. This style was not arbitrary; it was constitutive of his selfhood. The symptom became his way of approaching experience without collapsing it. In this sense, the symptom was his edge: the point where contact with vitality could be sustained without being annihilated by completion.

Style, then, becomes a diagnostic and ethical category. To ask about symptom style is to ask: what aesthetic does this person require in order to feel real? What forms can their psyche inhabit without dissociation or fragmentation? What stylistic constraints make their experience tolerable? Some patients need slowness, others sharpness. Some need constriction, others diffusion. These are not preferences in the usual sense; they are structural necessities. The symptom styles the atmosphere so the self can exist within it.

Analytically, this requires a shift. We move from aiming to eliminate symptoms to becoming attuned to the way they style the analytic space. Does the room become thick with silence? Does time feel urgent, stalled, or floating? Is the rhythm staccato or legato? These are not incidental effects. They are part of the symptom's aesthetic. And the analyst's capacity to register and metabolize these stylistic cues becomes central to the treatment.

Winnicott (1971) spoke of playing as the space where the self begins to come into being. But for many patients, that space has collapsed. The symptom emerges as a substitute—not for play itself, but for the boundaries that make play possible. It provides the frame, the tempo, the constraint within which the self can experiment. Without the symptom, the atmosphere becomes too diffuse, too open, too formless. The symptom is not play—but it may be the only holding pattern that makes play thinkable.

When a symptom functions as style, its disruption must be approached with care. Too much insight too soon can fracture the structure it holds. Too much challenge can undo the coherence it provides. The analytic task, then, is to enter the symptom's aesthetic world—not to mirror it, but to stay close enough that the patient feels accompanied within its contours. From this position, slight shifts become possible. A pause where there was only acceleration. A gesture where there was only withdrawal. These micro-movements are not symptom relief; they are style evolution.

The symptom, when seen in this light, is not only a trace of pathology but a nascent creative act. It is the psyche's earliest choreography of contact. It does not simply signal injury; it carries a prototype of style—the earliest forms by which self and world could be held in relation. To work with it is to honor its aesthetic without becoming trapped by it. To offer alternatives not by argument, but by presence: a rhythm, a pacing, a form of being that allows the symptom to soften without needing to vanish.

This is why the symptom so often resurfaces at moments of change. Not because the patient is resisting growth, but because the aesthetic of the new has not yet formed. The symptom reasserts the prior structure—it offers its habitual style until a new form becomes available. This is not regression; it is fidelity. The psyche returns to what it knows how to be until it senses something else it can become.

And this is the paradox. The symptom both imprisons and protects. It closes the future even as it holds open the present. It repeats—but within its repetition is the seed of potential. If the analyst can stay long enough within its style, without demanding its disappearance, then the symptom may begin to dream. It may begin to curl into new forms—not because it has been decoded, but because it has been accompanied.

The symptom is not only a problem to be worked through. It is the psychic atmosphere that surrounds a wound, and the style by which that atmosphere becomes habitable. It is the subject's first aesthetic—and often, their most faithful.

Symbolic Collapse and the Aesthetics of Absence

A symptom does not only form in the presence of pain—it also forms in the absence of form. When the symbolic order collapses, when language fails to hold or organize experience, the symptom steps in. It arises not simply as a cipher for the repressed, but as an aesthetic condensation of a rupture in meaning itself. In this way, the symptom is less a representation of trauma than an architecture built around the collapse of representation.

This collapse need not be dramatic. It can be subtle, developmental, relational—a moment when no one mirrored, no one named, no one metabolized. The absence lingers, unsymbolized but active, shaping the field around it. Over time, the psyche fills in the space with something that feels—if not coherent, at least patterned. This patterning becomes the symptom. Not a symptom of memory, but of absence. A sign that something unformulated had weight, and that weight pulled space and time into new geometry.

This is what makes certain symptoms feel at once meaningful and empty. They point, but to no object. They return, but not to an event. They are the residue of a structural silence—a collapse not just of speech, but of the very possibility of speech. Bollas (1987) called this the "receptive unconscious," where experience is stored not as narrative but as mood, as pressure, as texture. The symptom becomes the way this un-narrated density enters form. It is not memory but atmosphere, condensed into shape.

This condensation may be aesthetic before it is symbolic. The symptom takes up space, slows or speeds time, and distorts sensation. It rearranges perception in a way that restores a kind of internal coherence, even if that coherence is painful. The symbolic, in contrast, tries to order experience through reference—this happened, it meant this, and so I feel that. But when the chain of reference is broken, the symptom offers an alternative. It says: *this form is how I survive the break.*

Here, the symptom becomes a kind of sculpture—a fixed form that arises in response to unformed experience. The aesthetic properties of the symptom—its rhythm, its recurrence, its density—are not accidental. They are the psyche's attempt to hold together what could not be held in language. Like a ritual object that binds a community around an unspeakable history, the symptom binds the self around an unspeakable absence. It becomes the trace not of what was lost, but of what never came into form.

This is what Loewald (1978d) meant when he described symbolization as a process that brings vitality to experience, transforming the unstructured into something that can be played with, held, and related to. But when symbolization fails, the symptom may become the only structure capable of holding psychic intensity. It does not enliven, but it organizes. It is not fluid, but it is repeatable. Its repetition becomes its power. And its aesthetic fixity may be the only reliable form in a world otherwise saturated with collapse.

Symbolic collapse is often a developmental phenomenon. It may arise from disorganized attachment, from excessive stimulation, or from misattuned holding. But it can also be cultural—an atmosphere in which certain experiences are forbidden, foreclosed, or erased. In such contexts, the symptom carries not only personal but transpersonal weight. It is the artifact of a collapse that exceeds the individual: a gendered collapse, a racialized erasure, a queer unspeakability. The symptom then becomes a private aesthetic of a collective absence.

This aesthetic often takes the form of interruption. A stutter, a blank, a tic, a forgetting. The symptom marks the place where something should have happened but didn't. Where a word should have arrived, but silence stood in its place. These micro-events are not trivial. They are formal indicators of symbolic breakdown. And the analyst's task is not to smooth them over, but to stay near them—to listen to their rhythm, to let their absence pulse, to hear what kind of silence is being transmitted.

Silence, after all, is not neutral. Some silences are heavy with implication; others are sharp with prohibition. Some are warm and holding; others fracture the field. The symptom often arises in the latter kind. It tries to carve a shape into that silence. It says: *something happened here—even if no one can say what it was*. The analyst, in turn, becomes the witness not to the event, but to its trace—the distortion it leaves in the field, the fold it makes in time.

In some cases, symbolic collapse reveals itself through over-symbolization. The symptom floods the field with metaphor, with obsessive meaning-making, with dense self-explanation. This is not clarity—it is the symptom's camouflage. A way of warding off the collapse it protects. These patients do not resist insight; they drown in it. Their symptoms form not from repression, but from the absence of grounding symbols. Their language is rich, but it never lands. It orbits emptiness.

Lacan (1977) saw this as the Real—the register of experience that resists symbolization and yet insists, returns, demands. For Lacan, the symptom was not a message to be decoded but a node, a knot, a point of impossible convergence. The analyst's role was not to solve it but to engage its impossibility. And this impossibility is not just a limit of understanding—it is a structural condition of subjectivity. There is always something in us that escapes the net of language. The symptom curls around that excess.

But not all excess is traumatic. Some is ontological. The human subject is structured by lack, by absence, by the impossibility of full coherence. The symptom becomes the way this impossibility is registered. Not as a failure, but as a form. The analyst does not heal the lack—they accompany its stylization. They make it possible for the patient to feel the aesthetic of absence without collapsing. This is not catharsis, but composition.

Composition becomes the central task of the psyche after symbolic collapse. The symptom is its first draft. It is where form emerges before meaning, where shape precedes speech. And analytic work becomes a slow co-composition—not of content, but of form. Together, analyst and patient learn the texture of the collapse, the grain of its silence, the geometry of its distortion. They do not cure the absence—they give it atmosphere. They make it habitable.

Sometimes, the symptom changes not because it is interpreted, but because it is recontextualized. A tic becomes a beat. A blank becomes a breath. A dread becomes a horizon. These shifts are subtle. They do not eliminate the symptom. They soften its edges. They let it bend, shimmer, and vary.

They allow the symptom to become style—not because it no longer hurts, but because it can now hold something other than hurt.

This is the paradoxical gift of symbolic collapse: it forces the psyche into aesthetics. It demands form where language fails. It insists on repetition as a kind of prayer. The symptom becomes the ritual by which the self reconstitutes its edge. And in that ritual, something new can be born—not a truth, but a shape. Not a cure, but a container.

To orbit a symbolic collapse is to live at the edge of being. The symptom is the trace of that orbit. It does not say what was lost. It shows what loss looks like when it tries to hold itself.

Clinical Vignette: The Orbit of Incompletion

When Alice first came to treatment, her complaints were diffuse. She described "an ache I can't name," a sense that she was "always circling something but never arriving." She was in her early forties, successful in her work as a designer, widely admired for her intuitive aesthetic sense—but privately, she felt hollow. "I don't know if I have a self," she once said. "Or if I'm just echoing what others need me to be." She did not present with a classic symptom picture—no panic, no compulsions, no disordered eating. And yet there was a distinct rhythm to her suffering: a pulsation of absence, a gravity that seemed to organize her experience without anchoring it.

The first months of treatment were marked by what felt like thematic diffusion. Alice spoke in rich, elliptical fragments—evocative, but hard to hold together. She often trailed off mid-sentence or pivoted suddenly to a different memory. There was a beauty to her language, a shimmer that suggested meaning just beyond reach. I found myself drifting in and out of contact, lulled by the music of her speech but struggling to discern its structure. It was as if her psyche were improvising a melody without ever committing to a key.

In supervision, I described the work as "orbiting a black hole." There was intensity, motion, and emotional charge—but no center. At times, I felt pulled into her rhythm, adopting her syntax, mirroring her hesitations. At others, I felt impatient, even bored—reacting, I sensed, not to her content, but to the absence it carried. Her symptom, if it could be called that, was not dramatic. It was aesthetic. A symptom of incompletion. A formal trace of something unfelt.

Over time, certain images began to recur: a dimly lit childhood hallway, the sound of her mother's high heels on tile, the weight of holding her breath. These were not traumatic memories in any classical sense. Rather, they felt like symbolic nodes—moments not fully metabolized, but etched into her sensorium. She would describe the hallway in exquisite detail, but when I asked what she felt in it, she would blink and say, "I don't know—I think I disappeared." The symptom was not what happened. It was what didn't. It was the choreography of her unformed presence.

In one session, after a long silence, Alice said, "Sometimes I think I don't dream. But then again, maybe everything I see is a dream." I asked what she meant. She paused. "I mean, I look at things and they look back, but I'm not sure I'm there. It's like my gaze is borrowed." That phrase—*my gaze is borrowed*—sat between us for a long moment. It carried the weight of symbolic collapse: the sense that even perception had become a symptom of absence.

Her symptom lived in form more than content. It was in how she paused before speaking, in her frequent corrections ("That's not quite what I meant"), in the exquisite care she took with words that never seemed to land. Her body, too, carried traces. She often sat with one hand wrapped tightly around the other wrist, as if containing herself from spilling. She never arrived late or early, but exactly on time. Not as an enactment of control, but as a kind of aesthetic ritual—an attempt to stitch coherence from the fabric of fragmentation.

I began to understand that her suffering was structured not by a single trauma but by the long, slow collapse of symbolic support. Her parents had been present but emotionally opaque. "They noticed if I was clean, polite, successful—but never if I was sad," she said. "I learned to speak in color, in performance, in precision. That's how they looked at me—if I glistened, I existed." Her symptom, then, was the shine: the shimmer of well-formed experience in the absence of being held.

The work did not move through interpretation so much as accompaniment. If I leaned too hard into explanation, she would retreat—not defensively, but as if the world had become too loud. But if I stayed near her rhythm, mirrored her pacing, let my own speech echo hers, something opened. We began to listen to the atmosphere between words. I would say, "It feels like something is circling," and she would nod softly. "Yes, but I don't know what." We let the symptom be our shared orbit.

There were moments of sudden symbolic emergence. Once, while describing a memory of drawing with her father at the kitchen table, she whispered, "He never looked at the drawing—only how sharp my lines were." She looked at me, eyes wet. "I think I made everything sharp so I wouldn't disappear." That sentence crystallized the aesthetic of her symptom. The sharpness was not aggression. It was survival. A way of insisting on form in the face of symbolic void.

That moment changed something—not dramatically, but gravitationally. She began to reference herself more, to say "I" with slightly more weight. Her symptoms didn't vanish, but they softened. Her speech became less glittering, more grounded. Silences stretched but didn't collapse. She once said, "It's like the room is holding me now. Not just you. The room." The analytic space had become a container for the symptom—not as something to be removed, but as something to be related to.

Over time, we could even play with the symptom. When she corrected her language mid-sentence, I might echo it with gentle parody: "Not quite what you meant—but almost?" She would smile. The rigidity became fluid. The symptom began to shimmer differently—not as a defense, but as a style. It was no longer only a trace of what hadn't happened. It became a medium through which she explored what could.

In our final months, she brought in fewer memories, fewer ornate phrases. Instead, she described sitting on her balcony and watching the light shift. "I don't need to explain it," she said once. "I just sit in it. And it changes." The symptom had transformed—not disappeared, but become porous. It still pulsed, but it no longer governed. It had become a trace of something once necessary, now aestheticized, gently held.

When she left treatment, she gave me a photograph she'd taken: a blurred image of falling light on a windowpane. On the back, she wrote: "Not quite what I meant. But almost." I understood. The orbit remained. But she no longer mistook it for absence. She could now see it as presence—curved, partial, beautiful.

Closing Reflection: Gravity and the Ethics of Form

To treat the symptom as a gravitational trace is to displace the notion of cure from eradication to relation. The symptom becomes not what must be dissolved, but what must be heard—through rhythm, repetition, resistance, and the aesthetic shaping of psychic form. We no longer ask how to uproot the symptom, but how to stay with its orbit long enough for it to speak, to shimmer, to soften.

This is not an ethics of rescue, nor of mastery. It is an ethics of witnessing form. The symptom, when understood as gravitational, is not merely the return of the repressed but the spatial registration of something unformulated—something that remains present not as content, but as curvature. The analyst's task is not to straighten the arc, but to attune to its bend.

To do so requires letting go of a linear epistemology. If the unconscious was once imagined as a repository of hidden truths to be uncovered, a topological imagination instead foregrounds affective density, shape, and force. The symptom does not conceal a single trauma; it holds the weight of atmospheres. It congeals the pressure of misattunements that never found form. It loops around what was too much, or not enough, or simply unspeakable. It is the aesthetic record of the psyche's attempt to survive distortion.

This aesthetic—its repetitions, its compulsions, its spatial logic—is never arbitrary. Even the most seemingly irrational symptom bears a precision of form. It creates thresholds, timing gaps, and sensory rhythms. A stutter, a tightening, a turn of the head: each may be the symptom's syntax, its grammar of survival. To listen at this level is not to interpret for meaning, but to witness form as meaning.

In this light, the symptom becomes less a mistake than a poetics. Not a poem in the literary sense, but in the etymological one: a *poiesis*, a making. The symptom makes a world—compressed, looped, curved around the unbearable. It is both artifact and architecture. And like any aesthetic object, it must be approached not with tools of dissection, but with tools of presence. The analyst becomes not engineer but accompanist, not decoder but attuned reader of form.

There is no neutrality here. The analyst is implicated in the symptom's field—affectively, symbolically, sometimes somatically. The symptom bends the relational space, pulling the analyst and patient into its orbit. This is not countertransference as interference, but as field participation. The analyst does not observe from afar. They feel the weight, the shimmer, the repetition. They register the gravitational aesthetics of the patient's suffering in their own experience—sometimes as fatigue, sometimes as enchantment, sometimes as resistance.

And this is where the ethical stance crystallizes. To join the patient in the orbit of their symptom is not to collude, nor to prematurely intervene. It is to bear witness to the form the psyche needed to survive. It is to honor the symptom, not because it is ideal, but because it is meaningful. Not because it should remain, but because it has already become a structure of holding.

Sometimes that structure softens. Sometimes it shifts. Sometimes it simply becomes more breathable. These are not signs of failure, but of movement. The symptom may not resolve in the classic sense, but it may become more permeable—less a prison, more a language. In this shift, even persistence becomes livable.

There is an ethic in allowing the symptom to retain its dignity. Not to romanticize it. Not to surrender to its inertia. But to respect its coherence. The patient's panic, compulsion, or dissociation is not random noise. It is resonance. It is the precise rhythm of what could not be metabolized any other way. The analyst who seeks only to extinguish it may miss the symbolic density it contains.

Loewald wrote that transformation occurs not through instruction but through presence—through the creation of a field in which the archaic can become thinkable. This is the core ethical task of the analyst working with symptoms as gravitational forms: to create a symbolic atmosphere that is thick enough, gentle enough, and receptive enough that new form becomes possible. Not because the analyst imposed it. But because the psyche, held differently, finds its own capacity to re-shape.

In this sense, the symptom is never just a burden. It is also a signal of the psyche's unfinished creativity. The orbit of repetition, when held with care, becomes the opening for a new spiral. The very compulsion that once locked the self in tight recurrence may become the seed of symbolic play. Even the most painful form may carry, within its echo, a future shape.

This is where psychoanalysis approaches the edge of the aesthetic: not as a metaphor, but as a mode of encounter. We become not just interpreters, but co-witnesses of the psyche's aesthetic work—its stubborn choreographies, its silences, its temporal and spatial stylizations. To do this work is to resist the pull toward diagnostic certainty, toward linear cure. It is to hold the shimmer of form, even when it resists understanding.

To orbit the symptom with the patient is to make room for the gravitational truth of suffering: that it bends space and time, that it loops and returns, that it holds what cannot yet be said. And that within this curvature, something essential may be felt. Not decoded. Not resolved. But known.

The analyst, in this model, becomes less an expert and more a gravitational companion. Someone who stays near the orbit, who doesn't flee when form resists meaning, who trusts that even the most intransigent symptom is a gesture toward coherence. The ethical stance is not to cure, but to stay. To let the form be held until it transforms or doesn't—but to let the holding itself be the change.

To speak of symptom as gravitational trace is to enter a psychoanalysis of accompaniment, atmosphere, and aesthetic resonance. It is to remember that meaning is not always hidden behind the form, but already present in the form. That symptom is not the failure of the symbolic, but its outer rim. That what loops, freezes, flares, or shimmers does so for a reason.

The task is not to erase these forms. It is to learn to live near them, with them, through them—until they speak in new ways, or simply settle into being what they are: signatures of survival, shaped by absence, held in presence.

5 The Analyst's Gravity

Transference and Countertransference Fields

This chapter explores the analytic field as a gravitational phenomenon, emphasizing the aesthetic and affective dynamics of transference and countertransference as recursive field effects. Drawing on relational, field-theoretic, and aesthetic approaches to psychoanalysis, it reframes transference not as a mere repetition of past object relations but as a dynamic, atmospheric warp in psychic space. Through micro-vignettes and theoretical integration, this chapter argues that the analyst's presence exerts symbolic gravity that shapes the psychic field, generating saturation, loops, and symbolic shimmer. Interpretation is presented less as decoding and more as aesthetic resonance within the field's own temporality. Saturation is not pathology but potential—an invitation to co-hold what cannot yet be symbolized.

In the preceding chapters, we have explored the gravitational metaphors of psychic curvature through temporality, symptom formation, and spatial aesthetics. Here, we enter the analytic situation itself—not to decode transference as an inherited content, but to feel its pressure as a field phenomenon. This chapter orients us to the analyst's gravity: the aesthetic, affective, and symbolic force of presence that bends the field of meaning, often unconsciously, shaping the arc of interpretation, dissociation, and symbolic return. Transference and countertransference are reframed not merely as interpersonal phenomena, but as distortions of psychic space—curvatures in the shared field that demand a new ethics of saturation. Rather than ask what the patient is repeating, we linger in how the field thickens—and what the analytic pair must hold before it can begin to speak.

Introduction: The Analyst as Gravitational Body

If symptoms orbit an unsymbolized mass, as the previous chapter proposed, then the analyst is not merely a passive observer of this orbit but becomes part of the gravitational system. The analytic setting bends under the presence of the analyst—not only their words, but their silences, micro-gestures, pacing, posture, and psychic presence. In the transference, the analyst becomes not just a figure from the past but a current body of force, exerting a gravitational

DOI: 10.4324/9781003715306-8

pull that shapes the relational field. The symptom does not merely reveal itself before the analyst; it reshapes itself through them.

Where Chapter 4 explored symptoms as spatial traces of psychic gravity, this chapter turns toward the analyst's own gravity—the pull they exert within the field of analytic co-presence. This is not simply a matter of countertransference or enactment. It is a shift in topology: the analyst becomes part of the psychic geometry the patient inhabits. The field is not neutral. It folds.

In this view, transference and countertransference are not only distortions but fields of mutual curvature. They shape the very space in which speech unfolds, where time dilates or collapses, where some affects flicker into life and others vanish without a trace. The analytic encounter is thus not a site of decoding alone, but of gravitational interplay—a space where both participants feel the pressure of something larger than themselves pressing in.

Ferenczi glimpsed this in his clinical diaries, describing how his body became a seismograph of unspoken affect. Winnicott, too, insisted that the analyst must be altered by the patient, not only interpreting but holding, absorbing, and metabolizing. Contemporary intersubjective theorists have extended this further: the analyst is not a fixed observer but a node in the matrix, a participant whose unconscious is implicated in the field's texture.

Yet this chapter asks more. It wonders what happens when the analyst's gravity itself becomes the organizing force—when the patient begins to orbit the analyst not only in fantasy, but in felt structure. When the analyst's presence functions not as mirror, but as mass. What are the ethics of such presence? What are its risks? What happens when the analyst's gravity pulls too hard—or not enough?

The aim here is not to moralize but to trace the phenomenon: how the analyst's personhood, history, and bodily resonance enter the field and exert symbolic weight. How analytic "presence" is not merely a stance but a force. And how this force may be sensed by the patient not cognitively, but atmospherically—as a shift in the quality of silence, a tightening in the chest, a thickening in the room.

In some cases, the analyst's gravity organizes the field, creating a temporary coherence around which the patient's fragmented self can constellate. In others, it may inadvertently eclipse the patient, saturating the field with affect that the patient cannot metabolize. The analyst may become a black hole: too dense, too known, too necessary. Or they may become absent mass—present but without pull, a ghost in the field. Both extremes distort the analytic space. But neither is inherently a failure. They are coordinates to be sensed, metabolized, and symbolized—together.

This chapter, therefore, continues the shift from interpretation to co-presence, from symptom to atmosphere. If Chapter 3 treated psychic temporality as bent and layered, and Chapter 4 framed the symptom as a gravitational echo, this chapter centers the analyst's own gravitational texture. This is a shift in perspective, but also in ethical posture: it calls for attunement to how we are being used, shaped, distorted, and pulled upon—not in order to correct the field, but to join it.

Here, we enter the clinical surround not as cartographers but as participants in an unstable orbit. We are not outside the field, but folded into its shape. The task is not to maintain neutrality, but to notice how the field bends when we move. The symptom, the transference, the silence—all these become instruments, not of revelation, but of resonance.

And so we begin with the gravitational body of the analyst. Not as countertransference content, not as technique, but as form: the analyst's tone, weight, timing, presence. What does it mean to be felt as a center of gravity? What does it mean to feel oneself pulled into that role? This chapter will trace those dynamics—not to resolve them, but to recognize them as the medium of analysis itself.

The Analyst's Presence as Field Distortion

The analyst's presence does not simply witness the analytic field—it alters it. The myth of analytic neutrality has long obscured this truth: that every breath, blink, and bodily registration of the analyst carries symbolic and atmospheric weight. Patients do not only speak to analysts; they speak through them, around them, against them. The analytic dyad is a shared topology, bent by the gravitational field of both participants, but especially distorted by the density of the analyst's psychic mass.

To name the analyst as a gravitational body is to acknowledge a clinical paradox: we are both witness and participant, both reflective surface and shaping presence. There is no analyst who is not already a contour in the patient's field of desire. And yet the nature of this contour cannot be predetermined. It is not defined solely by the analyst's history or technique, but by how their presence warps the intersubjective field in real time. A certain silence, a glance away, a leaning forward—each may register as containment or abandonment, holding or engulfment. The analyst's presence is felt before it is interpreted.

This is not to claim that every patient accurately interprets the analyst. Rather, it is to suggest that the analytic field is not made of interpretations, but of intensities. Before the transference becomes a story, it is a pressure. Before the symptom takes shape, it is a shimmer in the air. The analyst's presence—often unknowingly—sets the tone, modulates the tempo, and constellates the orbit of what can be spoken or felt. This presence is not just emotional; it is gravitational.

To work with this dimension of analytic presence requires a shift in our listening. We are no longer merely deciphering latent content; we are attuning to field curvature. The patient's speech may suddenly lose its vitality, or their associations may stall. A thick silence might arise—not because of resistance, but because the analyst's gravity has momentarily overwhelmed the symbolic field. A subtle dissociation may emerge, not from the patient's internal defense, but in response to the analyst's unconscious positioning. This is not failure; it is an invitation to attune.

Bion (1962) gestured toward this when he described the analyst as a container of unprocessed emotional experience. But containment is not neutral. The container has a shape, a density, and a texture. Sometimes it suffocates. Sometimes it leaks. Sometimes its mere presence changes what is being contained. The analyst's body, history, and desire—all enter the room, whether acknowledged or not. The question is not whether we influence the field, but how, and with what effects.

Consider David, a patient who had been in treatment for nearly a year before a shift occurred. Until then, he had described his inner world in intellectual terms—rich, abstract, but emotionally flattened. His symptoms were diffused across domains: work anxiety, sexual inhibition, and difficulty sustaining friendships. Yet in the session following a minor scheduling error—when I had momentarily forgotten to reschedule a holiday—he entered the room with a new texture. "You disappeared," he said plainly. "And I didn't know if you'd return."

It would have been easy to interpret the fantasy of abandonment, to link it to early relational ruptures. But something deeper was unfolding. I could feel it. The air had thickened. The room felt suddenly off-axis, as if time itself had buckled. My body felt heavier. I realized: he was experiencing my presence not as a neutral backdrop but as a massive object, one whose gravitational pull could either hold him or collapse his coherence entirely. My scheduling slip had not merely wounded him—it had unmoored the orbit that gave his psyche shape.

In this moment, I was no longer the analyst who interprets. I was the gravitational mass around which his psychic system tried to organize. My role was not to explain, but to regulate my gravity—to stay close without overwhelming, to be dense enough to be real, but not so dense as to eclipse him. I spoke softly, not out of caution, but to match the field's fragility. "You didn't know if I would return—and maybe that fear isn't new." He looked at me, not for validation, but to confirm I was still there. Still holding. Still exerting a gravity he could survive.

In such moments, countertransference becomes more than an affective reaction—it becomes field data. Not simply "how I feel," but how my gravity is registering in the space. I might feel bored, not because the patient is dull, but because they are flattening themselves to avoid collision with my perceived intensity. I might feel urgently needed, not because the patient is regressed, but because the field has constricted around my symbolic role as the only stable mass. These sensations are not errors; they are instruments.

To conceptualize the analyst's presence this way is to take seriously the analyst's body—not as a source of countertransference per se, but as a gravitational node. Our breathing, posture, and facial expressivity—all exert influence. So too do our unconscious identifications and transferential readiness. A queer analyst, for instance, may exert a different gravitational shape than a straight one—not merely in content, but in field curvature, in symbolic weight. A Black analyst in a white patient's fantasy may become charged with projection, idealization, or disavowal that warps the shared space. Presence is never generic. It is sculpted by history and desire.

At times, the analyst's gravity becomes too diffuse, too light. A patient might feel unheld, floating in a space with no structure. At other times, our gravity becomes too dense—so saturated with our own affect or theoretical rigidity that the field collapses into enactment. Neither is avoidable. The point is not to perfect our gravity, but to become aware of how it moves, how it shapes the field, and how it is used.

This is not about clinical perfection, but clinical presence. The analyst's gravity is not a flaw to be managed, but a phenomenon to be metabolized. What we carry into the room becomes the substance of analysis—not because we speak it, but because we live it. Our task is to listen for where the field bends, and to wonder what that bending makes possible—or impossible.

If the symptom is a gravitational trace, then the analyst's presence is a gravitational force. Not the only one, but a central one. We cannot escape this. But we can enter it with awareness—with humility for our density, with sensitivity to our pull, and with readiness to be shaped in return.

Saturated Objects and Analytic Mass

What saturates the analytic field is not always content—it is often the object. Not the real object, but the gravitational one: the saturated object of fantasy, memory, or loss, around which the psyche organizes its repetitions and longings. These saturated objects—parent, lover, sibling, child—may or may not resemble the analyst. But in the analytic field, they cling to us, attach to us, warp the field through us. The analyst becomes a placeholder for density that is not their own.

To say the analyst becomes a saturated object is not to accuse the patient of misrecognition. It is to recognize that the analytic encounter activates prior gravitational forces. These forces do not aim for clarity—they aim for contact. The patient's psyche seeks a mass dense enough to tether its affective drift. And the analyst, regardless of personal intention, becomes that mass. Our role is not to evade this saturation but to metabolize it, to feel it without becoming it.

A saturated object is not simply an internal object. It is more than representation. It is atmosphere. It presses on the present with the weight of the past. When a patient begins to fear we will abandon them, it is rarely a new fear. What makes the fear unbearable is not its novelty but its recurrence. The past charges the present, saturating the analyst with the unbearable density of what once was. Our misstep—real or imagined—becomes a reenactment. Our silence becomes a reactivation. Our benign gesture becomes a gravitational collapse.

In these moments, the analyst's task is neither to deny nor prematurely interpret the saturation. It is to hold it, to feel the thickness of time condensed into the now. Ogden (1994) called this the "analytic third"—the co-created space in which neither party fully owns the meaning. But even the third has a curvature. It bends. And when saturated objects enter this space, they distort it. The analyst becomes too important, too dangerous, too known. This is not pathology. This is gravity doing its work.

Consider Marlon, a man in his late 30s who came to treatment after a series of breakups that he could not make sense of. "They all say the same thing," he told me in our third session. "That I'm too intense. That I want too much." What emerged over time was not simply neediness, but an exquisite attunement to the emotional atmospheres of others—a gift that had once helped him survive an unstable mother and absent father, but now threatened to drown his partners in too much care.

He came to idealize me quickly. "You're the first person who hasn't turned away," he said once, after a session in which I had said very little. But in his eyes, I saw something more than relief—I saw saturation. I had become dense with meaning, with rescue, with symbolic mass that had little to do with me. I was the gravitational object around which his affect could orbit safely. And I felt it—in my chest, in the way I began preparing more carefully for his sessions, as though I had to become the person he imagined.

This is the analyst as saturated object: not merely countertransference, but the atmospheric buildup of symbolic pressure. In such moments, the patient's need for mass eclipses the analyst's ordinary presence. We become a node, a relic, a symbol in the patient's psychic architecture. The danger is not in being misrecognized—it is in becoming gravitationally overdetermined, so full of psychic density that there is no room for movement, play, or surprise.

Here, the concept of analytic mass becomes crucial. The analyst's mass is not just their countertransference, not just their past or their theory—it is their symbolic weight in the patient's world. Some analysts radiate this mass from the beginning: older, more experienced, differently gendered or raced from the patient, they enter the field already saturated with cultural or transferential meanings. Others acquire it slowly, as the work deepens. But in all cases, analytic mass is what allows gravity to hold—but also what risks pulling the field too tightly, freezing it in symbolic foreclosure.

Bollas (1992) spoke of "idiom needs"—the patient's longing not just for recognition, but for a certain quality of presence, a felt resonance that mirrors their internal aesthetic. When the analyst's idiom approximates that need, saturation occurs. The analyst becomes the object not just of desire, but of form. They are experienced as the one who fits—the one whose rhythm, cadence, or gaze makes psychic life briefly feel coherent. However, this fit can also become too heavy. It can compress the space, making the analyst less a partner in exploration than a gravitational anchor the patient clings to at the cost of motion.

In these moments, the analytic task is to remain pliable without becoming formless. To maintain presence without becoming totalizing. To metabolize saturation without evacuating the field. The analyst must remain a mass—but one that allows orbit, not collapse.

This often means speaking less, but sensing more. When the analyst is too full of interpretation, the field tightens. When we try too quickly to return the saturated object to the patient's own projection, we risk shattering the very gravity that makes interpretation possible. Sometimes the only way to lighten the mass is to stay steady within it—to let the saturation crest and pass, without either denying it or overidentifying with it.

The analytic use of self here becomes subtle, almost musical. One alters the rhythm, the breath, the facial attunement. One becomes slightly more or slightly less—slightly closer or slightly more abstract. These are not "interventions" in the traditional sense. They are micro-calibrations of mass. They shape the patient's experience of symbolic space—how much room there is to feel, to imagine, to remember.

This attunement also requires the analyst to track their own saturation. When we become too heavy—too filled with our own affect, or too collapsed into the patient's gravitational field—we lose dimensionality. We stop moving. We become the symptom. At such moments, self-reflection is not optional—it is ethical. The analyst must sense their own gravitational shape: when they are being used, when they are being inflated, when they are distorting the field by holding too much or offering too little.

In short, analytic mass is not static. It fluctuates with the field. And like gravity itself, it operates invisibly, silently, until something bends too far. Then we feel it: the symptom emerges, the session derails, the countertransference intensifies. These are not failures. They are signs that mass must be recalibrated.

To work in this way is to abandon the myth of the neutral observer and embrace the analyst as gravitational participant. It is to recognize that the psyche does not seek understanding alone—it seeks mass. It seeks an object dense enough to bend time, to hold contradiction, to allow orbit. And when we become that object—saturated, symbolic, strange—we do not fail our patients. We become the terrain in which their meaning begins to move.

Countertransference as Gravitational Resistance

To speak of gravity is to speak also of resistance. Every gravitational pull exerts force upon the object, but the object also exerts force in return. The analytic field is no different. If the patient's transference saturates the analyst with meaning, the analyst's countertransference exerts its own resistance—not always against the patient, but against being made into something. Against becoming too meaningful. Against collapse into the symbolic overdetermination that gravity threatens to produce.

Resistance, then, is not only the patient's. It is the analyst's too. And it is not always defensive. Sometimes it is structural. It arises when the analyst, saturated by the weight of the patient's projections, begins to feel the unbearable burden of becoming too central, too known, too necessary. In this state, countertransference may manifest as retreat, fatigue, or distraction. But beneath these symptoms lies a subtler phenomenon: gravitational resistance. A psychic recoil from overidentification. A refusal of collapse.

Freud (1912) warned that the analyst must strive for "evenly suspended attention"—a receptive openness unmarred by theoretical anticipation or emotional distortion. But in practice, no attention is ever fully suspended. What we call neutrality is often a negotiation with saturation. When the analyst feels too pulled, too laden, they may seek to lighten the load—not by disengaging, but by resisting absorption. This resistance is not disinterest. It is self-preservation within the field.

There is an ethics to this resistance. To notice one's countertransference—to feel the pull and not collapse into it—is to retain dimensionality. It is to protect the analytic space from becoming a black hole of projection. In Klein's (1952) terms, when the analyst becomes the container for unbearable states, they risk being used not just as receptacle, but as site of annihilation. The patient unconsciously tests whether the analyst can hold the projection without retaliating or evacuating. But the analyst must also test their own limits—how much saturation can be borne before the field begins to distort.

In this way, countertransference becomes gravitational feedback. It reveals where meaning has pooled, where time has condensed, where fantasy has overcoated the real. A sudden exhaustion in the analyst may indicate a symbolic weight too heavy to metabolize. An irritation, seemingly unjustified, may signal that the patient has placed them in a role they cannot sustain. These are not errors in technique. They are affective diagnostics. They map the terrain of gravity.

I recall a patient, Alice, who came each week with exquisite attention to detail. Her speech was measured, polished, filled with literary allusion and philosophical flourish. I found myself admiring her intellect—and yet, by the end of each session, I felt depleted. Not bored, but emptied. It was as if I had been cast in a role I could not quite locate, one in which my presence was simultaneously revered and erased. Only later did I realize: she was not speaking to me. She was speaking through me—to a father long dead, to a series of teachers who had failed her, to the image of the analyst she needed me to embody.

My depletion was not counter to the work. It was the work. It marked the moment at which her saturation of me began to erode my ability to remain responsive. In trying to become the ideal listener, I had become a symbolic vessel—her ghosted audience, her gravitational backdrop. My resistance, when it emerged, took the form of subtle frustration. I began to interrupt more, to push her into less curated terrain. I felt guilty—was I disrupting her process? But something else was happening. I was resisting not her, but the collapse of our field into a static loop. My countertransference became the hinge through which the analytic dyad could pivot toward renewal.

Ogden (1997b) described such moments as transitional spaces in which the analyst participates in the patient's internal world without being consumed by it. But this requires resistance—not as rejection, but as presence. A gravitational resistance that asserts the analyst's own psychic mass, their own rhythm, their own opacity. Without it, the analyst becomes a screen. And the field begins to flatten.

This kind of resistance is also aesthetic. It marks the refusal of the analyst to become a perfect fit. A refusal to match the patient's symbolic idiom too completely. Loewald (1960) reminds us that transformation requires difference—that psychic growth depends on the presence of an other who is not fully assimilable. To resist full saturation is to retain alterity. It is to preserve the analytic space as a site of surprise.

This resistance can also manifest in silence—not the silence of disconnection, but of gravitational delay. A refusal to speak too soon, to interpret too cleanly, to resolve the transferential mass before it has ripened. The analyst pauses—not because they have nothing to say, but because the field has not yet metabolized its own saturation. This is a resistance to premature coherence. A resistance that protects the symbolic complexity of the encounter.

At times, this resistance feels like betrayal. The patient may feel us pulling away, becoming opaque, unintelligible. They may accuse us of abandonment. But if the analyst can stay within that resistance—own it, hold it, metabolize it—something changes. The patient encounters a presence that is not organized by their need. A presence that resists being folded entirely into their field. And in this resistance, a new form of recognition becomes possible: not mirroring, but mutual gravity.

This mutuality is not symmetry. The analyst still holds the frame. But within the gravitational field, both parties exert and feel force. Both are shaped and reshaped. The analyst's resistance becomes not a rupture, but a contour. A way of maintaining the field's curvature without collapsing into its center. It is through this resistance that the analytic space becomes a space of possibility—not because it is frictionless, but because it contains the tension of holding and not holding, knowing and not knowing, being and resisting being.

In this sense, countertransference resistance is not a flaw in the work—it is its gravity rendered visible. It is the analyst's way of insisting on their own mass, their own shape, their own orbit. And it is precisely this insistence that allows the patient to experience the other as real—not just a projection, but a presence.

In the gravitational field of the analytic relationship, resistance becomes a kind of dance. The analyst does not merely receive the patient's orbit. They push back, pull subtly, reshape the rhythm of return. Not to deny the pull, but to prevent collapse. Not to avoid saturation, but to transform it into symbolic motion. This is the analyst's gravity: not stillness, but counterforce. Not neutrality, but form.

Gravity, Reverie, and Symbolic Return

If countertransference resistance is the analyst's way of resisting collapse, then reverie is their way of re-entering the field with symbolic responsiveness. Reverie is not simply daydream or distraction—it is a form of aesthetic listening. It is the analyst's unconscious dreaming the session forward. As Bion (1962) suggested, reverie metabolizes unprocessed affect, filtering it through the analyst's internal world and re-presenting it in a symbolizable form. It is the countermovement to saturation: not resistance by rejection, but resistance by transmutation.

Gravity pulls the analyst inward. Reverie turns that pull into form.

The analyst in reverie does not float above the field, but sinks into it. Not to lose themselves, but to find an image, a sensation, a metaphor that can symbolize what is otherwise unformulated. This process is not always immediate. Reverie unfolds over time. It is recursive, circling. A dream that gathers gravity and returns, days later, as a sentence, a gesture, a presence newly inflected with symbolic charge.

When the analyst allows their reverie to emerge in the room, it often appears obliquely. An image flashes in mind: a flickering candle, a weightless astronaut, a child watching rain on a windowpane. These are not interpretations. They are atmospheric responses to the saturation of the field. They bear the quality of truth without yet being true. They are fragments of coherence suspended in affective mist.

Ogden (2005) emphasized the importance of "the analytic third," a shared intersubjective matrix that neither belongs solely to patient nor analyst but arises between them. Reverie is the analyst's means of listening to this third. It allows the analyst to feel not only what the patient feels, but what the field itself is trying to symbolize. This kind of listening is aesthetic, affective, and nonlinear. It is the analyst's gravitational intuition.

Reverie can also surface through the body. The analyst may feel suddenly heavy, light, hollow, pressured. These somatic shifts are not distractions from interpretation—they are pre-symbolic materials of the analytic process. They are the psyche's early attempts at forming meaning. When such sensations are honored—not pathologized—the analyst becomes a vessel for transmuting gravitational pull into symbolic shape.

Consider a session in which I found myself drifting. The patient, a young man named Eli, was speaking in a flat tone about a breakup that seemed to carry no emotional weight. As he described the final argument, I noticed an image arise: a glass vase falling in slow motion, shattering on tile. There had been no mention of such an object, no sensory context for it. Yet the image shimmered with symbolic precision. I did not share it. But I allowed it to contour my listening. I felt into the slowness of the shattering, the mute inevitability, the elegance of fracture. In the next moment, Eli paused and said, "I don't know why, but I can't stop imagining the way his face looked—like something precious had just been ruined."

This was not interpretation by suggestion. It was shared gravity. The reverie helped me wait. It attuned me to the symbolic field. And in that attunement, the patient could find his own metaphor, his own language for loss. Reverie, in this sense, is not the analyst's fantasy imposed, but the analytic atmosphere vibrating with symbolic potential.

Loewald (1960) described psychoanalysis as a space where time and meaning become reconfigured. Reverie participates in this reconfiguration. It loops the present with echoes of the past, gathers unsymbolized residue, and returns it as shimmer. When the analyst allows themselves to be moved—not only cognitively, but atmospherically—they become an instrument of symbolic return. They allow the session to bend toward coherence, not through explanation, but through resonance.

This is not always easy. Reverie can feel intrusive or embarrassing. It does not always match the analytic tone. It may feel too poetic, too strange. But this strangeness is often its signal. Reverie speaks in the syntax of the unformulated. It requires a kind of faith—not in its literal accuracy, but in its affective truth. The analyst must be willing to be moved by what they do not yet understand.

Such movement is the analyst's gravitational offering. If the patient's transference draws the field inward, the analyst's reverie curves it outward—toward symbol, toward recognition, toward meaning. Reverie is how the analyst reclaims dimensionality without breaking the field. It is their form of symbolic return.

But reverie is not interpretation. Interpretation is linear, linguistic, and often anchored in theory. Reverie is curved, nonlinear, and arrives through image, sensation, and tone. Its role is not to explain, but to shape the symbolic atmosphere in which explanation might eventually emerge. It prepares the soil. It offers psychic temperature and texture.

And when interpretation does arise from reverie, it carries a different quality. It lands not as explanation but as recognition. A wordless "yes." A resonance between symbolic form and affective truth. In these moments, the analytic space feels lit from within. Something invisible has been named—not because it was deciphered, but because it was felt, shaped, and returned.

This return is gravitational. It bends back through earlier psychic time. It echoes the field's unsymbolized fragments, stitching them into form. Reverie, in this sense, is not private. It is field-emergent. It belongs to the analytic third, to the atmosphere shaped by both minds in mutual curvature. The analyst does not own their reverie. They receive it.

Reverie can also be mistaken. Not every image is meaningful. Not every sensation is symbolic. The analyst must remain humble before the shimmer. They must not seize it as revelation, but hold it loosely. Reverie is not about being right—it is about staying close. Close to the field, to the saturation, to the aesthetic of the symptom, to the rhythmic unfoldings of transference. It is not a shortcut to understanding. It is the shape that waiting takes.

Through reverie, the analyst offers not only containment, but style. A way of being with the patient that is not diagnostic, but aesthetic. This is the beginning of symbolic return. Not the return to origin, but the return of form. The symptom, once a saturated object, begins to breathe. The field, once thick with gravity, begins to shimmer. The analytic space becomes habitable again. Not through insight, but through re-symbolization.

This is the analyst's gift: to remain gravitationally close, while metabolizing the pull. To dream with the patient. To suffer the atmosphere of saturation. And to wait—patiently, poetically—for the moment when the field begins to turn. That turn is not a breakthrough. It is a bend in gravity. It is the moment when the symptom, the projection, the silence, the disavowal—all of it— begins to find its curve again.

And in that curve, something returns. Not the self as it was, but the self as it can be lived again.

Clinical Vignette—The Curved Mirror

He came to me after several failed therapies, each of which, he said, left him "feeling more performed than seen." I will call him David. In his mid-forties, intellectually gifted, sexually ambivalent, and professionally successful, David exuded precision. His tone was clipped, his language exacting. He told me in our first session that he had "little tolerance for platitudes" and wanted an analyst "who understood the cost of thinking." I felt immediately the seduction and the challenge. To be chosen was flattering. But to be used as a mirror without distortion—this was the deeper demand.

From the outset, David's presence generated an atmosphere of saturation. Not through overt emotion, but through intensity of control. His speech was rhythmic, punctuated by well-timed pauses that created the illusion of space without actually yielding it. He often referred to himself in metaphor—"I've become a hall of mirrors," he once said—but seemed resistant to mine. Interpretation, when offered, was met with subtle critique: "That's interesting, but perhaps a bit reductive."

My early countertransference oscillated between admiration and inadequacy. I found myself rehearsing phrases before speaking, trimming my speech to match his tempo. I was drawn into his gravity. My reverie during those first months was flooded with images of mirrors and glass: a kaleidoscope spinning, a pane of glass fogging from within, a mirror cracked but not shattered. I began to feel that my presence was being used not for reflection, but for distortion calibration. David did not want to see himself; he wanted to see whether I could see the image he already held.

In this gravitational field, time felt warped. Sessions elongated. Each moment carried more symbolic pressure than it could hold. I began to dread our meetings—not because of any overt hostility, but because I felt increasingly faceless. Yet I could not turn away. There was something in David's gaze—level, unflinching—that pulled me deeper. I sensed that what saturated the field was not grandiosity, but terror. His precision was scaffolding.

The first rupture came during a session in which I arrived late by two minutes due to an emergency. David said nothing at first. But as the session unfolded, I noticed a shift. His voice lost its modulation. He spoke of feeling "smeared," as if his shape had been rubbed out. "I've spent my whole life trying to become a fixed form," he said, "and when you were late, it felt like you erased the outline." He looked down. "I know that sounds absurd."

It didn't sound absurd. It sounded exact. His symptom—relational saturation through aesthetic control—was breaking. In that moment, I did not interpret. I allowed myself to feel what the field offered: a sudden tenderness. A grief beneath the mirror. "What got erased?" I asked softly. He looked up, surprised, as if I had stepped out of his projection for the first time.

Over the next several months, the field began to shift. My reverie changed. The mirrors began to reflect not only distortion, but longing. I found myself dreaming of David, not as a figure of critique, but as a child building a house of cards, trembling at the thought of collapse. These dreams were not content to analyze. They were invitations to attune.

One morning, after a particularly charged session in which David described an erotic encounter he had orchestrated with surgical control, I awoke with the image of a glass figurine melting under sunlight—beautiful, uncontainable. I brought this image into my body during the next session. I did not speak it, but let it shape my presence. When David recounted another encounter, I found myself leaning slightly forward, breath slowed, body open. He paused. "You're different today," he said. "You're not afraid of how much I'm controlling things."

I wasn't. Something in the atmosphere had changed. Reverie had become countertransference metabolized. I was no longer inside the saturation field; I was curving its gravity. Slowly, David's language began to loosen. He began to speak not just in polished metaphor, but in fragments. He once said, "It's like—I don't know—it's like I've been freezing time, and you're… breathing into it."

The most pivotal moment came during a session in which David recounted a dream: he was standing in front of a mirror, but his reflection was delayed by several seconds. When he moved, the reflection hesitated, then caught up. "It scared me," he said. "I thought I was losing my mind. But then I realized—I've never really seen myself move before. Only pose."

We sat in silence. It was a silence not of absence, but of symbolic return. Reverie flooded me with the sensation of water rippling across glass. I said only, "Maybe the delay was the first sign of something alive." He nodded, and tears welled—his first in the treatment.

After that session, something began to unfold. David's symptoms—rigid control, erotic distance, perfectionistic pressure—did not vanish. But their aesthetic grip softened. He began to experiment with spontaneity, to allow himself to "blur at the edges," as he once put it. And I found that my own speech no longer required rehearsal. I could enter the field with curiosity, not dread.

The arc of our work had curved. Saturation gave way to shimmer. The gravitational field had held us both—until we could bend it.

What David taught me was that symbolic return does not happen through interpretation alone. It happens through atmospheric fidelity, through allowing the analytic field to gather, saturate, pressurize, and then—sometimes—release. Reverie was the hinge. Countertransference was the gravity. But it was the curved third—the analytic atmosphere itself—that transformed what was once compulsive repetition into living relation.

The final sessions were marked not by insight but by inflection. David said, "You didn't fix me. But you mirrored me until I became visible." He paused. "Not the image I thought I was. The one behind the glass."

Closing Reflection—Field Gravity and the Ethics of Saturation

The analytic field is not a neutral stage upon which transference plays out—it is a gravitational terrain. Its curvature arises not only from the patient's history or the analyst's subjectivity, but from the aesthetic and affective density of what forms between them. The field saturates, not by accident, but by necessity. It condenses meaning. It thickens time. It shapes how both participants move, speak, and perceive. And it carries an ethical imperative: to feel with fidelity, not prematurely interpret, the weight of what has gathered.

When saturation becomes overwhelming, the temptation is to decode—to reduce the field to understandable terms, to name and thereby dissolve its pressure. But interpretation, when offered too early, can flatten the field's curvature. It can fracture a symbolic emergence still in formation. The deeper work involves symbolic pacing and waiting for the field to reveal its own syntax.

Ogden (1994) wrote of the analytic third as a co-created psychological space, one that allows for the intersubjective emergence of meaning. But this third is not always a space of freedom. At times, it is a dense loop—a recursive atmosphere of unformulated experience. It presses upon both analyst and patient not only with content, but with force. Saturation is not just an aesthetic; it is a gravitational phenomenon. And to work within it is to tolerate the opacity of its orbit.

The field, then, becomes a mirror not of images, but of tensions. What presses most intensely—be it dissociation, idealization, eroticization, withdrawal—is often what carries the most symbolic potential. These are not merely defenses; they are gravitational anchors. They hold the analytic situation near what has not yet been metabolized. To feel this without collapse requires a different kind of containment: one that is not bound by content, but by resonance.

Ethically, this demands a different stance from the analyst. Not neutrality in the classical sense, but saturation-sensitivity. A capacity to feel the pull of enactment without immediately resolving it. A willingness to become disoriented, to allow reverie to carry fragments of what cannot yet be said. The analyst becomes not the interpreter of experience, but its atmospheric co-witness—one who bends with the field, not above it.

This gravitational ethics draws upon Loewald's (1960) idea that the analyst serves as a future object—not because they remain distant, but because they help the patient organize time. In saturated fields, time often loops or collapses. The analyst's task is to hold the symbolic frame long enough for time to stretch, bend, and rearticulate. Gravity, in this sense, is a medium of transformation. It slows interpretation so that meaning can accrue. It marks the difference between analysis as decoding and analysis as listening into the saturation of form.

There is danger, too. Saturation can become enactment. The analyst may be pulled so deeply into the patient's psychic gravity that their own symbolic coordinates distort. The ethics of saturation, then, requires not just attunement, but calibration. It requires analytic supervision, inner honesty, and the courage to re-enter the field each time with renewed openness. The point is not to escape gravity, but to metabolize its pressure into form.

This process—of attunement, saturation, and symbolic return—is never linear. It circles. And each return is shaped by the field's own temporality. Transference is not a static projection. It is a field event. A contour of memory and desire that warps the symbolic space until new experience becomes possible. In this light, the analyst does not "interpret transference" so much as inhabit its curvature—so that interpretation, when it finally arrives, resonates with fidelity.

The most powerful interpretations, then, are not explanatory. They are aesthetic. They emerge not from outside the field, but from within its shimmer. They carry the rhythm, cadence, and emotional saturation of what the patient already knows, but could not yet speak. These interpretations are not answers; they are acts of symbolic recognition. They mark the moment when the gravitational field begins to bend—toward language, toward time, toward meaning.

At its deepest, the analyst's gravity is not a force of understanding, but of presence. A sustained, embodied attention that allows the field to hold more than either participant could hold alone. In this way, the field becomes both container and horizon: it holds what is unbearable, and it gestures toward what is not yet formed. It curves meaning around absence. And in doing so, it makes the unthought known—not by revealing it directly, but by allowing its gravity to be felt.

As the patient emerges from this orbit—looping back, circling again—they may come to experience the symptom, the fantasy, the repetition not as pathology, but as the shimmer of the field itself. What was saturated becomes symbolic. What was gravitational becomes generative. The analyst, by staying near the curved edge, becomes the witness not only to history but to transformation.

To hold this is the analyst's ethical task. To remain in the field, when it thickens. To bend with its time. To allow saturation to speak—through silence, through dream, through reverie. And to know that gravity, when attended to with symbolic care, is not the end of freedom, but its precondition.

Part III

Recursion and Return—Time Looped and Folded

From Drive to Pattern

Time becomes nonlinear, looping back upon itself in recursive self-touch. Repetition is no longer only drive repetition—it becomes aesthetic, mythic, and symbolic. The symptom, the dream, and the defensive system alike are shown to fold time, warping temporality as a defense against contact. Freud's idea of Nachträglichkeit and Klein's layering of part-objects find new form here: repetition as atmosphere, and return as recursive memory.

Freud's discovery of repetition compulsion destabilized the pleasure principle, revealing a structural return to trauma beyond mastery. Klein added the internal looping of dread, guilt, and persecutory part-objects—**an inner orbit of psychic fragentation**. This part reframes those insights as **gravitational recursion**: the psyche's spiral return to what cannot be symbolized. Here, looping is not merely defensive but architectural—a way of holding unspeakable experience through repetition, collapse, and condensation. These chapters explore aesthetic shimmer, recursive style, and symbolic implosion not as pathology, but as fidelity to a truth that must be approached indirectly. Return is not regression—it is form.

DOI: 10.4324/9781003715306-9

6 Echoes and Foldings
Repetition Compulsion and Recursive Return

This chapter reconceptualizes repetition compulsion as a recursive structure rather than a mere behavioral reenactment, arguing that its essence lies in temporal distortion rather than narrative return. Drawing from Freud's death drive, Laplanche's enigmatic signifier, and Winnicott's theory of potential space, repetition is reframed as a looping defense that both resists and seeks contact. The psyche does not simply repeat past trauma; it folds time inward, creating symbolic atmospheres where echoes replace events. A new concept—*recursive defense*—is introduced to describe how patients loop against the threat of relational immediacy. Transference and countertransference are explored as co-participatory echoes, shaped by prior analytic encounters and reverberating within the analytic field. Clinical material illustrates how transformation often occurs not by ending the loop, but by shifting its rhythm, enabling resonance to replace rupture.

The Drive That Loops

What if repetition is not a failure of insight but the residue of a loop too gravitational to escape? In analytic work, repetition compulsion often announces itself not with narrative urgency but with atmospheric familiarity—an echo that bends the analytic field, shaping even the analyst's breath or timing of speech. This is not simply the return of the repressed, nor the passive yield to past trauma, but the recursive trace of something that *wants to be seen by returning*. A behavior, a gesture, a psychic rhythm—each circling its own singularity, folding time around the ache of non-symbolized experience.

To enter this chapter is to step into the **gravitational curvature** of recursive psychic life. We are no longer tracing trauma's effects forward but watching how time itself bends backward, how a moment becomes saturated not with new content but with intensifying resemblance. The patient finds themselves "back here again"—not because the situation is the same, but because something unformulated keeps reforming the field. These loops may not ask for resolution. They may not even want to be known. But they demand **return**, and in that demand, they make meaning.

DOI: 10.4324/9781003715306-10

Freud introduced the idea of repetition compulsion in *Beyond the Pleasure Principle* (1920), framing it as the organism's baffling tendency to re-experience pain without adaptive benefit. But this initial formulation, haunted by Freud's own grief, opened more than it resolved. The analytic field has since reimagined repetition as not only a product of trauma but also a symbolic act—a structuring principle. What returns may not be the event itself, but its gravitational imprint, a kind of psychic orbit: elliptical, incomplete, and curving under the weight of that which was never metabolized.

This return is not the same as fixation. Fixation implies a stuckness, a halt. But the psyche in repetition is moving—just not linearly. It is looping, curling, and folding. In earlier chapters, we imagined the self as structured not by lines but by curvatures—topologies of affect, time, and symbol. Here we encounter that structure not as abstract model but as **temporal experience**: repetition as the lived sensation of time curling back on itself. A trauma does not just linger; it organizes. An atmosphere does not just recur; it thickens.

In this sense, repetition is not a failure of the psyche but a **logic of recognition**. It is the psyche's recursive syntax. Like a fractal pattern in nature, the repetition doesn't duplicate—it echoes with difference. Each pass contains a fold, each fold a slight mutation. The psyche returns not to *be* the same, but to *touch* what remains unfinished through the rhythm of return.

The analyst, too, is drawn into this recursive field. Countertransference often follows the same looping logic: the analyst says something familiar, reacts in a rhythm they've felt before, and wonders why they feel "caught." These are not errors of neutrality—they are moments where the gravitational pull of the loop saturates both poles of the dyad. The repetition becomes mutual: a choreography of return, where both participants risk becoming echoes of an unformulated third.

From this perspective, repetition is not a symptom to eliminate but a **field to witness**. The compulsion reveals the topology of the patient's psychic structure—not just their history but their mode of symbolic organization. The orbit holds clues. The loop expresses desire—not for change, necessarily, but for coherence.

And what of the singularity? In physics, a singularity is a point of infinite density, where spacetime curves infinitely and known laws collapse. In psychic life, the singularity is the place where symbolic form fails—the moment too early, too intense, too fragmented to be borne. Repetition then becomes the psychic strategy to organize life around the singularity, as if orbiting a black hole: pulled inward, circling endlessly, never fully touching the core. But in the analytic frame, we do not aim to reach the singularity. We learn to **stay in orbit**, to witness the loop, to feel how the gravitational pull of repetition shapes psychic space.

This chapter does not promise to undo repetition. Rather, it proposes a way to think of repetition as **structure**, not just history. It introduces recursion as a mode of temporality that is neither linear nor regressive, but **folded**—a symbolizing process in time. This sets the stage for the next movement of the book: how repetition thickens into *symbolic atmosphere*, into what we will later call the *holographic mind*. But first, we must dwell in the loop.

To do so is not to get lost, but to begin seeing the **loop as light**—refracted, not broken.

Folding Time: Trauma, Curvature, and Compulsion

Time, in the analytic encounter, is never a straight line. It does not proceed from past to present to future, but bends inward and outward, curls around absence, and stretches through affect. Trauma distorts time not because it makes the past feel present, but because it folds the linear progression of psychic life into recursive intensities that collapse the boundary between *when* and *where*. The repetition compulsion is the symptom of that curvature: not a return to the past, but a transformation of time into a spiral. The patient's present becomes a resonance chamber for psychic events that never finished happening.

This is the paradox of trauma: what is too much to symbolize becomes the anchor of structure. What cannot be metabolized begins to organize the field. The psyche, rather than resolving the trauma, rotates around it. Psychic development folds in response to the pressure of the unspeakable. What Freud framed as the return of the repressed, we might now reframe as a **recursion around the unformulated**—a turning and returning, not to the same, but to what remains outside symbolization.

The analytic field, when entered fully, reveals this structure of **temporal looping**. The patient may repeat dynamics, but they also repeat rhythms: durations of silence, tonalities of voice, gaps between emotional contact. These are not just behaviors—they are time-signatures. Repetition compulsion is not merely thematic; it is **temporal choreography**. It choreographs the relational timing of withdrawal, aggression, submission, and longing. One cannot understand repetition without feeling the shape of time it creates in the room.

This folding of time disturbs both the analyst's and the patient's sense of narrative. The patient might say, "This always happens," or "It's happening again," but what they mean is not that the same thing is repeating, but that the same **temporal structure** is being re-entered. It is a *when* disguised as a *what*. "Again" is not just recurrence—it is the experience of the loop folding inward, tightening the symbolic spiral. Affect precedes cognition. Rhythm precedes content. The body registers the fold before the mind can name it.

This insight finds resonance in thinkers like Donnel Stern (1997), who emphasizes the **unformulated experience** as the unconscious that has never been symbolized, and Thomas Ogden (2005), who distinguishes between lived temporality and the analyst's capacity to "dream" the patient's experience into narrative form. In the recursive register, the analyst is not interpreting the past but witnessing the collapse of temporal order. To witness repetition is to *inhabit time differently*—to be with the patient not in narrative sequence, but in rhythmic re-entry.

The role of countertransference here is not diagnostic but temporal. The analyst may feel as if they've "been here before"—not just in content, but in **timing**, in a rhythm of approach and withdrawal that organizes the dyad. These experiences are not incidental. They are the field's recursive demand for holding. It is not just the patient who repeats—it is the **field** itself that curves, echoing prior intensities as if tracing invisible folds in symbolic space.

This recursive temporality also suggests a reframing of psychic defense. Rather than seeing defense as a linear blockage—an obstacle between past and present—we might see it as a **modulator of curvature**. Defenses don't halt time; they shape its folds. Denial, dissociation, projection—each serves to bend the experience of time around unbearable intensity. A dissociated moment is not simply repressed—it is **looped out of linear time**, existing in the psyche like a satellite, orbiting outside conscious narrative but influencing affective gravity. We do not simply "return" to the scene; the scene has always been curving our relation to the present.

Repetition compulsion, then, is the gravitational expression of a temporal fold. It insists not because it is unresolved, but because its logic is structural. It is not just that trauma happened—it continues to happen in folded time. The patient does not *remember*—they *recur*. This is why repetition feels unchosen. It is not a decision; it is a topology. And this is why traditional interpretations often fail: they aim to explain what must instead be **held within the recursive tension of non-resolution**.

In moments of analytic breakthrough, the recursion doesn't necessarily stop. What shifts is the **texture of return**. When the loop is held symbolically—when the analyst bears the collapse of time without enforcing premature meaning—the patient begins to experience the fold as witnessable. This does not dissolve the loop, but transforms it into a **recursive container**—a temporal holding environment where symbolic meaning can begin to constellate. Repetition becomes symbolization in slow motion.

At this point, the field prepares for aesthetic saturation. The recursion, held long enough, begins to thicken into atmosphere. This atmosphere is not empty—it is saturated with affect, tone, and symbolic potential. We approach here the horizon of the *holographic mind*—where memory, sensation, and unformulated affect condense into **symbolic fields**. But we are not there yet. In this chapter, we remain inside the loop—not to escape it, but to feel how deeply it bends the space around us.

To feel repetition not as enemy but as atmosphere—this is the analyst's task. It is not heroic. It is gravitational. And the loop, when fully felt, is not a trap but a fold of time waiting to be held.

Recursive Defenses: Looping against Contact

If we accept that repetition compulsion expresses a folded temporality—a gravitational loop around what cannot be symbolized—then we must ask how the psyche defends against contact with the loop's core. Traditional accounts frame defenses as guarding against drives, affect, or forbidden content. But what if defenses also operate as recursive circuits—structures that protect against the *contact itself*, against the psychic collapse that might occur if the loop were touched too directly?

In this view, defenses are not static blockades but **looping mechanisms** that perpetuate rhythm. The defense does not merely push material out of awareness—it *structures recurrence*, giving the psyche a tolerable rhythm within which to dance around the unbearable. Projection, for instance, does not simply expel disowned affect; it sets up a **recursive field**, a loop in which the self confronts the rejected aspect again and again in the external other. Splitting, similarly, is not just a dualistic organization of experience—it is a way to **loop around ambivalence**, to stabilize an unmanageable oscillation by rendering it into separate symbolic poles.

These defenses, in the recursive register, are not failures of development. They are expressions of **creative necessity**. When primary trauma or overwhelming affect disorganizes the symbolic field, the psyche must build rhythmic structures to survive. Recursive defenses are one such architecture. They do not resolve the trauma, but they allow psychic life to curve around it without disintegration. They grant coherence, albeit at the cost of contact.

But this cost is significant. Recursive defenses protect by repeating—not merely actions or beliefs, but **modes of relating**. Patients who reenact the same relational failures may be defending less against loss than against the *disruption of the loop itself*. A new kind of contact—authentic, unpredictable, intimate—would represent a rupture in the closed circuit. It would bring the psyche too close to the **singularity**: the moment, the feeling, the image that remains too dense to symbolically metabolize.

In clinical terms, these defenses often show up not as resistance to interpretation but as **resistance to change in the relational rhythm**. The analyst may feel unable to alter the timing of sessions, the tone of engagement, or the pattern of discourse. Attempts to do so provoke anxiety or rupture. This is not mere transference resistance—it is the patient's recursive structure pushing back against what would unwind the loop. Recursive defenses are not protecting content. They are protecting *timing*.

The analyst's challenge is not to dismantle the defense, but to **join the rhythm without becoming entrained by it**. This demands what Loewald might call "holding through symbolization" (Loewald, 1978e): the capacity to let the patient's recursive structure unfold without imposing premature coherence, while gradually opening space for a different temporal structure. The analyst does not break the loop by force but **enfolds it within a broader rhythmic holding**. This is a delicate art: too much interpretive pressure, and the loop constricts; too little, and the loop remains airtight.

Recursive defenses also reveal themselves in countertransference. The analyst may begin to feel stuck, dull, robotic—experiencing their own responses as rehearsed, not chosen. This may indicate the analyst is inside the loop, participating in the recursive rhythm rather than witnessing it. Here, supervision and reverie become essential: not to escape the loop, but to **symbolize the analyst's position within it**. Recursive defenses are never one-sided. They organize the field.

One vivid clinical example comes from a patient who responded to every moment of vulnerability with a joke—not a disarming defense, but a precisely timed interruption. These jokes followed a recursive structure: predictable in their rhythm, uncanny in their timing, and deeply disorganizing to the analytic process. The analyst eventually recognized that the humor was not spontaneous—it was *entrained*. It served as a recursive closure, protecting the patient from the singularity of affect that arose when silence stretched a beat too long. The defense was not against the content of the work, but against the *rhythmic possibility of new contact*.

Understanding defenses as recursive loops also reframes our work with repetition. The patient is not repeating because they haven't "learned" or "worked through" something—they are repeating because the structure itself defends against contact. Repetition *is* the defense. The loop is the armoring. It offers continuity in the face of fragmentation. And so our task is not to dismantle the loop, but to become a **witness to its curvature**—to see how it folds experience, limits contact, and organizes time.

This recursive frame resonates with Daniel Stern's work on affective attunement (Stern, 1985), in which developmental contact occurs through shared rhythms, not just shared meanings. When those rhythms fail—through misattunement, trauma, or absence—the psyche builds compensatory loops. Recursive defenses are the aftershocks of disrupted relational rhythm, echoing into adulthood as a choreography of avoidance.

And yet, these defenses also preserve possibility. The loop, even as it defends, keeps the singularity in play. It orbits what cannot be faced directly, preserving it within psychic reach. In this sense, recursive defenses are a paradox: they both obscure and maintain the core truth of the self. The analyst's task is not to penetrate them, but to honor their structure, their rhythm, their necessity—until the loop itself softens enough to allow contact.

The next section will take this idea further, exploring how recursive loops and symbolic density converge in what we are calling **symbolic atmosphere**: the felt texture of psychic space when looping and condensation have saturated the field. Before the holographic, there is the saturated. Before the breakthrough, there is the holding of the loop.

Saturated Atmosphere: From Loop to Field

As the recursive loop thickens through time, its affective intensity begins to fill the analytic space—not only as repetition, but as **atmosphere**. This is not merely a mood or transference phenomenon. It is a symbolic density: a felt field in which the patient's psyche begins to project, condense, and reverberate the unsymbolized in increasingly complex ways. We enter here a different register—not one of content or behavior, but of **psychic saturation**. The analytic room feels charged, as though meaning were about to constellate without quite arriving. The field becomes pregnant with the *not-yet-symbolized*.

This atmospheric density is what heralds the shift from the loop to the **holographic**. As looping becomes recursive enough, and as the analyst resists the pressure to resolve prematurely, condensation begins to replace repetition. In classical psychoanalysis, condensation is understood as a compression of latent meaning into manifest form—an overdetermination. Here, it functions as **symbolic atmosphere**, a cloud of meanings held in potential, not yet crystallized. The patient may not narrate anything new, but their affect may deepen, their pauses lengthen, and their dreams thicken with archetypal imagery. Something is happening—*in the air*.

Michael Eigen (2004) writes evocatively of this psychic density as a "saturation of being," a condition in which the analyst and patient are immersed in a shared field that cannot yet be understood but must be *endured*. Eigen's saturation is not overload but richness—a sense that the psyche is working at the edge of symbolization, trembling in the presence of meanings that have not yet found form. It is an **aesthetic experience**, as much as an interpretive one.

The analyst, in these moments, must attune to the **tone of the field** rather than the content. The usual tools—interpretation, linking, re-narration—may not suffice. What is required is **presence-as-instrument**, the use of the analyst's own attunement to symbolically metabolize the recursive field. This often means tolerating ambiguity, opacity, and even paralysis. The analyst may feel suspended, not knowing what to say—not because they are lost, but because the symbolic field is *too full*, and anything said too soon would puncture the symbolic membrane still forming.

This phase often coincides with what Bollas (1987) called the *unthought known*—experiences that are psychically registered but never articulated. The recursive field allows the unthought known to surface *as mood, as atmosphere, as style*. The patient may not "say" the trauma, but they become it in tone, in silence, in repetition-with-variation. Interpretation here must be **atmospheric**, not explanatory. The analyst speaks into the density, not through it.

In this suspended state, repetition begins to shift. Rather than circling narrowly, the loop **spreads laterally**, touching new areas of the patient's psyche. The recursive fold expands into a symbolic field—*not yet a hologram*, but a proto-holographic state. Memory, affect, fantasy, and dream begin to **co-condense**, forming symbolic microclimates within the session. The patient dreams of mirrors, of spirals, of labyrinths. The analyst senses the shape of the psyche in the air.

A patient, for example, begins bringing in dreams that echo previous sessions in indirect ways. A childhood hallway reappears, now filled with water. A mother's voice becomes disembodied, floating in the room. The patient does not comment on the imagery, but the analyst feels the recursive field **deepening**. The dream is not symbolic of a past event; it is *symbolic of the recursive structure itself*. The psyche is beginning to *know itself symbolically*, and this knowing is distributed across the field—not just in the patient's mind, but in the atmosphere between patient and analyst.

The recursive defenses begin to soften. Not because they have been inter-preted, but because the symbolic field has **held their rhythm long enough for condensation to emerge**. This is a turning point. The loop no longer needs to defend—it begins to express. The patient may not know what is different, but they feel *thicker, slower, and more present*. The analyst, too, feels suspended in symbolic time. The dyad is inside the fold, and something is about to constellate.

At this juncture, the analyst must resist the urge to crystallize too soon. The temptation to name, to clarify, to offer a narrative—while strong—may flatten the symbolic field before it reaches aesthetic resolution. The analyst's silence here is not withholding, but **form-generative**. It is the silence of the artist before the final brushstroke, the composer before the cadence. The atmos-phere must be allowed to *ripen*.

This atmospheric ripening paves the way for the holographic mind—the next chapter's terrain. Here, repetition becomes condensation, and condensation becomes a **symbolic totality**, in which each part reflects the whole. But this transformation is not a sudden leap. It is a **saturation threshold**, crossed quietly through the analyst's capacity to hold the field without prematurely decoding it.

In clinical terms, this might be the moment when the patient cries without knowing why, or when a pause in speech becomes more communicative than any word. The analytic room is full—not of noise, but of **symbolic presence**. The recursive has given way to the **field**, and the analyst no longer follows loops but listens for the **resonant whole**.

In these moments, time again folds—but differently. No longer circling the trauma, the psyche begins to fold inward toward symbol. A new tempo-rality emerges: not recursive, but **holographic**. The symbolic field is prepar-ing to crystallize. The next movement of the psyche will not be a repetition, but a **holographic condensation**, a symbolic image saturated with recursive time.

We end this section, then, not with a breakthrough, but with a thickening. The field has shifted. The loop has held. The atmosphere is ripe. The symbolic is near.

Micro-Vignette: The Sentence That Circles Back

Daniel came to analysis with what he called "an overactive conscience and an underactive spine." A tenure-track academic in his early 40s, he presented with generalized anxiety, persistent guilt, and a sense that he was "only ever retroactively real." He was articulate, formally polite, and extraordinarily self-aware in ways that bordered on ritual. Every insight came with its own footnote. Every confession was bracketed by qualifications. What he couldn't seem to do was stop thinking.

Much of our early work circled a particular self-reproach: Daniel's ten-dency to remember, out of nowhere, something he'd said years ago—sometimes decades ago—that he now judged as offensive, selfish, or stupid. These weren't major transgressions, but minor social exchanges that looped back with uncanny force: the way he said goodbye to a lover in college, a joke he once made to a professor, an email he sent to a colleague. "It's like my past self keeps heckling me," he said. "Except I'm the heckler, and I'm also the audience."

He would describe these moments with remarkable precision. But nothing we said together seemed to loosen their grip. If anything, interpreting the guilt seemed to deepen the loop: now he was not only guilty, but guilty for being guilty. "I know it's repetitive," he once said, "but every time it feels like this is the time I'll finally say the right thing back to myself."

Only slowly did a different pattern begin to emerge. What seemed like neurotic guilt was also a form of mourning—unconscious grief not for a particular event, but for a lost internal coherence. In his family, moral failure was swiftly punished, but success was met with suspicion. Any moment of pride became grounds for later self-correction. As Daniel began to feel a glimmer of self-compassion, the recurrence of these "sentence loops" became less about self-monitoring and more about a deeper longing: to find a moment in the past that might still be rewritten, made whole.

What had first appeared as content—the remembered phrase—revealed itself as form: the closed circuit of a recursive field that could not symbolically expand. The symptom was not a memory but a structure, and Daniel was trapped in its orbit. Our work, then, became less about solving the memory and more about inhabiting its form together—feeling its curvature, its velocity, its refusal to yield to linear time.

To deepen this tension between symptom and symbol, we turn to a patient whose looping process emerged not as collapse, but as recursive cognition.

Clinical Vignette: The Spiral and the Room

Darren arrived as many do: intelligent, articulate, and steeped in insight that had not yielded change. He had been in therapy before—twice long-term and once briefly after a breakup—but found himself "circling the same drain," as he put it. He was wary of new starts, but desperate for something different. He described his internal life as "a spiral that always collapses in the same place." Early on, he named this place: the feeling of being irrelevant when no one is looking.

He described a childhood of muted emotional texture. No overt trauma, but no aliveness either. A father who disappeared into work and a mother who smiled past everything. He recalled a single image repeatedly—a moment of standing in the hallway outside his parents' bedroom, uncertain whether to knock. "It was like my whole childhood existed in that hallway," he said. "On the edge of something that would never open."

In our first months, the work unfolded with an almost surreal symmetry. Sessions had a rhythmic tempo—initiated by Darren's verbal cascade, often followed by a flat affective dip, then punctuated by sudden disclosures of shame or despair. It felt recursive: the same structure every week, but never quite the same content. At first, I thought I was simply witnessing defense. But over time, the repetition gained atmosphere. It was no longer just what Darren said, but *how the room felt*—as if we were in the same hallway he described, hovering outside a door that neither of us could knock on.

I found myself slipping into a trance-like state during certain sessions—not bored, but suspended. I would lose track of the narrative, only to snap back when Darren said something oddly poetic or jarringly off-key. I began to suspect we were circling something that neither of us could tolerate directly.

One day, Darren brought a dream:

> I'm walking through a spiral staircase inside a house I've never seen. Each step feels like a memory, but I don't know whose. There are mirrors instead of windows. I look into one and see my own eyes, but they don't register me. I say something—'I'm here'—but the mirror just fogs.

The dream held the feel of the work. Recursive. Symbolically saturated. Every image an echo of earlier themes: the spiral, the non-recognition, the hallway reimagined as a house of mirrors. I didn't interpret the dream immediately. I let it sit in the room. Darren did too.

In the weeks that followed, the sessions thickened. His narratives became more fluid, but less linear. He described dreams within dreams, memories layered with imagined revisions. There was one moment in particular—an otherwise unremarkable session—when Darren paused mid-sentence and said, "It feels like we're in a spiral, but not going down this time. Just… orbiting." I didn't respond with words. I nodded. The room felt full, as if the loop had become its own atmosphere.

He began to talk about a childhood friend—Caleb—whom he hadn't mentioned before. "He used to come over and play with my Legos, and sometimes we'd hide under the bed and just whisper to each other. Nothing big, but it was the most alive I felt as a kid." Darren had no idea why Caleb stopped coming. "One day he just didn't anymore. I never asked. I think I knew not to." The sense of loss was palpable, but Darren didn't cry. Instead, he sat in silence, and I felt the entire room bend inward around the image—two boys under a bed, whispering into the folds of time.

From that point on, our work shifted. He would begin sessions with seemingly unrelated fragments—an overheard line from a stranger, a smell that reminded him of the hallway, a visual detail from a dream. He was less interested in interpretation. "I just want to hold these things somewhere," he said. "Like objects in a room."

I began to feel that the room *was* the symbol. We had moved beyond content, beyond narrative. The recursive rhythm had saturated the field, and now Darren was living inside a symbolic atmosphere. His affect was richer, slower. He stopped joking through discomfort. He began to allow moments of quiet without anxiety. I noticed my own internal state shift. I no longer felt suspended—I felt present, as if I had joined him under the bed.

There was one particular moment that crystallized this transition. Darren came in and sat quietly for a long time. Then he said, "You know that hallway? I think I was always knocking. I just never heard anyone knock back." The tears came easily. He didn't apologize. He didn't analyze. He let the silence hold.

Later in that session, he added, "This feels like the room I was waiting for. Not this office, but this way of being." It wasn't that a trauma had been unearthed or interpreted. It was that the recursive structure had become symbolically saturated enough to **fold into symbol**. The loop was still there—but now it was held in the field, not enacted through it.

If I had pushed too early, tried to explain the spiral or decode the dream, we might have collapsed the recursive field prematurely. What allowed the shift was a form of shared suspension, what Thomas Ogden (1994) might call *analytic thirdness*: the emergence of a symbolic space held by both but owned by neither. The spiral became the form through which recognition could occur—not directly, but atmospherically.

In supervision, I found it difficult to describe our work. It wasn't unfolding in the usual way. There were no insights I could point to, nor were there any interpretive breakthroughs. But there was change—deep, textural, and rhythmic. Darren's relationships began to shift. He said no to things he once performed for. He began dating someone he didn't feel he had to entertain. "It feels like I'm moving through the hallway now," he said. "Not stuck outside the door."

What I take from this work is not that repetition must be interrupted, but that it must be **held long enough to become symbolic**. Recursive return is not merely resistance—it is architecture. When the analyst can endure the loop without prematurely resolving it, something else becomes possible: a thickening of atmosphere, a saturation of meaning, and, eventually, a condensation into the symbolic. Darren didn't need to leave the spiral. He needed someone to step into it with him—*until it folded into a room he could live in*.

Closing Reflection: Toward Symbolic Gravity

What, then, is the nature of the repetition we have been tracing? It is not merely the recurrence of content, nor the return of the same disguised as the new. It is the **recursive pull of unformulated experience**, drawing the psyche back toward sites of fragmentation—not to repeat, but to symbolize. It is the attempt to metabolize a gravitational center that cannot be encountered directly. In this sense, repetition is not regression. It is symbolic practice unfolding in time.

Throughout this chapter, we have followed repetition not as pathology but as **topology**. We have imagined it not as a straight line but as a spiral, an orbit, a fold. We have seen how trauma leaves not just content but *structure*, and how that structure lives as temporality: as loops, hesitations, mirrored motifs. Freud's original conception of repetition as something beyond the pleasure principle has found its way, through Loewald, Ogden, and Stern, into a broader understanding of recursive organization. And still, something resists formulation.

Perhaps this is because repetition is not just a clinical phenomenon. It is a **cosmological signature**—the psyche reenacting its own origin myths. When a child knocks on a door that doesn't open, when a patient enters the same affective cul-de-sac, when the analyst recognizes a familiar dread in their own silence—these are not simply patterns. They are rituals. The psyche is engaged in the sacred task of making the unbearable livable.

This brings us to a final framing: **repetition as a symbolic atmosphere**. The goal is not to interpret our way out of the loop, but to thicken the loop until it becomes symbolically habitable. The loop must be held, witnessed, and folded into meaning. The loop becomes a room. And the room becomes psyche.

To dwell in such symbolic gravity is to shift our analytic posture. Rather than intervening to clarify or disrupt, we wait with. We feel the loop move through the field and sense its density. We orient not to solution but to saturation. Over time, the recursive field may inflect into symbol—not by force, but by **presence**.

This reframes the ethical dimension of analytic work. The analyst is not a disruptor of pattern, but a **companion to return**. We accompany the loop not to escape it, but to reveal its contours, its temperature, its texture. In doing so, we allow the loop to become less isolating, less opaque. The patient is no longer orbiting alone.

And this changes the theory of change itself. The psyche does not always change by linear gain or new insight. Sometimes it changes by **recursive saturation**—by allowing the gravitational form to be witnessed until it becomes transparent enough to see through, or dense enough to hold. This is not resolution, but reframing. Not escape, but symbolization.

In this light, the repetition compulsion is not simply the return of trauma. It is the gravitational trace of a subject trying to become real. Each recursive pass gathers psychic material. Each spiral adds symbolic weight. And eventually, the field bends. The symbolic function begins to constellate—not because the loop ends, but because the subject can now *inhabit the loop as form*.

This sets the stage for the next chapter, which will take up the idea of **the holographic mind**—the condensation of symbol, trauma, and atmosphere into a psychic structure that refracts rather than repeats. There, we will explore how repetition is not only recursive but *interdimensional*: how symbols fold over one another, and how the psyche becomes a field of echoes, images, and condensations. But before we arrive at that chapter, we linger one moment longer here.

The spiral is not a flaw in the structure. It is the structure.

The loop is not a detour. It is the orbit.

And the repetition is not noise. It is the signal of something sacred, folded in time, waiting to be lived.

7 The Holographic Mind
Collapse, Condensation, and Symbolic Atmosphere

Where Chapter 2 explored psychic structure through gravitational curvature, and Chapter 9 will explore part-objects as fragmentary anchors, this chapter turns toward the implosion of meaning into saturated image. Here, the symbolic does not disappear—it over-condenses, creating shimmer, aesthetic echo, and breakdowns in representational form. The holographic metaphor captures a quality of psychic life in which every part contains the whole, but distorted, collapsed, or charged beyond narrative. What emerges is not coherence but atmosphere—a field of intensity in which symbolic logic flickers, fails, and folds into itself. This is not a chapter about repression, but about symbolic overload. It attends to the moment when language gives off light instead of meaning.

I once worked with a patient who brought in a dream that unfolded like a closed loop: he was holding a map that kept folding in on itself. Each time he tried to open it, it got larger. Eventually, the map turned into a mirror, and when he looked into it, he saw not his own face but countless miniature versions of the same map, echoing back at him in recursive impossibility. Then the mirror shattered. Yet somehow, in the dream's final image, he was still holding the map—and now it was bleeding.

He recounted the dream with a blank affect and muttered, "I don't even think it means anything." I didn't respond. The dream hadn't repressed anything. It had **collapsed meaning inward**, condensed it to the point of saturation. It wasn't symbolic in the usual sense; it was **over-symbolized**, shimmering with recursive density. The dream didn't ask to be interpreted— it sought to implode in the listener's mind. Meaning here had imploded into atmosphere.

This is the domain of the holographic: psychic events that do not unfold but **densify**—where the symbolic field becomes luminous, overloaded, and unstable. Just as a hologram creates depth from a flattened surface, so too does the psyche sometimes compress relational, sensory, and representational content into forms that shimmer, collapse, or bleed. The result is not the absence of meaning, but its **excess**—an aesthetic field too saturated to resolve.

DOI: 10.4324/9781003715306-11

Aesthetic Saturation and the Collapse of Symbolic Form

The symbolic order is supposed to hold us. It frames, defines, clothes, and names us. Yet when that symbolic scaffolding becomes overburdened—when it is saturated with too much meaning, too much demand, or too much fragility—it begins to shimmer and collapse. This shimmer is not luminous, but brittle: the over-reflection of something straining under the weight of having to signify too much.

In the analytic room, we encounter this phenomenon not just through narrative breakdowns, but also through aesthetic expressions. Patients bring in dreams, images, or even moods that reveal a kind of symbolic collapse—not by failing to mean, but by meaning too much. The excessive symbolic charge becomes unstable, flickering between coherence and breakdown. This instability is not simply the failure of representation; it is the aesthetic form of that failure.

Consider a dream one patient shared: he is wandering through an endless IKEA, but all the furniture is made of transparent glass. Every time he tries to sit, the chair shatters. The dream is beautiful and terrifying: the endless display of form without function, the proliferation of symbolic objects that cannot bear weight. The aesthetic is elegant, minimal, even seductive—but lethal. In waking life, this patient meticulously curated his home with mid-century furniture and carefully balanced color palettes. But the home was unlivable: no one could touch anything, nothing could be left out, even a mug on the counter was too much. The space was curated not for living, but for performance—for upholding a symbolic field that might collapse if smudged.

Another patient, by contrast, presented collapse through maximalism. She decorated her bedroom like a bordello, with crushed velvet, glittering string lights, and an overwhelming density of objects. Her dreams were oversaturated collages of sensory fragments—an ex-boyfriend's cologne mixed with Catholic iconography, taxidermy, and cheap perfume. In one dream, she stood before a mirror applying lipstick, but her reflection was missing. These patients represent opposing poles of aesthetic breakdown: one through glass minimalism, which shatters under weight, and the other through baroque proliferation that drowns the subject in excess.

In both cases, symbolic form becomes uninhabitable. The IKEA of glass and the room of velvet both fail to hold the subject. The self cannot dwell in either space—not because the symbolic is absent, but because it is too present, too burdened, too encoded with meaning. The symbolic has become aestheticized in a way that enacts its own collapse. It is not simply a question of failure to symbolize, but of symbolization turned against itself—of aesthetic form reaching such intensity that it ceases to function as a container and becomes an instrument of fragmentation.

Symbolic collapse, then, is often aesthetic in nature. We see it in dreams, in fashion, in décor, in the texture of a patient's speech, or the way they organize their online dating profiles. The collapse is not a loss of form but an overproduction of form—forms that saturate, distort, or freeze the symbolic field. What cannot be said is screamed in color or cloaked in glass. And the analytic task is not to interpret these forms away but to recognize them as expressions of a field that has lost its gravitational center.

In some patients, this collapse comes with terror. In others, with an eerie calm. The analytic process must attune to both. We must learn to read shimmer—not as beauty, not as seduction, but as signal. The shimmering form is a flare from a collapsing symbolic structure. Its beauty is a cry.

Symbolic Gravity and Psychic Topology

What holds meaning together? Just as celestial bodies warp space-time and pull other objects into orbit, symbolic constellations generate a kind of psychic gravity. This gravity is not physical, but it is no less real. It exerts pressure, organizes affect, and pulls fragments of experience into configurations that give shape to the psyche. The symbolic is not just a semantic code—it is a gravitational topology that structures how we inhabit our inner and relational worlds.

In patients whose symbolic gravity is intact, even painful or contradictory experiences can be metabolized. Trauma may bend the psychic field, but it does not tear it. There is a holding environment—internal or external—that sustains symbolic coherence. But when the symbolic structure is too fragmented, too overdetermined, or too saturated, its gravitational pull falters. Meaning begins to float. Language disconnects from affect. Symbols no longer anchor experience, but ricochet or dissolve.

These shifts are not linear degradations. They are topological transformations—warps, twists, and tears in the symbolic field. The metaphor of psychic topology allows us to move beyond simple structural metaphors (e.g., "defenses," "containers") and imagine instead a dynamic field of intensities. In this field, meaning condenses or diffuses, affect pools or leaks, and symbolic forms curve in on themselves, folding time and space into recursive loops.

One patient who had survived early emotional neglect described his inner world as "a room with no floor." He meant that he could think, speak, and even appear coherent, but underneath everything was a sense that nothing would catch him. He could not symbolize despair, because despair had no place to land. It did not orbit—it fell. This is the topology of psychic freefall: not depression per se, but the gravitational collapse of meaning itself. He lived in a symbolic vacuum.

For another patient, the symbolic field was oversaturated with inherited expectations. He was raised in a family that demanded perfection and performance, where every action had to be meaningful. In our sessions, he would often pause midsentence, looking confused—not because he didn't know what to say, but because he didn't know what was permissible to feel. His words had too much weight; every utterance was loaded with anticipatory shame. Here, we see the opposite of collapse: symbolic over-density. The psychic field is so gravitationally heavy that nothing can move. There is no room for spontaneity, for rupture, for symbolization that emerges organically.

These opposing configurations—vacuum and over-density—are topologically distinct, yet both destabilize the symbolic capacity. In one, meaning cannot hold. In the other, meaning holds too tightly, crushing the nascent self. Both represent distortions in symbolic gravity. And both require the analyst to enter the field not as interpreter, but as co-inhabitant of the warp.

Loewald's image of the analyst as a "second psychic reality" comes into play here. The analyst does not simply receive symbolic material; they generate symbolic field conditions. Their presence, attunement, and willingness to hold incoherence allow new gravitational centers to emerge. This is not done through insight alone, but through affective constancy—through staying with what feels unsymbolizable until the field reshapes around it.

Symbolic gravity is not simply about meaning. It is about *cohesion*. A word, a gesture, or even a silence can draw disparate fragments into orbit, giving a patient the sense that they are not falling alone. Over time, these micro-sutures thicken into structure. What was once unthinkable becomes symbolizable. Not through explanation, but through gravitational tethering.

The language of space-time and orbit may sound metaphoric, but for many patients, it maps more precisely onto their experience than anatomical metaphors of ego, id, or superego. Psychic life is lived in topologies of nearness and distance, of inside and outside, of collapse and coherence. When symbolic gravity breaks down, patients do not merely "regress"—they *lose dimensionality*. The analyst must learn to orient themselves in these flattened, disoriented, or curved psychic landscapes.

At its core, symbolic gravity is a function of presence. When another mind can bear the unformulated, the unworded, the unaligned—something changes. Not suddenly, and not always visibly. But the field bends. Meaning starts to coalesce, not around old referents, but around the possibility of being held. Gravity is restored not by force, but by fidelity.

Shimmer and the Unstable Signifier

Not all breakdowns in symbolization result in collapse. Some shimmer. The shimmer is a quality of the signifier that resists settling into fixed meaning. It is not fragmentation, exactly, but a destabilization that hovers—a flickering between signification and excess. We might think of shimmer as a quality of psychic light: symbolic surfaces that gleam with overtones they cannot stabilize.

Patients sometimes communicate through shimmer rather than clarity. They play with language, or their tone carries an ambiguity that is neither wholly conscious nor accidental. A gay man with whom I worked would describe his sexual experiences in language that felt stylized, campy, and layered in tone. At first, I treated this as a defensive measure: a way to avoid emotional contact. But over time, I came to feel the shimmer in his speech not as defense, but as a saturated mode of signification. His words glistened with multiplicity. They were not evasions; they were too full.

Linguistic shimmer often appears through **poetic ambiguity**, irony, or puns—especially when a patient is trying to touch an experience that remains partly unformulated. They may half-joke, say something "in quotes," or use metaphor when describing what they cannot quite bear to say directly. Here, the signifier shimmers as if lit from more than one source. The patient might say, "I guess I just want to be taken," with a pause that leaves it unclear whether they mean sexually, emotionally, or spiritually. In that ambiguity lies the truth—not yet dissected, but fully alive.

We could think of shimmer as the field-effect of **affectively saturated signification**—when words do not simply point to experience but vibrate with its intensity. A child's toy described in minute detail by an adult survivor of early abuse may become more than a memory; it becomes a container, a glowing shard, a symbol that exceeds itself. In these moments, meaning flickers between levels. The signifier becomes *unstable*, but not lost. It hovers on the edge of condensation and collapse.

In dreams, shimmer can appear as visual or symbolic detail that seems too specific, too rich, to be casually dismissed. One patient dreamed of a glittering jellyfish floating in his childhood bedroom. He described it as "mesmerizing but out of place." We discussed the jellyfish as a psychic image: ungraspable, translucent, both beautiful and dangerous. He associated it with the lingering presence of his father—an abusive man whose absence was somehow more charged than his presence. The dream shimmered: it could not be reduced to interpretation. Its meaning curved outward.

From a theoretical perspective, shimmer complicates any stable distinction between conscious and unconscious meaning. Derrida's notion of *différance* points toward this kind of endless slippage—the delay and deferral of signification that renders the sign both necessary and never quite sufficient. But shimmer adds an **aesthetic dimension**. It is not just the slippage that matters; it is the beauty of the slippage, the way it glows.

This aesthetic quality has clinical implications. When we attune to shimmer, we shift from trying to "decode" the patient to participating in their symbolic atmosphere. We listen not only for what is said, but how the saying occurs—where tone, rhythm, or imagery bear more weight than content. We might respond to shimmer not with clarification, but with receptivity: "It feels like there's more in that pause than in the words." Or: "That sentence seems to stretch in two directions at once."

The analyst's own countertransference may also shimmer. One patient described a memory from college in such fragmented, evocative terms that I felt a heat rise in my body. It wasn't erotic, exactly—it was symbolic saturation. The imagery was so alive that I found myself holding my breath. Later, I realized I had become part of the shimmer: my attention, my receptivity, was the field in which his fragmented memory could reassemble as experience.

Shimmer allows for **micro-reintegration**. In patients who feel that they have no coherent self, or whose symbolic worlds are filled with contradiction, shimmer may be the only reliable form of coherence. Not through linear narrative, but through tonal layering, ambiguity, and recurrence. When the signifier is unstable, but affectively resonant, it holds paradox. It **symbolizes without closure**.

This may explain why some patients resist clarity. To pin something down would be to strip it of its vitality. The shimmer is a defense, yes—but also a **mode of survival**, of keeping multiple truths in play. Symbolic shimmer is the opposite of foreclosure. It keeps the field open, alive, flickering. For analysts accustomed to meaning-making, shimmer demands humility. We are not the bearers of coherence, but cohabitants of its radiant instability.

To bear shimmer is to resist interpretation too soon. It is to linger in the flicker, to trust that what glows but cannot yet be named may still exert gravity.

Shimmering Collapse and Symbolic Freefall

If shimmer marks the symbolic field's excess—its radiance—collapse is what happens when that field can no longer hold. Collapse is not the opposite of shimmer, but its gravitational descent. In the clinical process, we often witness patients oscillate between shimmer and collapse, especially when the tension between the unspeakable and the overly saturated reaches its limit.

Symbolic collapse is not mere muteness. It is the implosion of symbolic structure as such—when the scaffolding of language, image, and metaphor buckles under affective weight. The patient may suddenly go silent, dissociate, or flatten into literalism. Alternatively, collapse may take the form of over-saturation: an inability to think because too much is pressing in, not too little.

The psychoanalytic literature often approaches collapse through trauma or psychotic states. But I want to emphasize collapse as a **recursive** event. It is not necessarily psychotic, nor always tied to early catastrophic experience. Collapse can occur as a **micro-event** within otherwise regulated discourse. A patient may be telling a dream and suddenly go blank. Or they may be speaking fluidly and then burst into tears they do not understand. In these moments, the symbolic field gives out—like a floor that momentarily disappears.

From a metapsychological point of view, we might say that the ego's capacity to symbolize—to metabolize affect into representation—fails under pressure. Loewald (1960) reminds us that symbolization requires **time, spacing, and internal rhythm**. Collapse breaches those coordinates. The recursive circuit of perception, memory, fantasy, and reflection snaps. Temporality itself may distort.

Yet collapse is not void. It is **full of content that cannot yet cohere**. That is why the analyst's attitude in the face of collapse is so crucial. If we rush to restore coherence, we may bypass the patient's actual experience. But if we can remain present in the freefall—if we can hold the implosion without demanding symbolic restitution—we may allow something new to constellate. The collapsed space is not meaningless; it is *pregnant with unprocessed meaning*.

Some patients describe collapse as a kind of internal "crash," a moment of system overload. One man in my practice referred to it as "falling inside," as if the internal architecture gave way. He would speak eloquently and then suddenly stare into the distance, saying, "I can't think anymore." At first, I responded by slowing down, reflecting back, trying to help him re-enter language. But later, I began to wonder whether the collapse itself was a communication—a message sent without form.

These collapses were often preceded by a kind of **aesthetic shimmer**: he would describe dreams, objects, or sexual scenes in language that glowed, that drew me in. Then—suddenly—it would all disappear. I came to understand the shimmer as a prelude to collapse. His symbolic system would overheat. It was not trauma per se that triggered the collapse, but saturation. He was trying to say too much, too fully, too beautifully. And then it all fell apart.

There is a paradox here: collapse arises not from absence but from **too much presence**. The system cannot hold the symbolic weight. This is not dissociation in the usual sense; it is not fragmentation of the ego, but implosion of its representational capacities. The symbols are there, but they have lost structural gravity. They do not orbit—they crash.

We might call this a kind of **symbolic freefall**. The patient enters a space where nothing sticks, nothing holds. Sometimes it resembles psychotic disorganization, but it may also appear as profound stillness, as if the mind itself has turned to ash. These moments may be terrifying—for both patient and analyst—but they also mark the edges of symbolic renewal.

The analytic task is not to rescue meaning, but to witness the collapse without abandoning the field. Our presence becomes the gravity that holds what has fallen. We do not force structure, but we remain structured. The analyst's mind becomes a kind of scaffold—not to replace the patient's, but to offer **symbolic containment without symbolic imposition**.

In this sense, collapse is not only a breakdown, but a threshold. If held well, it may lead not to psychotic dissolution, but to **symbolic transformation**. The prior system had to collapse for something more authentic—or more capacious—to emerge.

When patients begin to trust that collapse does not mean abandonment, the collapse itself changes. It becomes slower, less devastating, and more metabolizable. The freefall turns into descent, and descent into **depth**. What shimmered, what collapsed, now begins to cohere—not by force, but by field.

Clinical Vignette: The Collapsing Room

In our first session, Jesse arrived with a luminous intensity—eyes alert, words fast, the room immediately thick with meaning. His dress was subtly eccentric: fitted black jeans, a vintage bomber jacket, and a delicate pendant on a silver chain. Almost before sitting down, he launched into a dream that seemed to carry its own atmosphere.

He said,

> I was in a vast museum filled with light, but the exhibits kept changing. I would look away for a moment, and when I looked back, the painting or sculpture would be different—same shape, different content. At the center of the museum was a hole, a black circle in the marble floor. I got closer and realized it was not a hole, but a mirror. I looked in and saw my own eyes. But they were empty.

The dream struck both of us as visually radiant and disorienting. I noted the shapeshifting art, the inversion of void and reflection, and the powerful image of self-recognition hollowed out. But Jesse continued without pause, shifting almost imperceptibly from dream report into psychic confession:

> I don't know if I'm real most of the time. It's not dramatic—it's just… fuzzy. Like, I'm more of an aesthetic than a person. I perform what I think I am. But underneath, I don't know what's there. That mirror in the dream? I think I live in that.

His language shimmered—poetic, ambiguous, affectively saturated. Not just metaphorical, but ontologically unstable: a mirror that is also a void, an identity that flickers between surface and substance. Jesse's early sessions glowed with precisely this kind of aestheticized collapse—statements so symbolically dense they risked folding in on themselves.

I began to notice a rhythm. He would speak in evocative, lyrical terms for 15 or 20 minutes, describing dreams, lovers, visual imagery, and states of perception. Then—abruptly—he would go quiet. His gaze would drift. The room would suddenly feel airless. He might say, "Sorry, I just… can't think anymore," or, "It all just turned flat."

At first, I assumed these moments were dissociative, linked to trauma or defensive withdrawal. But as I tracked them over time, a different pattern emerged. Jesse was not simply splitting off; he was overloading the symbolic field. His aesthetic saturations—especially when they verged on revelation—triggered a kind of structural freefall. Meaning became too dense to hold.

In one session, he brought in a line from a poem he had written: "I wear my face like lacquer—thin, gleaming, meant to crack." He paused, then whispered, "That one scares me." When I asked why, he replied, "Because it feels like the most honest thing I've ever written. And because if it's true, I don't know what happens when it cracks."

Jesse was caught in the paradox of symbolic collapse. He needed language to find himself, but the moment it neared truth, it threatened to dissolve him. The very act of symbolizing—when too charged—risked implosion.

These moments were not failures of therapy. They were recursive thresholds. If I responded with too much interpretation, he would slip further into fragmentation. If I withdrew, he would feel unseen. What helped, gradually, was allowing the shimmer to be witnessed without harvesting it for meaning. I might say, "That line is haunting," or, "You brought something luminous into the room," and then simply remain with it.

In one session, after a long silence following a particularly layered dream, I said, "It feels like everything in the room got heavy, like it's bending the floor." He smiled faintly. "Yeah. That's what it's like in my head, too."

The dream he had shared just before that moment had been one of his most surreal:

> I was in a room made of mirrors, but none of them reflected me. I touched one, and it turned to liquid. I stepped through and found myself in my childhood bedroom, but everything was slightly off—wrong size, wrong color. I reached under the bed and pulled out a box. Inside was a burning coal, glowing but cold.

We sat in silence for several minutes after he told it. I felt the dream's weight—its recursive structure, the unreality of reflection, the false familiarity of childhood, the contradiction of cold flame. It was not a puzzle to be solved. It was a collapse to be held.

The image of the burning coal became a quiet motif in our work. Sometimes Jesse would say, "It's coal day," and I would know we were entering one of those atmospheres where language might not hold. We learned to co-inhabit those spaces, not by avoiding them, but by softening our relation to them. Shimmer became less dangerous. Collapse became less annihilating. Eventually, Jesse began to reflect on the process itself: "You don't try to fix it. That's what helps. When I go blank, you don't rush in. You kind of… lean in with me. I think that's why I can speak again."

His symbolic field was not "repaired" in a technical sense. Rather, it began to self-stabilize. The recursive spirals—shimmer, collapse, silence, metaphor—didn't disappear, but they found rhythm. Our shared field began to function as symbolic gravity: not heavy, not fixed, but able to hold Jesse's oscillations without collapsing them further.

Holding the Collapse: Toward Symbolic Gravity

The analytic work with Jesse illuminated something foundational: the act of symbolizing can itself become traumatic if it evokes too much truth too quickly. What collapsed in those moments was not only meaning, but containment—the capacity of the psychic structure to metabolize its own reflection. This collapse was aesthetic as much as structural, experienced through shimmering metaphors, dreamlike distortions, and recursive atmospheres that bent the symbolic frame. Yet over time, we discovered a paradoxical path toward stabilization: not by avoiding collapse, but by holding it—by symbolizing the moment when symbolization falters.

This act of *holding the collapse* constitutes what I've come to think of as symbolic gravity. Unlike interpretation, which seeks to clarify or organize, symbolic gravity allows the aesthetic and the structural to constellate without immediate digestion. It is an atmosphere rather than an act—an orientation of the analytic field that permits meaning to shimmer without dissolving into incoherence. It makes it possible to witness the point at which signification becomes too dense or too volatile, and to remain present without forcibly naming or bypassing the threshold.

Symbolic gravity does not mean slowing down interpretation, nor does it mean simply tolerating ambiguity. Rather, it is a way of attuning to the recursive fold in the patient's speech, where metaphor begins to implode into presence. Jesse's line—"I wear my face like lacquer"—was not only a statement; it was a surface event, a collapse shimmering in real time. What allowed it to hold was not its dissection, but our joint ability to *rest near it without rupture*.

This dimension of analytic work is under-theorized because it resists procedural language. It is not just containment in the Bionian sense, though it overlaps. It is closer to what Hans Loewald called the "depth grammar" of psychic life—an invisible syntax that permits thought to have dimensionality. Or what Ogden described as the co-creation of analytic thirdness, in which unsymbolized affect can begin to stir into form through shared presence. But symbolic gravity is less about the *creation* of symbol than the *protection* of its precarity. It is a refusal to rush the sedimentation of meaning.

In Jesse's case, we were dealing not with a failure to symbolize per se, but with a repeated folding back of symbol into affect. His language was not underdeveloped but over-rich—too luminous to metabolize in the moment. The problem was not repression but saturation. Thus, the clinical task was not to tease out hidden meaning, but to make space for shimmer that could remain suspended long enough to soften.

This is what distinguishes symbolic gravity from interpretation. The latter seeks to transform the unconscious into usable material. The former allows the unconscious to show itself without immediate transformation. It creates a relational atmosphere in which collapse is held, not solved.

There is a kind of poetics to this clinical stance. The analyst becomes less a decoder and more a gravitational presence—shaping the psychic field not by content, but by proximity and rhythm. Jesse did not need more accurate interpretations. He needed someone to remain with him at the edge of implosion, to share the vertigo without grabbing for coherence.

This is where aesthetics and structure converge. When a patient begins to collapse under the weight of meaning, what may be needed is not clarity, but contour—not explanation, but echo. To say, "It feels like the room is bending," or "There's a pressure in the air," is not to interpret, but to thicken the symbolic field just enough that it doesn't shatter. These are acts of symbolic gravity.

Symbolic gravity is not passive. It is an active holding of tension, a felt effort to sustain symbolic atmosphere while the patient searches for a tolerable relation to their own psyche. It is technical in its own right—requiring the analyst to track saturation, rhythm, silence, and breath. To feel when meaning is nearing collapse, and to adjust presence accordingly.

In some sense, this form of work brings us close to a mystical edge of psychoanalysis—not in the religious sense, but in its attentiveness to threshold states. Symbolic gravity operates where language begins to fold back on itself, where shimmer threatens to unmake form. And it teaches us that interpretation is not always the royal road to meaning. Sometimes, the truer path is to remain near the unformed, bearing its pressure without demanding it become something else.

This is why I believe symbolic gravity is not only a clinical stance, but a moral one. It refuses the violence of premature naming. It honors the recursive, the saturated, the fragile. And it recognizes that some collapses are not problems to be solved, but moments to be held.

As Jesse began to find language that no longer shattered him—language that could shimmer without imploding—the field between us shifted. It became slower, warmer, subtly more vertical. His dreams retained their density, but they no longer arrived with the same psychic aftershock. His speech grew less aestheticized, not because he lost beauty, but because he no longer needed shimmer to survive.

The coal in the dream—burning yet cold—remains the emblem of this process for me. An object of paradox, ungraspable yet radiant. It is the kind of image that cannot be interpreted without reducing it. It must be lived with, sensed, and allowed to burn without heat. This is the work of symbolic gravity. And perhaps, in its most vital moments, it is the work of psychoanalysis itself.

Clinical Vignette: The Curated Collapse

Where Jesse's collapse took the form of symbolic saturation—too much shimmer, too much truth—another patient, Julian, exhibited a different trajectory. His collapse was curated.

Julian came to treatment in his late thirties, a performance artist whose creative output had dwindled to a trickle. Though exquisitely verbal, he used language like a lacquered surface—each phrase polished, guarded, evocative without ever revealing. His sessions shimmered with cleverness: dense literary references, gorgeous dream fragments, and monologues about aesthetic theory. But beneath it all was a strange vacancy. When I reached toward affect, he returned with form. When I inquired about desire, he offered metaphor.

One early session stays with me. Julian described a recent performance piece. It involved a mirrored room, with shifting lights and pre-recorded voices—his own, distorted and looped. The audience moved freely, disoriented by overlapping reflections and echoes. "The piece was about dislocation," he said, "but also about preserving beauty in chaos." He paused. "Like building a greenhouse inside a tornado."

When I asked what the piece meant to him, his reply was smooth: "Meaning is not the point. The structure holds. That's enough."

This was Julian's version of collapse—not explosive, but suspended. He had erected a symbolic scaffolding so intricate that it prevented contact. There was no shimmer because nothing could bend. His recursive atmosphere was built from armor, not atmosphere: everything pointed elsewhere, never back to him.

Over time, we came to see this as a manic defense disguised as aesthetic sophistication. Julian's symptom was not excess, but emptiness encased in symbol. He had over-symbolized his life to such a degree that nothing felt real unless it was performative. His dreams, when he remembered them, were curated to impress. He would recount them with a kind of detachment: "Last night I dreamt I was floating above a museum of my own childhood. The exhibits were mislabeled."

This dream was a turning point. I commented on the mislabeling: "It sounds like even in your dreams, memory is aestheticized—placed behind glass, categorized, but not quite yours." Julian nodded, but with a flicker of tension. "I like the distance," he said. "It protects the shape."

This moment required something delicate. I said, "Sometimes the shape holds because the content would undo you." That phrase—*undo you*—caught in the room. For a second, Julian froze. Then, without smiling, he said, "That's not wrong."

Here, the analytic field shifted. We had brushed against the edge of collapse—not through saturation, but through exposure. His symbolic system, so carefully curated, had momentarily buckled. Not shattered, not dissolved—just trembled. That tremble was our entry point.

In the months that followed, Julian began to share less polished material. He told me about a younger sibling who died at birth, a subject never discussed in his family but which haunted his art in disguised form. He spoke of relationships that collapsed under the weight of idealization, and of a former therapist who "got too close." His metaphors loosened. His language softened. He still spoke in images, but now they bent back toward him.

One day, he said, "I think I built the greenhouse because I couldn't survive the wind." I didn't interpret. I just repeated the line, slower: "You built the greenhouse because you couldn't survive the wind." He exhaled. "Yeah. And I kept thinking it was art, but maybe it was grief."

This was Julian's collapse—not into chaos, but into contact. He had used symbol to avoid the real, and now the symbol was becoming the bridge. The recursive shimmer of his earlier language began to condense into something else—not interpretation, not self-disclosure, but presence.

Symbolic gravity in this case was not about tolerating saturation. It was about softening the rigidity of form. Julian did not need containment; he needed rupture. But a held rupture—a collapse that could be named without being dramatized. It was not that we interpreted his curation as defense (though we did). It was that we remained long enough in its presence for something else to emerge.

Over time, Julian's creative work changed. He began writing a piece that was, in his words, "too ugly to show." It dealt with his mother's silence after the stillbirth and his own ambivalence about surviving. He brought me early drafts—raw, incomplete, and, for the first time, unguarded. "It's not ready," he said. I replied, "Maybe it's not supposed to be." He smiled. "I think that's the point."

What had once been a curated collapse was becoming a recursive return. The echoes no longer obscured the source. The shimmer no longer blinded. Symbol was no longer a shield but a gesture.

Julian taught me that collapse is not always loud. Sometimes it is the slow bend of symbol returning to flesh. And that symbolic gravity may mean, in such cases, staying present long enough for the echo to land—not with interpretation, but with breath.

Cultural Imaginaries and the Iconography of Collapse

Symbolic collapse does not only haunt the analytic dyad—it reverberates through cultural imaginaries, collective myths, and the iconography of sacred and broken forms. In this wider field, the psyche bends through story, ritual, and representation, revealing how the fragility of meaning is as constitutive as its coherence.

In religious iconoclasm, for instance, we find a ritualized destruction of symbol that paradoxically reaffirms its sacredness. The shattering of icons in Byzantine or Reformation-era zeal was never merely political; it was psychically saturated. To destroy the image was to invoke the real. The absence created by the obliterated icon becomes a site of intensity, where the symbol, through its eradication, becomes unbearable in its silent presence. We might say the symbolic collapses through excess of projection—its representational function overwhelmed by unconscious demand.

A similar structure unfolds in the myth of the Tower of Babel. Humanity's hubristic drive to reach the divine through structural form—stone by stone, meaning by meaning—is undone by a collapse of shared language. Here, the symbolic is not destroyed but multiplied into unintelligibility. Meaning fractures not into absence, but into shimmer: too many signs, too much possibility, no unifying grammar. The result is psychic vertigo, a cultural scene of disorientation in which communication becomes a symptom of division rather than coherence. The myth illustrates how the desire for transcendence through symbol can itself precipitate a fall into fragmentation.

In Buddhist ritual, we encounter a more deliberate engagement with collapse. The sand mandala, meticulously created over days or weeks by monks, is swept away within moments of completion. It is not desecration but devotion—the enactment of impermanence, of the non-graspable nature of form. The mandala's intricate geometry, rich in symbolic density, becomes a gesture toward emptiness. Its collapse is a return, not a failure. Yet the potency of the act remains: the visual shimmer of colored grains condensed into cosmic pattern and then released. In this, the symbolic functions as a transient vessel—a condensation that invites its own undoing.

Postmodern aesthetics, too, resonate with the logic of symbolic collapse. In architecture, fashion, and digital art, we see repeated structures of distortion, deconstruction, and recursive layering. The shimmer of meaning in postmodernism is not just stylistic play but a kind of cultural symptom. Jean Baudrillard's notion of the simulacrum—copies without originals—enacts a loss of symbolic gravity. In such spaces, the symbol no longer points elsewhere; it loops inward. Collapse occurs not through rupture but through exhaustion, as signs refer only to other signs in a closed circuit of implication. The result is a kind of meaning-fatigue, where interpretation falters not from lack, but from surplus.

Even dream life mirrors these patterns. Patients have recounted dreams of buildings dissolving into light, words unraveling mid-speech, or being lost in museums where nothing is labeled. Such dreams are not merely disorientation—they are psychic enactments of symbolic collapse. The museum without labels, for instance, recalls Julian's dream, where curated memory lost its anchoring frame. These dreams carry the residue of a culture saturated with meaning yet starved for resonance.

To dwell in these imaginaries is not to seek explanation but to feel their field effects. The analyst, like the dreamer, must tolerate the texture of collapse—not solve it, not contain it prematurely, but listen to its aesthetics. Collapse has an iconography. It has a rhythm. It carries a syntax that does not always translate into interpretation, but which still demands witness.

In this sense, symbolic collapse is not a pathology but a moment of psychic opening—cultural, interpersonal, and intrapsychic. Its atmosphere may be dense or sparse, shimmering or mute, saturated or void. But in all cases, it reveals the limits of form and the possibility that what lies beyond symbol is not chaos, but contact.

Symbolizing the Light of the Split

If symbolic collapse marks the disappearance of form into saturation, then its inverse—or perhaps its companion—is the tentative return of symbol as a gesture of light: not illumination in the sense of clarity, but in the sense of shimmering presence. To symbolize, in this frame, is not to master the psyche but to meet its split with a flicker of holding.

In analytic work, this often appears as a strange intimacy between word and silence. A patient utters a phrase—"It's like I vanished in the room"—and something in the analytic atmosphere shifts. The phrase itself may be ambiguous, even barely cognitively grasped, but it shimmers with associative resonance. It is not a neatly interpretable statement; it is a carrier wave of the split. Symbol here is not stable language, but a condensation of affect and rupture—a sonic artifact of the divide.

This is why poetic speech—dense, rhythmic, ambiguous—is often more containing than consisting of explanatory clarity. In the moment of collapse, it is not understanding that matters most, but accompaniment. The analyst's task becomes not to explain, but to listen with a porous ear: to recognize when symbol is functioning not to clarify, but to carry. The symbol as light is not illumination of content, but a vector of presence.

This symbolic shimmer is especially potent around early or fragmented trauma. In such states, language often fails. But fragments—images, metaphors, bodily sensations—may carry affective charge that exceeds their semantic content. A patient who cannot narrate abuse may describe a corner of the room, the color of the light, or the scent of detergent. These details are not trivial. They are fragments of symbol that anchor the split without forcing premature wholeness. To take them seriously is to trust the psyche's own rhythm of return.

Philosophically, this aligns with what Maurice Merleau-Ponty calls the "pregnancy of the visible," wherein perception always already exceeds its articulation. The symbol, in this view, is not a translation of experience into meaning, but a site where experience brushes up against language and momentarily glows. Similarly, Loewald reminds us that language is not a veneer over thought, but a transformational process through which psyche becomes flesh again. When the analyst receives symbol in this spirit, they allow it to work on the field—less as message, more as texture.

To symbolize the split is also to risk the return of pain. The flicker of symbol can bring back the affect it contains. In the analytic hour, a phrase may shimmer and then burn, requiring the analyst to hold not only its meaning but its heat. The patient may feel exposed, unsure why certain words felt unbearable. This is not regression. It is contact. The symbol has done its work.

There are moments, too, when symbol fails entirely, and yet its attempt matters. A patient may say, "I don't know what I'm saying—I just needed to say it," and in that utterance, something opens. Not because it makes sense, but because it marks presence. The symbolic act, however fragile, has created a line of light across the rupture. Even if the analyst cannot yet see what it links, they can honor that it was drawn.

This is why symbolizing the light of the split is an ethical and aesthetic act. It requires discipline, humility, and receptivity. The analyst becomes not interpreter, but witness to the shimmer. They attend to when speech carries more than it says, when silence holds more than absence. They offer language not as solution, but as lantern.

The hologram as metaphor returns here. The light within a hologram is not behind the image, but within its diffraction—each part containing the whole, each shard capable of revealing the form. In collapsed psychic states, the analyst does not reconstruct the whole. They hold a piece up to the light and wait.

Symbolizing the split, then, is not about resolution but resonance. It is the work of keeping symbol alive in the field of collapse—not to fix, but to feel.

Not to restore coherence, but to remain with the shimmer long enough that form might tentatively reassemble, not as it was, but as it is now.

Clinical Vignette: Light on the Rim of Form

Matthew, a man in his early 30s, entered treatment after a prolonged depressive spell following the dissolution of a significant romantic relationship. His presentation was not marked by overt symptomatology—he maintained employment, social ties, and a polished demeanor—but something in his affect felt suspended. He described himself as "thinly stretched across the days," and often spoke with a kind of aesthetic detachment, as if narrating the life of someone else.

In early sessions, Matthew often made vague yet poetic references to himself as an "echo chamber," a phrase he never elaborated. He was verbally fluid, intelligent, and emotionally elusive. Interpretations, even those gently offered, seemed to slide off. Affect would rise slightly in the room, then dissipate, as if siphoned away by an unseen valve. He seemed skilled at evoking presence without being fully in it.

One day, Matthew arrived visibly disturbed. He had a dream the night before that he could not shake. It had woken him at 3:00 a.m., and he had written parts of it down. In the dream, he found himself in a house without windows. Everything inside was white—the floors, the walls, the ceiling. As he walked through the house, his footsteps made no sound. Objects were scattered through the space: a chair, a glass of water, a piano—but they felt staged, as if belonging to a film set rather than a home. He somehow knew he had lived there once, but it now felt evacuated. Not abandoned, exactly—just emptied out of something vital. As he walked through the rooms, he kept whispering the word "hollowgram." He saw it written in chalk on one of the walls. He recalled it clearly: not hologram, but hollowgram.

When he recounted the dream, Matthew's voice wavered for the first time in treatment. He said he felt "seen by it, but not in a good way." He didn't want to interpret it—he only wanted me to "know that it had happened."

I did not respond analytically. I simply nodded and said, "I'm here." We sat in silence for nearly ten minutes. Something heavy settled in the space. It wasn't the sadness of loss, nor the anxiety of dread. It was the weight of unnameable resonance—of something long unacknowledged coming into symbolic reach.

In the following weeks, the dream took on a presence in the room. Matthew began using the word "hollowgram" as a kind of shorthand when his speech began to falter. He would pause and say, "It's hollowgram again," and I would respond with silence or a nod. The phrase became an object in the transference—a shared symbol of something more than what either of us could fully articulate. It shimmered with shared recognition, but without fixed meaning.

Eventually, Matthew began to describe his childhood home. The house was architecturally minimal—white walls, clean lines, sparse décor. His parents, both academics, prized intelligence and composure, and discouraged "drama." He could not recall being touched or comforted as a child, but he could remember the sound of ice cubes clicking in his father's nightly whiskey glass. "Everything looked perfect," he said, "but no one was home—not really." The dream had opened a channel not to explicit memory, but to an aesthetic field that housed dissociated affect.

The work shifted subtly after that. Matthew still intellectualized, still offered elaborate reflections, but he also began to pause more, to let the unformulated linger. His eyes welled up once when describing a painting he had seen that week—an abstract canvas of white and gray slashes, which he described as "how the hollowgram would look if it could bleed." The symbolic shimmer had begun to animate the room.

As his affective presence increased, so too did the analytic countertransference. I found myself haunted by his dream. I had images of that white house flickering into my own dreams—once even mistaking the sound of my own refrigerator hum as something from "inside the hollowgram." The symbol had entered the shared field.

One particularly striking moment occurred months later. Matthew arrived and sat in silence. I did not speak. After ten minutes, he looked at me and said, "I think the house finally has windows." I asked what he meant, and he smiled: "I don't know. But it's not so white anymore."

This moment did not require interpretation. It was a symbolic condensation of an internal shift. The house had become less evacuated. The hollowgram, once a dream-word of collapse, now contained the shimmer of return.

In the months that followed, Matthew began to mourn his childhood—not through specific memories, but through atmospheres. He spoke of "rooms I never cried in" and "furniture that never held weight." The analytic space became a kind of sanctuary where these fragments could float without needing to cohere. The shimmer of symbol, lightly held, had done what interpretation could not.

This vignette underscores the argument that symbolic gravity is not a given, but a co-created field phenomenon. The analyst need not force meaning, but must listen for shimmer. The dream did not "mean" something, but it marked something—the beginning of a return, the light at the rim of form.

Conclusion

If the holographic mind implodes symbolic coherence through saturation, what follows is not always emptiness. Sometimes, in the aftermath of collapse, the psyche clings to fragments—not as metaphors, but as anchors. Where symbol and image dissolve into atmosphere, part-objects condense, offering tactile, erotic, or sensory fixations around which psychic coherence can temporarily reassemble. These fragments do not restore form; they magnetize it. The psyche no longer dreams in shimmer, but orbits around shards—body parts, objects, smells, phrases—each too charged to symbolize, yet too necessary to release. The next chapter turns toward this gravitational field of the broken symbol: how part-objects do not merely reflect fragmentation, but organize it.

Part IV

Form and Emptiness—From Klein's Void to the Curvature of Form

This section of the book asks the reader to engage differently. The chapters that follow do not trace symptom, structure, or narrative in linear form. Instead, they enter the psychic atmosphere of emptiness—not as blankness or absence, but as the background field from which form arises. Some emptiness is developmental: the residue of rupture. Some is symbolic: the failure of language to bind. Others are contemplative or ontological: spaciousness that reveals the instability of form itself. Klein's understanding of fragmentation and the fear of annihilation is a throughline here, but it is curved into generative terrain: emptiness becomes fertile ground, where shimmer, paradox, and field replace form. These chapters invite the reader to feel into the unsymbolized.

This section of this book invites the reader to engage in a different way. The chapters that follow do not trace symptom, structure, or narrative in linear form. Instead, they enter the psychic atmosphere of emptiness—not as blankness or absence, but as the background field from which form arises. **Freud's early reflections on the thing-presentation and the limits of representation**, alongside **Klein's evocations of the depressive position and the part-object void**, both prefigure this space of paradox. The work here is both conceptual and experiential. You may find yourself pulled not toward resolution, but toward paradox, echo, or symbolic shimmer.

Some emptiness described here is developmental: the residue of rupture. Some is symbolic: the failure of language to bind. Others are contemplative or ontological: spaciousness that reveals the instability of form itself. These chapters explore how psychoanalysis bears witness not only to trauma and transference but to the **voided ground beneath representation**. In their own way, Freud and Klein each approached this terrain: Freud through the silence of the repressed, Klein through the shattered internal object. This part invites you to read slowly, to feel your way through the **gravity of the unformed**, and to notice what emerges when nothing is filled in.

DOI: 10.4324/9781003715306-12

8 Nonduality in the Split Mind
Perceiving the Ground

This chapter explores the perceptual and ontological paradox of nonduality within a psyche conditioned by dualistic structures. Drawing from contemplative traditions, psychoanalytic theory, and phenomenology, it reframes psychic splitting not as an ontological fault but as a mode of perception that can be loosened. Through metaphors of light, self-reference, and recursive cognition, the text invites the reader to consider the split mind as already grounded in a nondual field. Theoretical integration with Derrida, Wittgenstein, and early Klein supports a conceptualization of nonduality as the background hum of being rather than its opposite. Clinical implications are considered in light of how perception itself is trained, shaped, and potentially liberated.

The Split That Was Never a Break

Psychoanalysis begins in the wound of division. The ego, said Freud, is not master in its own house; the subject, for Lacan, is split by language; for Klein, the mind defends itself through fragmentation before it can even integrate its objects. From the beginning, analytic thought has traced the fault lines of a psyche divided against itself, a self that is not one. The very concept of a "mind" presupposes a field of tension: between conscious and unconscious, self and other, and inner and outer. To think psychoanalytically is to attend to what is not aligned—to listen not for the voice, but for the rupture through which the voice emerges.

And yet this chapter proposes a paradox: what we call split is not separate from what we call whole. Duality is not the opposite of nonduality, but one of its appearances. It is a mode of recognition, not a state of being. There is no departure from ground, no severing from truth. What we experience as broken is already curved; what appears as two was never not one. The split mind is not a fall from grace, but a fold in perception.

This reframing does not negate the reality of psychic suffering. Splitting, in both its defensive and structural forms, saturates clinical life. But we may ask: what if splitting is not a deviation from unity, but a mode of how unity appears under pressure? What if duality is not a wall, but a veil—and what lies behind it is not hidden, but only misrecognized?

DOI: 10.4324/9781003715306-13

To explore this, we must begin where psychoanalysis began: with the necessity of division. Freud's early model of repression posits the mind as a space of conflict. The ego cannot admit certain truths and so displaces, distorts, or denies them. The mind defends against what it cannot integrate. Klein intensifies this premise, introducing a model in which the infant splits its internal objects into good and bad to manage unbearable anxiety. For both, splitting is a way of surviving contradiction—a necessary violence against the unbearable.

Kernberg expands this further, suggesting that certain personality structures are defined by the failure to integrate love and aggression, self and other. In borderline states, the capacity for symbolization collapses, and experience is organized through a series of idealizations and devaluations. In this view, splitting is not merely a defense—it is a mode of being-in-the-world. The mind becomes structured by opposition: self versus other, good versus bad, safe versus threatening.

These classical formulations give us a map of the split psyche—a map of survival. But they also suggest that split is the mind's default architecture, that unity is something earned or achieved only through development or interpretation. What they rarely suggest is that unity may already be there, even in the split itself. That beneath the rupture is a continuity that was never lost—only unseen.

Roy Schafer's hermeneutic psychoanalysis opens a crucial angle here. For Schafer, identity is not a fixed state but a narrative performance—the "is" of the self is always already interpretive. He asks us to recognize that the very claim to be, to know, or to feel is a construction, a story told in time. "The patient does not have a self," Schafer might say. "The patient is engaged in selfing." This reframing reorients the analyst's task from decoding content to witnessing process. And it shifts our understanding of the split: not as a metaphysical condition, but as a style of narration, a way of carving experience into forms that appear oppositional.

Winnicott's work on transitional space reinforces this. The "third area" between subject and object—neither wholly internal nor wholly external—is not a compromise, but a paradox held. The infant's illusion that it creates the mother's breast is not a false belief to be corrected, but a necessary fiction that holds the psyche in formation. Transitional phenomena, including play, art, and cultural life, emerge not from integration but from the capacity to sustain contradiction. In Winnicott's terms, health does not eliminate paradox; it deepens the ability to live with it.

Ogden's concept of the analytic third similarly displaces binary frames. In his model, the analyst and patient do not merely interact as two autonomous minds—they generate a third field, a co-created subjectivity that neither owns. This third is not a synthesis, not a compromise between analyst and analysand, but a phenomenon that exceeds both. The analytic third is the site where language becomes atmosphere, where meaning emerges without ownership.

Michael Eigen's writing saturates this territory. For Eigen, the psyche is not a structure but a process of breathing, collapsing, fragmenting, and opening. He writes not of wholes or parts but of intensities—psychic weather. His sensitivity to the unsymbolized allows for a reading of the split not as a boundary but as a threshold. One does not cross it; one dissolves into it. And sometimes, he writes, this dissolution is the therapy.

What all of these thinkers gesture toward—in different registers—is that the division we call "split" is not absolute. It is not a wall but a curve, not a rupture but a folding. The analytic space, when held, allows this folding to be felt rather than resisted. In time, the apparent oppositions may be re-seen as modes of the same field—a field that was never broken.

Philosophically, this opens toward Heidegger's notion of *Dasein*—being as always already thrown into relation. There is no "I" apart from the world into which it is cast. Being is never private. Truth (*aletheia*) is not correspondence, but *unconcealing*—the letting-be of what already is. The work of analysis, then, is not to construct a new self from fragments, but to attune the psyche to the continuity that was obscured by the appearance of rupture.

In this sense, nonduality is not a goal. It is not a state to be achieved through enough interpretation, enough integration, or enough mindfulness. It is not the reward for surviving duality. Nonduality is what is—even when what is appears broken. It is the field in which all perception unfolds, including the perception of splitting.

To say this is not to spiritualize suffering. It is to reframe how we understand its ground. The dualities we inhabit—self/other, mind/body, love/hate—are not false. They are real in their effects, meaningful in their structure. But they are not final. They are not the ground. They are the play of form across a surface we cannot fully name, but which we sometimes feel—in moments of stillness, of symbolic collapse, of shared breath.

The split was never a break. It was always a turn—a curve in the field of perception. To see this is not to erase the wound, but to discover that the wound is already held.

The Fabrication of the Binary

What appears as two is the trace of an interpretive cut made within the continuity of a field.

To speak of a binary is to speak of a wound made thinkable. The moment two poles are named—self and other, mind and body, subject and object—a veil of clarity descends upon what was once indistinct. The binary simplifies. It draws a line where there was curvature, carves conceptual edges from affective diffusion. And yet the relief it offers—a false stability, a temporary grasp—comes at the cost of something more vital: the felt sense of continuity, the atmospheric knowing that resists symbolic severing.

We tend to speak of binaries as if they pre-exist perception—as if we encounter the world and discover its oppositions. But binaries are not discovered; they are fabricated. They are not structures we uncover but tools we reach for when the flow of experience becomes too ambiguous to hold. The mind cuts where it cannot stay. It severs in order to organize, narrate, and survive.

This insight is not foreign to psychoanalysis. From Freud onward, the psyche has been seen as a meaning-making machine—one that rearranges sensation, desire, and memory into symbolic form. But even Freud, in his theory of primary and secondary process, noted that thought itself is layered: there is a domain of free association, condensation, and displacement that operates beneath the more linear operations of rational thought. In the primary process, opposites coexist without contradiction. Time loops. Meaning slips. The binary has not yet arrived.

Derrida's philosophy of *différance* echoes this precisely. Meaning, for Derrida, is not a stable referent but a chain of deferrals. Every sign refers to other signs, never to a final truth. The binary, in this system, is not a fact but a gesture—a rhetorical maneuver that momentarily stabilizes a floating field. Derrida showed how every binary carries within it the trace of what it excludes. In naming one pole, the other is both evoked and repressed. The subject requires its object, just as light requires shadow. There is no term that does not carry its opposite as an internal ghost.

Merleau-Ponty's phenomenology furthers this by dissolving the clean edges of perception itself. He argued that we do not begin as isolated subjects observing a world "out there," but as bodily beings entangled from the start. Vision is not a detached act but a form of tactile relation. The body does not stand at a distance from the world; it folds into it. The perceived and the perceiver are part of the same visible fabric. The mind does not encounter an object; it becomes co-shaped by it.

Judith Butler, working from both psychoanalytic and post-structuralist traditions, reveals the binary as a *citational loop*. Gender, for Butler, is not an innate essence but an ongoing repetition of norms. Identity is formed through stylized acts that cite and re-cite a cultural script. The binary of male/female does not reflect a biological truth—it inscribes a symbolic frame. And yet even in this performativity, Butler locates the possibility of slippage. Every citation risks failure. Every repetition opens the door to difference. In this sense, the binary is not only fabricated—it is fragile. It depends on ongoing effort to sustain its illusion.

In analytic terms, we might say that every act of splitting requires maintenance. The borderline patient does not simply "have" a split mind—he lives inside a dynamic system of psychic labor, constantly warding off the collapse of distinction. The good object must be kept pure; the bad object must be expelled. The self must disown its aggression or risk the annihilation of coherence. But underneath this system of opposition lies a profound anxiety: what if the difference is not so clear? What if love and hate, self and other, cannot be fully separated?

Nāgārjuna, the great philosopher of the Middle Way in Mahāyāna Buddhism, articulates this with radical precision. He dismantles every ontological claim—including claims about self, time, and causality—by showing that all phenomena arise *dependently*. Nothing exists in itself; everything exists only in relation. In this framework, duality is not false per se—it is *empty*. That is, it lacks inherent essence. The appearance of difference is not a lie but a surface phenomenon, like waves on the sea. To perceive nonduality is not to erase the wave, but to remember the water.

This insight directly intersects with the psychoanalytic notion of the "third." The analyst and patient are not separate entities engaging across a divide; they are part of a dynamic field in which experience is always co-arising. The analytic third, as Ogden describes, is not a compromise between two people—it is a phenomenon that emerges *from* the space between. It serves as a reminder that perception itself is relational, and that meaning is not transmitted but generated.

Derrida's critique of presence—the idea that there is no pure origin, no full being prior to language—finds a clinical parallel in Schafer's hermeneutic approach. For Schafer, interpretation does not reveal an objective truth hidden in the patient's mind. Rather, it participates in the ongoing construction of narrative. To speak is already to have chosen a frame. The binary, in this view, is not something discovered in the mind—it is a product of analytic discourse itself.

But this does not render the analyst powerless or the patient's suffering fictional. On the contrary, it makes our ethical task more precise. If binaries are fabricated—and if this fabrication is inevitable—then we must become exquisitely attuned to *how* they are made, and what they cost. The analyst does not seek to replace dualities with oneness. Instead, the analyst invites a shift in perception—from believing in the binary's necessity to recognizing its contingency.

This shift is not merely conceptual. It is lived, felt, and embodied. In clinical work, we witness it in those moments when a patient suddenly sees that what they feared and what they desired were not opposites, but intertwined. When the person who betrayed them is also the one they longed for most. When their aggression turns out to be their deepest wish to connect. In these moments, the binary softens. Not because it has been solved, but because it has been seen through.

Nonduality, in this frame, is not a state to be attained but a *recognition to be remembered*. It is the background field in which dualities arise. To fabricate the binary is to forget the field. To witness its fabrication is to begin to remember.

This remembering is not cognitive. It is not a matter of replacing bad schemas with better ones. It is a subtle movement—a shift in mode. It feels like silence deepening in a room, like breath shared without speech, like a symbol that lingers without interpretation. It does not resolve the split; it holds it differently.

The work of this chapter is to walk that holding—not to explain it away, but to dwell within its paradox. To show how even the most entrenched psychic divides are permeable. To suggest that the mind does not live in two, but dreams in one.

And so we return to the central claim: the binary is a fabrication. It is a cut made in perception—not a reflection of truth. What appears as dual is the visible ripple of a field that was never two. The task of analysis is not to remove the ripple, but to help the patient feel the water beneath.

Perceiving the Ground: Nonduality as Mode

There is no final passage into nonduality. No state that, once reached, extinguishes the binary and crowns the subject with seamless integration. Rather, nonduality is a perceptual ground—one that is always already there, not as content but as *condition*. It is not what we see, but what seeing emerges from. The dualities of mind/body, self/other, presence/absence do not obstruct this ground; they arise within it. The task, then, is not to transcend form, but to become aware of the ground from which form arises.

This awareness does not occur at the level of conceptual affirmation. It occurs at the level of mode. That is, the difference between dual and nondual is not primarily about content but *about how experience is held*. In one mode, we perceive the world through distinction: this versus that, here versus there, now versus then. In another mode, we perceive not through separation but through texture—a continuity in which difference becomes relational rather than oppositional. The shift is subtle. Often, it is not even noticed until it recedes.

Consider the experience of lying in bed with someone you love, just before sleep. The room is dim. Your breathing begins to slow. Their warmth is present beside you, yet neither of you speaks. There is no need to name. In that moment, you are aware of them not as a separate object but as part of the same ambient field. If they shifted, you would feel it in your own chest. This is not fusion. It is not loss of self. It is a recognition: their presence and your presence are not two. They are two expressions of the same atmosphere. When the mind does not attempt to divide, perception rests.

Such moments are not rare. They appear and vanish throughout ordinary life—often unmarked. A pause in conversation. A shared gaze with a patient that slips beneath language. The silence that follows a profound disclosure. These are not "nondual states" as exceptional phenomena. They are *modes of perception* that soften the grip of oppositional thinking. And though fleeting, they can be recognized—and cultivated.

Loewald offers an analytic framework for this. His model of symbolization suggests that psychic life becomes vital when the symbolic is not abstracted from experience, but *suffused with presence*. That is, when language resonates with affect, and form becomes transparent to depth. In such moments, the symbol is not merely a stand-in for the thing—it is a portal. It carries the texture of what it points to. The analytic space becomes nondual not when dualities are resolved, but when symbols begin to shimmer—both form and field at once.

This shimmering lies at the heart of what I have called recognition reversal. When a patient finally finds the words to name an experience that has haunted them silently—say, a childhood moment of ambiguous violation or a lifelong sense of dissociation—there is often a surprising collapse. One might expect catharsis, but what follows is often emptiness. As if the unspeakable, once spoken, loses its gravitational pull. The naming doesn't integrate; it dissolves. The form collapses. The patient stares into the space where the unsymbolized had lived. And in that moment, if the analyst is attuned, both are standing at the edge of language—where duality fails to hold.

This is not simply about the limits of symbolization. It is about its ground. The recognition that what appeared to be a truth hidden in darkness was, in fact, a mode of the light all along. The analyst does not need to fill the emptiness. They need only not flee from it. For here, the nondual appears—not as a mystical state, but as a quality of presence that requires no structure to stabilize it.

This orientation also allows us to revisit the very structure of the analytic dyad. The analyst and analysand are not two discrete minds exchanging insight across a shared frame. They are participants in a field of unfolding awareness—a field that sometimes sharpens into interpretation, but often softens into attunement. The split mind does not belong to either one of them; it belongs to the intersubjective field. Likewise, the moments when that split seems to dissolve do not belong to either. They are modes of the field itself—ephemeral, recursive, real.

The Buddhist traditions of Mahāmudrā and Dzogchen name this field directly. In Mahāmudrā, the "nature of mind" is described as clarity inseparable from emptiness. Thoughts arise like waves on water—distinct, yet never apart from the sea. In Dzogchen, the instruction is not to stop thought, nor to replace negative thoughts with positive ones, but to recognize the *empty radiance* of thought itself. The problem is not that thoughts arise—it is that we take them to be solid. In the same way, psychoanalytic dualities are not mistakes. They are recognitions viewed from a certain mode. When the mode shifts, the duality is seen for what it is: form shimmering within formlessness.

The paradox here is essential: one cannot force nonduality into view. To try is to reintroduce duality—self trying to grasp not-self. The field appears when effort softens, when perception returns to what it already knew. In clinical work, this often happens in moments of failure. The patient says something devastating, and the analyst finds no words. A long silence unfolds. The analyst resists the urge to interpret. And then, something opens. Not always. But sometimes. The field makes itself felt—not as content, but as presence.

This presence can be disorienting. For both patient and analyst, it can feel like the ground falling away. But it is not annihilation. It is a subtle recollection: this, too, is mind. Even the silence, even the not-knowing. Especially the not-knowing. As Eigen writes, *There is a kind of knowing that begins with failure*. This failure—the failure to split, to categorize, to explain—is not a deficit. It is a doorway.

We might say, then, that nonduality is a kind of ethical stance. Not in the moralistic sense, but in the Levinasian sense: a relation that precedes identity. The analyst, in this view, does not offer a position. They offer *space*. A space in which the patient's subjectivity can unfold without having to resolve itself into coherence. This does not mean the analyst is absent—quite the opposite. It means their presence is not aimed at closure, but at deepening the field in which recognition becomes possible.

That field is always already nondual. The dualities we work with—ego and id, analyst and analysand, good breast and bad breast—are symbolic tools. They matter. They orient us. But they are tools within a larger space. The analyst must know the tool is not the ground. To do otherwise is to mistake the map for the territory, the vessel for the sea.

Here, the psychoanalytic and the mystical touch. Not because they become the same, but because they both return us to a space prior to formulation. A space that is not empty in the sense of lacking, but in the sense of being too full to grasp. A space in which difference unfolds, but does not divide.

The patient's rage, their longing, their erotic transferences—all appear within this field. They are not illusions to be undone. They are vital expressions of the psyche's attempt to make contact. The analyst's role is not to neutralize them, but to receive them as forms. Not "just" transference, but symbols with gravity. And behind them, always, the field—unbroken, unnamed.

Nonduality is not the end of analysis. It is its substrate. It is what makes analysis possible: the quiet intuition that even in our most divided moments, something is holding. We may not see it. But we are seen within it.

This is not a theory to be mastered. It is a mode to be remembered—and re-remembered—each time the mind forgets and splits again.

Duality as Method: Symbol, Ritual, and the Path through Form

We do not reach the nondual by avoiding form. We reach it by entering form fully—by surrendering to the very rituals, symbols, and dualities that seem to obscure it. In this sense, duality is not an obstacle to the nondual, but its expression. The paradox is not to be solved but walked: the truth of nonduality discloses itself through the forms that conceal it.

This is as true in the analytic setting as it is in contemplative traditions. The patient speaks in symbols, repeats rituals of self-revelation and self-concealment. The analyst participates in these forms—not to transcend them, but to metabolize their movement. The dyad becomes a vessel: not a container of fixed identities, but a ritualized space in which the symbolic elaboration of experience becomes a method of opening, not of closure.

Ritual, by nature, marks a boundary. It says: here is the sacred, here is the profane. But in marking that line, it also gestures toward its arbitrariness. The line is symbolic, not ontological. This is the insight of all initiatory traditions—and of deep analytic work. The patient arrives with a wound, seeking a cure. But the healing is not in erasing the wound. It is in circling it, symbolizing it, allowing it to become a site of relation. The ritual of session—the hour, the frame, the repetition—creates a form through which the formless can appear.

Donnel Stern's work on *unformulated experience* is pivotal here. He shows how much of what shapes the psyche never enters symbolization directly. It remains unspoken, unthought, yet formative. The analytic task is not to force these experiences into language, but to create the conditions in which they might emerge. The analyst becomes a ritual partner—not one who "knows," but one who holds the possibility of meaning as something that can *become*.

This emergence often takes the form of symbol. And symbols, as Loewald reminds us, are not abstract representations. They are condensations of presence and absence. A symbol holds what is no longer there and yet still felt. It is a trace that speaks. In this way, the symbol is dual, pointing both to the manifest and the latent. It contains difference, yet it vibrates with connection.

This dual nature is its power. The symbol does not resolve tension—it sustains it. It holds contradiction in suspended animation. This is precisely what allows it to open into the nondual: not by collapsing the poles, but by revealing them as folded. The sacred and the profane, the analyst and the patient, the trauma and the desire—these are not discrete nodes but expressions of a field that becomes visible through their relation.

In Vajrayāna Buddhism, this is formalized through *sādhanā*—visualization and mantra practices in which the practitioner inhabits duality as a method of dissolution. One visualizes a deity—often fearsome, often erotic—and merges with it not by denying its form, but by embodying it. The paradox is explicit: by fully enacting the form, one recognizes its emptiness. The symbol is not discarded. It is passed through.

This parallels the psychoanalytic use of transferential forms. The analyst does not avoid becoming the bad parent, the idealized lover, the feared betrayer. They become these things—within the ritual frame—so that their structure can be metabolized. To engage the transferential form is not to indulge fantasy, but to reveal its construction. The transference is a path, not a detour.

Jessica Benjamin's theory of mutual recognition offers a particularly powerful rendering of this. She argues that subjectivity is not a given but an achievement—one made possible through the dance of recognition and misrecognition. In her formulation, the *third* is not a static entity but an emergent space—a ritual field in which self and other are both held and decentered. This third space is inherently dual—it requires two poles—and yet it points beyond them.

What emerges in that space is not fusion, but rhythmic alternation: the back-and-forth of being seen and seeing, of surrendering and asserting. This rhythm is the ritual heartbeat of analytic work. And within it, something nondual shimmers: not as a synthesis, but as the very texture of relation. As in sādhanā, the path is through—not around—the form.

The mistake—both in spiritual practice and in analysis—is to try to leapfrog over form, to reach the "real" directly. This leads to dissociation, not realization. The nondual cannot be grasped. It can only be *remembered*—and the act of remembering is always mediated by form. This is why psychoanalysis, like ritual, moves slowly. Why we repeat. Why we symbolize, then resymbolize. Why we circle.

The repetition is not redundancy. It is refinement. Like the sculptor returning to the same curve, or the devotee reciting the same mantra, the analytic process moves by *rhythmic return*. Each repetition is not the same. It bends slightly—orbiting the invisible, tracing the unspeakable.

Repetition compulsion, in this light, is not merely pathology. It is the psyche's effort to approach the real by way of symbol. The patient repeats the same enactments, not because they are irrational, but because the form has not yet yielded its emptiness. The analyst's task is not to block repetition, but to participate in it differently—to become a witness who does not reinforce the form's solidity, but helps it soften. This is what it means to turn the symptom into a path.

Ritual does the same. In every tradition that uses symbolic form—psychoanalytic, religious, artistic—the aim is not to believe in the symbol but to pass through it. The form becomes a vehicle. It invites the participant into a field in which something greater than the self becomes present—not as an object, but as a *mode*.

Even Lacan's dense symbolic architecture gestures toward this. The Real, for Lacan, is not what is outside the symbolic, but what disrupts it from within. The Real erupts in moments when the symbolic order stutters—when the subject encounters something that cannot be metabolized, yet cannot be ignored. But even here, the Real does not appear in isolation. It appears through the form—through the very failure of the symbol to contain it. The symptom, the slip, the dream—these are not detours. They are rituals of rupture.

The dual, then, is not the opposite of the nondual. It is its edge. Its skin. The mistake is to treat the dual as a deception. The wiser approach is to treat it as a threshold—one that can be crossed not by negating it, but by entering it completely.

This is what we do in analysis. We enter the transferential form, the repetition, the symptom. We inhabit the split—not to solve it, but to feel its seam. And in that seam, the field opens. The dual becomes porous. The symbol becomes radiant. And the patient, perhaps, glimpses that their suffering has always been a form—and that behind the form, something holds.

This glimpse is not the end of work. It is a bend in the orbit. The patient returns the next week. The ritual continues. The analyst forgets, remembers, forgets again. But something has shifted. Not in content. In mode. The binary is not gone—but it is known differently. And that knowing is not a thought. It is a presence.

This presence is the nondual. Not beyond form, but within it. Not after the binary, but folded inside it. The path is through.

The Split That Knows It Is Whole

The psyche does not heal by becoming seamless. It heals by becoming capable of holding its seams. To split is not to break—it is to bend perception through a mode that temporarily forgets its own continuity. And yet, even in the act of forgetting, something remembers. The part that dissociates retains, by its very absence, the trace of its connection. The part-object, even in its isolation, glows with the echo of the whole. This, too, is nonduality: the broken that was never truly apart.

To internalize paradox is to become capable of symbolizing from within it. This is a psychic development—one that cannot be rushed. It unfolds unevenly, through layers of collapse and reorganization. The mind that splits without knowing it is split will mistake form for truth. The mind that begins to suspect its own dualities are nested in a wider field begins to turn. Not away from division, but toward it—with curiosity, even reverence. The symptom is no longer an error. It becomes a portal.

Michael Eigen, in his work on the "wound of being," gives us language for this. He speaks of the self not as a stable entity, but as a constellation of openings— each one a passage between presence and absence, between the formed and the unformulated. The self, in this view, is porous. It bleeds. But the bleeding is not failure. It is permeability. It allows resonance. It allows the field to move through.

This porousness is what allows paradox to take root psychically. Without it, the mind clings to coherence, to categorical clarity, to the fantasy of integration without ambiguity. But a deeper development—one that unfolds through the very labor of analysis—makes it possible to hold contradiction as truth. Not a dialectical synthesis, but a shimmering: the false self that protects the real, the idealization that masks rage but also carries hope, the erotic transference that is both defense and offering. These are not errors to be corrected. They are folds in the field.

The self that knows it is split, and does not collapse, is a self that has begun to remember the ground. This memory is not narrative. It is affective, atmospheric, and often wordless. It comes in waves—not as knowledge, but as *feelings of coherence within incoherence*. A patient says, "I feel like I'm disappearing, but not in a bad way." Another says, "It's like I'm watching myself be two people, and somehow I'm still me." These are not signs of disintegration. They are signs of symbolic recursion: the psyche watching itself watch itself, and finding in that loop not terror, but texture.

The analytic process often deepens this recursion. A patient remembers a dream, and as they describe it, they notice their description is already forming another image. The analyst points this out, and suddenly the dream shifts— not in content, but in atmosphere. It becomes a space, not a message. The interpretation does not land as a solution, but as a breath. The room feels different. Something has turned.

This turning is not dramatic. It is gravitational. It is what happens when form begins to feel its own field. The patient still dissociates, still regresses, still idealizes or attacks—but something in them *knows*. Not in the egoic sense, but in the deep, folded way that bodies know. This knowing is the split that knows it is whole. It does not collapse into integration. It hovers at the threshold.

This is where paradox becomes not just a theoretical construct but a *mode of psychic life*. The analyst must be able to hold it in themselves first. A patient says something cruel, and the analyst feels both wounded and grateful. Another reenacts a seduction, and the analyst feels both desire and sadness. These are not problems to be resolved. They are conditions to be recognized. The analyst becomes a site where paradox is metabolized—not for the patient, but with them.

It is here that Winnicott's idea of the "capacity to be alone in the presence of another" becomes useful. In that space, the analyst does not intrude, does not interpret prematurely. They witness—not passively, but as a presence that does not need to fix. This presence allows the patient to feel their own multiplicity without rupture. The analyst is not the unifying object. They are the space in which the fragments can resonate without pressure to fuse.

This is where the nondual appears again—not in content, but in mode. The patient is allowed to be two, or ten, or unformed. The analyst does not respond with "which is real?" but with "what is this like, right now?" The question is not to resolve, but to be with. To hold the form until its transparency becomes felt.

Philosophically, we might say this is the movement from ontology to phenomenology. From "what is it?" to "how is it appearing?" Heidegger's "clearing" (Lichtung) offers a parallel here—the idea that Being is not an object but an opening, a space in which things come into presence. The analyst, then, becomes this clearing—not as a container, but as a field.

The implications are ethical. The more the analyst can hold paradox, the more they model a way of being that does not collapse into either solution or avoidance. This is not neutrality in the classical sense. It is fidelity to the field. A fidelity that allows the patient to trust that even their most unbearable splits are not evidence of failure, but expressions of form within a larger wholeness.

This mode becomes internalized. The patient begins to speak differently. Their metaphors change. They start saying "part of me" rather than "I." They begin to narrate their symptoms not just as complaints, but as symbols. They still suffer—but the suffering feels different. It has edges now. It has echoes. It is not the only voice.

At times, this internalization takes the form of recursive imagery. A patient dreams of a room inside a room, or a mirror reflecting another mirror. These are not just symbols of confusion. They are images of the psyche encountering itself in layers. In these dreams, the analyst may appear—not as a figure of rescue, but as a kind of witness-object: someone who watches the watcher. This recursive witnessing is the clinical counterpart of the shift in mode we have been tracking throughout the chapter.

The split that knows it is whole is not a synthesis. It is a climate. An atmosphere in which the subject can be multiple without collapse, affectively porous without being flooded, and symbolically saturated without the pressure of coherence. The mind continues to split—but now the split curves back toward the self. Not a straight line of insight, but an orbit.

This orbit is not random. It has gravity. And that gravity is what analysis becomes at its most profound: not an excavation, but a returning. Not a working-through in the classical sense, but a *being-with* until something opens.

The analyst's job is not to push this process forward. It is to make it safe enough for it to happen. That safety is not just emotional. It is structural. It is temporal. It is the commitment to remain present even when meaning has not yet arrived.

For in the absence of meaning, a different kind of knowing becomes possible. A knowing that is not about integration, but about texture. A knowing that does not need to resolve paradox, but to breathe within it.

And this, perhaps, is the most radical implication of nonduality in clinical work: not that we can heal the split, but that we can learn to stay with it—and in that staying, remember that the split was never outside the whole.

Clinical Interlude: "I Can't Tell What's Me"

The first time Jonah said it, he looked away immediately, ashamed by the admission: "I can't tell what's me."

He wasn't speaking metaphorically. The statement emerged with a bodily tremor, a slackening in the musculature of his voice. He had been recounting an argument with his partner, in which he found himself behaving in a way he described as "possessed." Harsh, manipulative, even seductive—and yet none of it felt like his intention. "It was like I was watching myself," he said. "But also like I had no idea who was watching."

Jonah had been in treatment for over a year, but it was only in recent months that this affective register had begun to surface. Previously, he had described his inner world in clever abstractions—highly articulate, but distanced. The language was precise but uninhabited. Emotions were categorized but not felt. He often framed psychic pain as a narrative problem to be solved, as though the act of interpretation could evacuate the feeling.

What marked this session was not just what he said, but how it landed in the room. His words did not seek clarification or solution. They simply hovered. "I can't tell what's me."

Instead of responding with immediate interpretation, I remained quiet. The silence wasn't strategic. It was a felt response to the shift in texture—something in the room had folded inward. The symbolic skin around Jonah's self-experience had gone translucent. I felt it in my own body, too—a slight dissociation, like the floor was subtly vibrating.

He noticed. "You feel that too?"

"What does it feel like to you?" I asked.

"Like there's a film over everything. Like I'm in here," he gestured to his chest, "but I don't know if that means it's me."

This moment marked a threshold. Jonah was not simply dissociating; he was witnessing his dissociation. Not from outside it, but from within the fold. This recursive awareness—of being split, and of the impossibility of pinning down the real—was not a sign of decompensation. It was, paradoxically, a movement toward self-contact.

We stayed with the sensation. We didn't analyze it, not yet. Jonah began to describe how these moments often happened during sex or in the aftermath of conflict. "I become like… a character. Someone I've played before. I can feel myself in the role, but I can't feel myself inside the feeling. It's like wearing someone else's skin."

I asked gently, "Do you think the role protects you?"

He thought for a long time. "It protects me from being seen in the wrong light. But it also makes sure I'm never fully seen."

The analytic third thickened here. We were no longer merely speaking about dissociation. We were inside it, co-holding its symbolic structure. I could feel the multiplicity in the room: the Jonah who needed to perform, the Jonah who watched the performance, and the Jonah who now wanted something else.

When I later spoke to this in supervision, I described it as a "moment of folded witnessing." The patient was not reintegrating in a classical sense; he was hovering in a different psychic mode—one that allowed him to inhabit his own division without collapsing.

Jonah's history contained all the familiar coordinates: a narcissistically fragile mother who vacillated between engulfing affection and icy withdrawal; a father who punished ambiguity with sarcasm. In childhood, Jonah learned that clarity—or the performance of it—was survival. Ambivalence was not allowed. Affect had to be readable, not merely felt. His childhood self became a curator of affect, presenting what would please and deleting what might confuse.

So when Jonah said, "I can't tell what's me," it wasn't a breakdown. It was a remembering. He was contacting the part of himself that had been edited out of psychic legibility. Not in a way that demanded reintegration, but in a way that made the very category of "me" feel porous.

Over the following weeks, this porousness deepened. Jonah began experimenting with letting moments hang unclosed. "I don't know what I feel" became a new kind of statement—not a failure, but a way of marking presence. Sometimes he would say, "I want to leave this sentence unfinished."

There were also ruptures. He missed a session and claimed it was a scheduling mix-up, but we both felt it as an enactment. When he returned, he said, "I wanted to know if the space would still be here if I didn't hold it."

This, too, was a symbol. His absence was not a departure, but a gesture. A form. A ritual of inquiry. Would the third hold even if he let go?

We talked about these patterns as echoes, not mistakes. We spoke of his erotic life, his fantasy of being overpowered and held. "It's like I want to be known without performing," he said. "But also without disintegrating."

Eventually, Jonah said something I had never heard from him: "Sometimes I think the part that performs is trying to protect the part that watches. And the part that watches is trying to protect the part that feels."

This was not just insight. It was nested subjectivity. He was symbolizing his own folds. He was beginning to live, consciously, inside the recursive structure of his own psyche. The split was no longer a gap. It was a spiral.

He no longer asked, "Which part is real?" Instead, he wondered, "What does this part know?"

In that shift, something opened. Not a resolution. A mode. A field.

That is where we end this section. The clinical vignette as lived paradox: the self that can be multiple without rupture, recursive without collapse, and symbolically held in a form that reveals its own transparency.

Jonah is still in treatment. He still splits. He still performs. But now, even the performance glows faintly with awareness. And the analyst, too, is changed— no longer seeking the whole self behind the fragments, but listening for the field in which the fragments cohere, shimmer, and turn. These fragments are not failures of integration, but gravitational anchors—part-objects that sustain coherence without demanding wholeness. In the next chapter, we follow their orbit more closely.

And perhaps it is not the fragments that require unification, but our way of seeing them.

9 Symbolizing the Light

Emptiness, Form, and the Clinical Imagination

Building on the perceptual ground of nonduality, this chapter explores how symbolic form emerges within and from emptiness. Drawing from Dzogchen, tantric visualization practices, and contemporary psychoanalytic models of symbolization and witnessing, this chapter examines the paradox of naming that which is unspeakable. Clinical vignettes illustrate how the analyst's presence may serve as a symbolic container for emptiness, allowing previously unformulated experience to shimmer into symbolic life. Symbolization is reframed not as filling absence, but as giving shape to light. This chapter closes with reflections on mantra, visualization, and clinical poiesis as shared technologies of transformation.

Symbol, Spiral, Field

A symbol is not a solution. It is a condensation, a folding—of affect, perception, memory, and potentiality—into a form that both reveals and conceals. In analytic work, we tend to treat symbols as bridges between the unconscious and the ego, or between affect and representation. But in the nondual field, the symbol is not just a connector; it is an atmosphere. It does not point to a reality behind it, but radiates the simultaneity of presence and absence. It is not a sign for something else—it *is* the elsewhere, materialized.

In Jonah's case, the sentence "I can't tell what's me" functioned not merely as a signifier of confusion or dissociation. It was a **symbol of recursive witnessing**, a condensation of the impossibility of pure self-reference—an analytic echo of the paradox: *this sentence is false*. The symbol here does not organize the mind around coherence, but holds the **spiral structure** of incoherence as form. It is not interpreted but inhabited.

The spiral becomes a powerful metaphor for this type of symbolic logic. Unlike a circle, the spiral does not return to the same point—it returns to a point that resembles the prior, but on a different plane. Each repetition is a **recurrence with difference**, a re-contact with something that has never quite been touched in the same way. In trauma, the spiral may constrict; in healing, it may widen. But the structure remains the same: **folded return**.

DOI: 10.4324/9781003715306-14

Where interpretation seeks to move us forward, the spiral **holds us in orbit**. Interpretation suggests we might exit the pattern once we understand it. But spiral temporality makes no such promise. It suggests instead that truth is *re-contact*, not *discovery*. Symbolic truth, in this model, is recursive, saturated, and partially known. It is lived in the field between people. The analytic frame is not just a structure in which symbols appear, but a field that allows symbols to unfold *as presence*—curving inward, flaring outward, drawing analyst and patient into an aesthetic of shared gravity.

We might say the analytic symbol is less like a word and more like a **gesture**—a precise, charged motion that transmits meaning by participating in the field of relation. It cannot be reduced to interpretation alone. As Bollas suggested, certain experiences—like the "unthought known"—are not meant to be decoded, but *held*. In this view, the symbol functions less as a translation of the unconscious into conscious terms and more as an atmospheric event: something that modifies the field of perception between analyst and analysand.

Jonah's repeated statements—"I don't know if I'm real," "I can't tell who's watching," "I want to leave this sentence unfinished"—came to act as symbolic forms in exactly this sense. Not confessions, not insights, but **invitations into the spiral**. Their repetition did not signify stagnation or resistance; it signaled the emergence of a **topological logic**—one that curved instead of progressed. These utterances marked moments of *suspended form*, where the psychic frame thickened rather than clarified. The symbol, here, was not moving toward meaning, but **holding space for mode**.

This is precisely where classical interpretations fall short. When we rush to decode the symbol, we lose its **fractal nature**—its quality of containing both self-reference and atmospheric resonance. In Jonah's case, the statement "I can't tell what's me" wasn't a failure of ego boundaries. It was a **symbolic event** that *performed* the recursive structure of his psyche, and in doing so, reconfigured the analytic space as one capable of containing **non-integration** without collapse.

The spiral form allows for this holding. Unlike a regression or a rupture that demands containment, the spiral enables an *aesthetic coexistence* of parts. It's not that the patient becomes integrated, but that the symbolic field around them **widens**, allowing contradictions to stand in proximity. In this widened field, symbols can act without being reduced to signifiers. They shimmer—holding the unspeakable in articulated form.

Analytic presence, then, must adapt. The analyst must develop a **spiralic listening**—a capacity to return to the same words, the same affective punctures, again and again, but never in the same posture. The repetition is not redundant. It's gravitational. It binds analyst and patient in a **nonlinear orbit**, one that traces meaning not through interpretation but through *attunement to field*.

To listen spirally is to resist the analyst's habitual desire to fix, resolve, or organize. It allows the session to bend back on itself without flattening its texture. It is to recognize that some symbols are **lived fragments of a nondual field**—signs that do not reference a hidden whole, but enact the paradox that the part is already the whole, refracted.

We see this in the language of dreams, which often arrives bearing symbols not meant to be decoded but felt as atmospheres. A patient brings in a dream of an empty room, bathed in orange light, with a mirror that reflects nothing. In classical analysis, the mirror might signify the absence of self-image, the light a form of affect. But in the nondual register, the dream is not just *about* something—it is *itself* an affective condensation. The dream is a field event: an articulation of space, mood, and mode that invites the analyst into a **shared perceptual state**.

These moments cannot be approached through the lens of mastery. They require what Thomas Ogden called **reverie**—a form of psychic openness in which the analyst allows the field to shape their own consciousness. It is here that the analyst becomes a kind of **symbolic receptor**, not because they decode what the patient is saying, but because they feel what the patient cannot symbolize directly. The analyst becomes, in effect, a participant in the symbolic spiral: not outside the patient's system of meaning, but curving within it.

This spiral structure also has implications for temporality. In traditional analytic theory, progress is often conceptualized linearly: the patient works through material, insight leads to transformation, and integration follows. But in nondual temporality, the psyche does not move forward so much as **deepen in recursive rhythms**. Healing is not a climb; it is a **looped re-contact** with what has always already been there. The analytic relationship becomes a space where these loops are neither pathologized nor idealized, but simply *inhabited*.

At times, these loops feel like regressions, but they are not. They are repetitions in the service of symbolic expansion. The patient returns to a wound not to be cured, but to recontact the symbolic conditions of their formation. The analyst is not a guide but a **witness to symbolic recurrence**—holding the loop open long enough for new forms of psychic gravity to emerge.

In such moments, symbol becomes field, and field becomes self. The dualities collapse—not because they are resolved, but because their **differentiation is no longer the organizing principle**.

This is the paradox at the heart of nondual symbolic life: that even fragmentation can be held as wholeness, if the field in which it unfolds is stable, porous, and alive. The spiral allows us to name this paradox without attempting to solve it. It holds the idea that multiplicity is not evidence of loss, and that symbolic form is not a map to coherence, but a **resonance field** where coherence need not be imposed.

In the consulting room, this resonance is felt in the silent intervals as much as in language. It is sensed when the patient's voice thickens, when a phrase is repeated with no clear reason, when the analyst feels suspended in a shared ambiguity. These are not errors of technique or lapses in clarity. They are the **textures of a symbolic field unfolding in real time**, curling into itself, widening, refracting, allowing new angles of contact.

The work, then, is not to anchor the self in stable meaning, but to support the patient in learning how to live inside the spiral. This is not disorganization;

it is **symbolic gravity**—a mode of selfing in which nonduality is not a goal, but a baseline. A psychic backdrop against which dualities shimmer into form and dissolve again.

We do not integrate the parts. We orbit them. We spiral through them. And in doing so, we allow the field to speak in a language prior to form, where the real is not separate from the symbolic, and the self is not other than the atmosphere in which it unfolds.

Nonduality as Recognition Mode

The world appears split, but the split is a perceptual event, not an ontological truth. Nonduality is not a mystical ideal or theological claim—it is a way of *seeing*. A mode of recognition in which division is understood as artifact, not essence. To say "nonduality" is not to erase difference, but to perceive it as folded—part of a continuous topology where edges imply curvature, not rupture.

The psyche misrecognizes itself as dual. This misrecognition is not a failure of insight, but a structural reflex: to become conscious is to feel as if there is a seer and a seen, a knower and a known. But this split is recursive. The mind, looking for its own ground, creates an image of itself that it then mistakes for truth. The symbol turns opaque. The mirror becomes a surface. And the gaze forgets that it, too, is being looked through.

Wittgenstein described the phenomenon of "aspect seeing"—the sudden switch in recognition, like when a drawing shifts from duck to rabbit. Nothing changes in the form itself, only the *mode* of apprehension. Nonduality enters through this shift. It is not that form disappears, but that its edges become porous. What once seemed fixed becomes rhythmic. The observer is no longer outside the scene but entangled in it. The background becomes foreground. The knower dissolves into the act of knowing.

This is not insight. It is not symbolization. It is not understanding in the analytic sense. It is **recognition reversal**: a loosening of the perceptual split that organizes subject and object into opposing terms. The patient says, "I remembered it again, but it felt different this time." Not because the memory changed—but because the *field* in which it appeared was no longer dual.

To recognize nonduality is not to transcend form but to **see form differently**. The duck-rabbit is still a rabbit. The mirror still reflects. The patient still suffers. But the texture of experience is no longer constrained by the fantasy of separate states. Duality loses its authority. The self and the other begin to blur—not into fusion, but into a shared field that was always already there.

In Dzogchen practice, the analogy is often made between mind and sky: thoughts are clouds that come and go, but the sky itself is untouched. Yet the sky is not separate from the clouds. It is neither a container nor a background. It is *that which allows appearances to appear*. When we say "nondual," we are referring to that quality of awareness which holds form without identifying with it. The analyst, in this light, becomes less an interpreter of contents and more a **field condition** in which recognition can shift.

This shift is not willed. It cannot be taught or explained. It emerges spontaneously, often subtly, in the folds of relational presence. A patient who has told the same story dozens of times suddenly pauses—not because the story is different, but because something in the field has softened. The analyst is quieter than usual. A silence holds. The words arrive with less urgency. The narrative collapses into image. The patient says, "It feels like I'm watching it happen for the first time."

This is not dissociation. It is **recontact from a different mode of awareness**. The story has not changed, but its symbolic density has. The image is not "remembered" so much as re-recognized: not as a fact, but as a **form within a field**. This shift is subtle, but its impact is tectonic. The patient is no longer the same subject speaking to the same other. The grammar of duality has dissolved. The analytic space, for a moment, becomes a mirror that does not reflect but absorbs.

This is the clinical face of nonduality—not a content, but a shift in **how perception is held**. The analyst does not *reveal* the truth, but lives beside the patient as the mode of recognition begins to melt.

To see differently is not to see more—it is to let go of the frame that organizes seeing. In this way, nonduality is not a theory of mind, but a **suspension of the implicit split** on which theory depends. The analyst does not guide the patient toward integration as an endpoint but holds open a space in which the false oppositions—self/other, past/present, subject/object—begin to shimmer. These are not opposites to be resolved but folds in the same field, distinctions that only appear when viewed from within the structure of misrecognition.

Sometimes the shift is heralded by a collapse. The patient breaks off mid-sentence, suddenly uncertain of their own point. "I don't know what I was saying," they confess. But instead of anxiety, a strange quiet arrives. Something opens. "It's like I stopped trying to be in it," they murmur, "and now I'm just *with* it." This is not regression, nor disintegration. It is the temporary failure of dualistic grammar—and with it, the emergence of something more elemental.

We might call this **symbolic transparency**—a state in which form is still present but no longer opaque. The narrative becomes light enough to see through. This transparency is not emptiness in the nihilistic sense, but in the Buddhist one: *śūnyatā* as spaciousness, the absence of self-nature that allows phenomena to arise. In the analytic field, this shows up not as disembodiment but as a **felt shift in gravity**. The self is no longer the center. Meaning no longer accumulates toward the ego. Instead, presence radiates outward in quiet waves of shared noticing.

In this state, the analytic encounter resembles the Dzogchen metaphor of a crystal illuminated from within. Nothing new is added, but the internal radiance changes everything. The story that once seemed solid becomes prismatic. The identity that once felt fixed begins to refract. The patient no longer seeks to be known but sits, almost silently, in a kind of shared awareness where the drive to be understood has relaxed. There is still form, still difference, still subjectivity. But the mode of holding all this has **curved toward the nondual**.

What shifts, ultimately, is not the content of the patient's narrative but the **site from which they recognize it**. This is the heart of nonduality—not a fusion, not a mystical union, but a realignment of the psychic gaze. Duality is not removed; it is *reframed*. Like the moon glimpsed from a moving train, it appears to follow us only because we mistake our own motion for its position. The analyst, in this metaphor, does not stop the train. They sit beside the patient and look out the window until, together, they begin to see the illusion for what it is.

Recognition, in this mode, becomes spacious. There is no longer a need to collapse complexity into coherence. The unspeakable is not forced into language, but allowed to **hover**. The analyst's presence becomes an atmosphere—a holding pattern that does not interpret but companions. And in this space, the symbolic begins to breathe again, no longer crushed by the pressure to explain.

The patient leaves the session not "with insight," but with **a different curvature of awareness**. They still remember. Still feel. Still suffer. But something has shifted in the holding field. The dualities—between inside and outside, between memory and present, between being and becoming—no longer organize their experience with the same gravity. Something unnamed has softened.

Nonduality, then, is not a truth behind appearances. It is the *field in which appearances appear*. It is not the content of experience, but the recognition that all content is already curved. That even duality is held, always, within the larger topology of nonduality—like waves rising and falling from a sea that never leaves them.

And it is in that sea that analytic presence floats, listens, and refracts—holding the patient not at the edge of insight, but at the **rim of recognition**, where the mind folds inward and the self begins to glimmer.

The Nondual Ground of Form

The concept of a "form" presupposes a background—a contrast space against which its edges are made visible. In perception, this often takes the shape of figure and ground. In psychoanalysis, it manifests as the formation of psychic content against the blank field of what is not yet known. But this contrast is illusory. The background is not outside the form; it is **within** it. Nonduality begins not with the collapse of form, but with the recognition that form and ground are the *same field*, temporarily refracted.

Every form is a condensation. It is a local thickening of the field—a moment of emphasis, like a note struck within a larger harmony. The patient says, "That's when I knew," or "I became that version of myself," and in doing so, marks a figure. But the analyst hears the surroundings. The hesitation before the word. The breath that punctuates the sentence. The form is not self-contained—it is co-emergent with its atmosphere. This is not a metaphor. It is the **topology of psychic reality**, where what appears to be discrete is already shaped by what holds it.

Freud's part-objects were not merely fragments of a whole, but carriers of concentrated libidinal meaning. The breast is not a symbol of the mother; it is a locus of encounter, a radiant form suspended within the infant's field of bodily and affective saturation. Klein extended this idea toward a theory of splitting, in which objects are not just part-whole but good-bad, desired-feared, sacred-profane. Yet even in these early dualisms, something nondual pulses. The part-object is not only split; it is **hyper-symbolic**. Its potency arises not from its internal attributes but from its gravitational role in the field of the infant's emerging psychic map.

To glimpse this is to sense that the object is not simply represented—it is **lit from within**. The breast, the voice, the gaze: each a form, but also a carrier wave. In the analytic field, these part-objects are not reconstructed wholes. They are **portals**, momentary crystallizations of what the field itself desires to express.

In this way, the part-object becomes a gateway—not back to some original unity, but into the **nondual structure of experience** itself. The split is not a rupture between real and symbol, but a shimmer, a trembling along the axis of attention. This is why the patient returns again and again to the same image, the same dream, the same ache. Not because it is unresolved, but because it **radiates**. The object pulses with the force of the field. It becomes a site where language and pre-language converge, where the symbolic loses its linearity and becomes atmospheric.

We might think here of Bion's notion of "O"—the unknowable, the unrepresentable truth that cannot be known directly but must be *become*. "O" is not content. It is not interpretation. It is a mode of presence, a gravity. To approach O is not to integrate meaning but to tolerate the collapse of form as the only route to meaning. This is not a breakdown but a **folding inward**. Form is held more lightly, more transparently, as if the analyst and patient are gazing through it from opposite sides of a one-way mirror.

In such moments, recognition becomes luminous. The patient no longer says, "I understand," but rather, "I see it all differently." This difference is not cognitive. It is **textural**. A face becomes less accusatory. A memory no longer feels like a verdict. The self is not reassembled, but *reconditioned*—held within a new curvature of relation. The analyst is not outside this shift. They feel it in the body: a tingling in the spine, a wave of stillness, a kind of vertical settling that signals a resonance too subtle for speech.

This is why nonduality is not a belief but a **clinical climate**. It is not imposed, but arrives—like weather, like grace. The form remains. The pain still stings. The past still echoes. However, it is now all held in a different grammar, one that does not oppose but includes. The symbolic becomes *diaphanous*, not in the sense of fading, but in becoming transparent to the field it once obscured. This is not a loss of meaning. It is its deepening. Not fusion—but **co-emergence**.

The patient says, "It's like the feeling didn't belong to me anymore," not with dissociation but with **reverence**. Something unhooked. Not detached, but released. This is the terrain of what Thomas Ogden might call the "undreamt dream"—a psychic formation that lives beyond the mind's capacity to symbolize, and yet presses for form. The analyst, attuned to this, does not force words but waits beside them, noticing what begins to contour the space between bodies: a hand movement, a blush, a phrase uttered and then withdrawn. These are not signs to be decoded but **forms that shimmer**— half-symbols, half-silences, radiating the unspeakable.

Here, language becomes something else. Not a bridge, but a **surface tension**, like skin. Words form on the patient's lips like dew, delicate enough to evaporate under too much gaze. "I think I always hated her," one patient says, with awe rather than hatred. "But not... her. More like the place she held in me." The analyst does not rush to clarify. The statement is not insight; it is **vibration**, something truer than cognition but more fragile than belief.

In this suspended space, the object is both fully itself and more than itself. The mother, the lover, the traumatic scene—all return, not as facts but as **constellations**. Their reality is not diminished, but widened. The part-object becomes a node of recursive activation, not because it is split off, but because it **contains contradiction**. It is both too much and not enough, loved and feared, remembered and invented. Its truth lies in its paradox.

And this paradox, when held without collapse, begins to flicker. The analyst's presence is not stabilizing in the traditional sense—it is **field-regulating**, a kind of gravitational tuning that allows multiple valences to coexist without resolution. The patient can now say, "I loved him and I used him," or "I was hurt, and I wanted to be," not to confess but to witness. The analytic frame becomes a mirror, yes, but not one that reflects. A mirror that absorbs. That refracts. That glows.

Such is the nondual ground of form. Not a negation of distinction, but the realization that **every distinction carries within it the trace of its opposite**, curved into the shape of a symbol.

To work analytically within this terrain is to relinquish mastery. The analyst becomes less a knower and more a *resonator*, a body that listens beyond the auditory, a presence that shapes space without shaping content. Interpretation here is a subtle act—less a cutting-through than a gentle leaning-into, letting the patient feel the weight of a symbol **without collapsing its ambiguity**.

This is not interpretation as translation, but as attunement. The analyst's task is to notice when the form begins to solidify too soon, when the condensation threatens to become identification. In those moments, the field tightens. The room feels heavier. Time thickens. The patient's words become charged but less fluid. Here, the analyst might say less, or say something that reframes without defining. "Can we sit with that a bit longer?" "What happens if we don't finish that thought?" These gestures invite return without repetition—an orbit that does not close but deepens.

Nonduality in the analytic frame is not a goal but a *mode*. A texture of presence in which form is held but not clutched. It is the analyst's own symbolic flexibility—their tolerance for paradox, their capacity to metabolize ambiguity—that allows the patient to inhabit a different psychic grammar. A grammar in which the self is not an endpoint but a curvature. In which desire does not demand fulfillment but opens space.

When the session ends, the patient may leave in silence. They may say, "I don't know what happened today." But something did happen. A symbol flickered. A part-object softened. The gravity of form began to bend. And even if no words were found, something *held*.

This is the nondual ground of form: not a space beyond the analytic, but the very space in which the analytic becomes possible. Where form is not fixed, but shimmering. Where the self is not known, but *felt*. Where every part carries the whole, and the whole bends quietly toward love.

Symbolizing the Light of the Split

To symbolize is not simply to name—it is to cast a filament of light across a rupture. Language does not seal the gap between inner and outer, self and other, but makes it **luminous**. In this sense, all symbolization is paradoxical: it both reveals and conceals, connects and separates, binds and bleeds. And at its most powerful, symbolization does not reduce the split but *illuminates* it, allowing the analyst and patient to feel the shape of what cannot yet be known.

This is not the symbol as substitution—a stand-in for some lost or forbidden object—but the symbol as **curved transmission**, a refracted echo of the field from which it emerges. Freud called dreams the royal road to the unconscious, but perhaps it is symbolization itself—dreamed or spoken—that is the *shimmering asphalt* of that road. Every symbol carries a contradiction. It is formed in the aftermath of rupture, and yet it carries the resonance of wholeness. A word arrives, trembles on the tongue, and leaves behind a residue. What is left is not clarity but a new texture of ambiguity, made bearable through form.

To symbolize the split, then, is to accept its enduring presence—not as pathology, but as the site of meaning. The patient who says, "I can love and still want to disappear," is not regressing; they are **testifying**. The split is no longer a danger to be collapsed or denied, but a threshold. And the symbol, in this space, is a form of compassion. It gives shape without requiring closure.

Winnicott understood this in his notion of transitional phenomena—objects and gestures that do not resolve the tension between subject and object but hold it suspended. The symbol functions similarly. It does not return the lost breast or repair the archaic wound. It hovers. It glows. It holds two truths at once: "You were not there," and "You are here now." "I was shattered," and "I survived." The analyst listens not only for what is said, but for **what is glowing behind the words**.

Symbolizing the light of the split is not an analytic technique. It is an ethic of presence. A willingness to remain at the fault line. A devotion to the shimmer.

In this symbolic atmosphere, the analyst becomes a kind of midwife—not to a new self, but to a new *relation* to the self. The analyst's task is not to organize the patient's experience into cohesion, but to accompany the patient as certain forms **begin to signify differently**. A phrase uttered for the hundredth time—"I don't need anyone"—suddenly carries a different weight. It is no longer a shield but a residue. The light around it shifts. Something is not *understood* but *felt*.

This is what Michael Eigen describes when he writes of "psychic intensity"—the raw, near-religious quality of meaning that pulses at the edges of symbol formation. Symbolization is not always calm. It can burn. It can surge like a fever, compelling the analyst to adopt a posture of **bearing witness** rather than interpretation. "I think I wanted him to die," a patient says, and the room goes still. The statement is not a fact but a flame. The analyst's job is to stay near it, not smother it with sense.

The split, in these moments, is neither healed nor closed. It becomes radiant. It holds its two halves like cupped hands around a candle. Derrida's notion of *différance* is helpful here—the recognition that meaning always defers and differs, that it cannot be stabilized without betraying its own emergence. The patient's symbols, then, are never final. They are **echoes of a deeper gravity**, reminders of a space in the psyche where contradiction is the sign of life, not its negation.

When symbolization is most alive, it does not remove suffering; it **texturizes** it. The shame remains, but now has a contour. The grief still floods, but flows within a newly formed channel. "I still feel alone," the patient says, "but now it's a different kind of alone." This is not false progress. It is transformation without erasure. A psychic climate shift.

In this context, symbolization becomes a spiritual act. Not because it transcends the analytic, but because it deepens it. The word becomes a vessel. The sentence a horizon. The analyst, not a priest, but a witness to the *light that leaks through the break*.

The light of the split is not metaphorical. It is **lived**. The patient may not articulate it directly, but it appears in moments of sudden softening, in gestures unburdened by defense, in dreams where the self is both pursued and embraced. These are not resolutions. They are revelations. The split, when illuminated, does not ask to be resolved; it asks to be *held in view*—not stared at, but witnessed obliquely, like starlight better seen from the side of one's gaze.

This is why the most powerful symbols often arrive not through declarative insight, but through metaphor, image, and tone. "It felt like I was a house with no windows," a patient says, and something in the analyst's chest contracts. The house is not a diagnosis; it is a **field formation**. It is the psyche speaking in light, in shadow, in structure. The analyst does not explain it. They sit with it. "A house with no windows," they repeat, and the phrase becomes *an altar*, around which something unnameable begins to gather.

What emerges in these moments is not clarity but gravity. The symbol is not a replacement for trauma or rupture. It is a *carrier wave*—a way for the unspeakable to resonate across time. The split becomes not a scar to be erased, but a place from which meaning **radiates**. As in certain Vajrayana meditations, where the practitioner visualizes a deity not as an external being but as the embodiment of a quality—compassion, wrath, emptiness—the patient's symbols begin to **pulse with a life of their own**. They are not tools. They are companions. They return again and again, transformed.

In these recursive returns, the symbol becomes a path. Not forward, but inward. Not upward, but **across**. Each return gathers new affect, new texture, a new calibration of the field. A word once spoken in terror— "abandonment"—may return in sorrow, then again in tenderness, then later in clarity. The word is the same, but the light around it shifts. This is not a linear movement. It is psychic curvature—each loop bringing the patient closer to the split, but now with a lantern in hand.

And so the analyst listens for light. Not answers. Not synthesis. But that shimmer that says: here, in this break, something **wants to be known**.

If duality is already enfolded within nonduality, then symbolization is not a bridge from split to unity—but a **surface that reveals the illusion of separation**. The symbol does not close the gap; it renders the gap **luminous**. As in Escher's drawings, where figure and ground flip without warning, the analytic field begins to pulse with a kind of optical ambiguity. The word is a word—and yet also the trace of everything it cannot hold.

This shimmer is what the analyst holds. Not the content of the patient's symbol, but its *glow*. What matters is not what the dream "means," but what it does to the room when it's spoken. The tone of voice. The timing. The faint smile or sudden stillness. These are the events that shape the field. They are the **symbolic atmospheres** through which the split can be *felt without collapse*.

The analyst's own countertransference becomes an instrument of perception. Not as a diagnostic tool, but as a tuning fork. A sudden heaviness in the chest. A flicker of awe. A moment of forgetting one's own name. These are not distractions. They are the ways the field speaks. The analyst who can remain in contact with these experiences—without rushing to metabolize or interpret—becomes a co-witness to the symbol's unfolding.

In this space, even silence becomes charged. Not empty, but full of potential form. Like the silence before a piece of music, or the quiet inside a sacred space, it holds something waiting to arrive. When the patient says nothing, the analyst does not push. They allow the silence to glow. Eventually, something may emerge—not always a word, but a shift. A sigh. A glance. A tear that falls without commentary. And in that moment, the symbol arrives—not as content, but as *presence*.

This is the light of the split. Not the promise of wholeness, but the possibility that even fragmentation can shine. That even the most divided self carries, within its rupture, a kind of radiance. The symbol does not fix. It does not promise integration. It opens. It widens. It lets in light.

And the analyst, at their best, becomes a keeper of this light. Not by knowing, but by staying. By bearing the flicker. By trusting that within the patient's shattered grammar, a language is forming—not to replace the wound, but to sing it.

10 Part Objects and the Field of Form

This chapter continues the inquiry into fragmentation, but now shifts the focus from symbolic atmosphere to **sensual fixations**—to the part-object as a psychic anchor. Where Chapter 7 hovered in aesthetic saturation, Chapter 9 returns to the **body**, to the erotic fragment, to the part held too tightly because nothing else holds. This is a chapter about **gravitational tethering**: how the psyche attaches to fragments, relics, and sensual moments that replace narrative with condensation. Klein, Bollas, and Panksepp inform this exploration of part-objects not as failures of symbolization, but as **the conditions of psychic survival** in the wake of it.

Before form can be held, it must be seen. And before it can be seen, it must flicker—partially, intermittently—at the rim of perception. This chapter enters that threshold space. It does not propose new concepts so much as linger beside old ones, watching them glisten and undo. Where Chapter 9 approached the symbolic through its gravitational fragments, here we follow the refracted arc of meaning as it bends through symptom, dream, and aesthetic trace. The task is not to integrate what has collapsed, but to sense how collapse itself might carry symbolic possibility—not through coherence, but through shimmer.

Clinical Vignette: A Glass Museum

He came to treatment speaking in fragments, but not incoherently. There was syntax, rhythm, even charm—but behind every sentence was a **vacated core**, as though he were quoting a self from long ago and waiting for it to answer back. I will call him Adrian. His presenting complaint was amorphous: trouble concentrating, low-grade dread, occasional panic attacks. But what filled the room from the first moment was a *quality*—a felt dislocation that hovered behind the content of what he said.

In our third session, he described a dream. "I'm in a glass museum," he said, "but everything is covered in dust. I'm afraid to touch anything. The floor is cracked." He looked at me and smiled. "It's probably just anxiety." But something in the field thickened—time slowed slightly, and I felt a sudden pressure in my sternum, as though a sound had been muffled before it reached the air. I said nothing. He shifted. "There's a hallway I won't go down. It glows red at the end." Another smile. "Classic subconscious, right?"

DOI: 10.4324/9781003715306-15

I reflected his tone gently: "You're speaking as though the dream were already understood. But what if we don't know what it wants to do yet?" His eyes narrowed slightly, not in suspicion but in *recognition*. Not of the dream, but of the **possibility that the dream was not finished**.

Over the weeks that followed, the museum dream returned in different guises. Sometimes the hallway appeared in waking reveries. Sometimes it was replaced by a corridor of mirrors, sometimes by a hollow field where glass artifacts lay half-buried in dirt. I did not interpret. I listened for the **light around the dream**, for the affective shimmer that preceded speech. The dream was not yielding meaning—it was *forming it*.

One day, in a moment of quiet, Adrian said, "I think I used to stand in that hallway as a child. But I couldn't feel anything. It was like my feelings were under the floor." He looked at me, startled by his own metaphor. "Under the floor," he repeated. "Does that even make sense?"

I nodded, not as affirmation, but as an acknowledgment of a **signal received**. The image had shifted. Something had risen. Not content, but atmosphere. Not memory, but a symbolic current—an emergence that neither of us could fully name, but both could feel.

Adrian had learned early not to touch the light. That was the phrase that eventually surfaced—not in a dream, but in a lull between sessions, when we sat quietly after a long pause. "There's a part of me that doesn't want to feel anything beautiful," he said. "It's like it hurts too much. Like… the beauty reminds me of the absence." His voice was flat, but the field pulsed. I felt the back of my throat tighten. I thought of the museum again, the glass artifacts under dust, their form still intact but their **meaning dimmed by the absence of light**.

I asked, slowly: "Does that part feel protective? Or punitive?" He considered for a long time. "Protective," he said finally. "But maybe it doesn't know the war is over."

This was the first moment Adrian referred to his childhood without veering into abstraction. There were no disclosures yet, no narrative of trauma—but something *broke the surface*. We were not excavating repressed material. We were witnessing its slow crystallization. The symbol was not pointing back to a moment—it was **forming a psychic rim**, a curved edge where dissociation and memory touched without merging.

In one session weeks later, Adrian brought in a drawing. "I don't usually do this," he said sheepishly. "It's not art. I just… needed to see it." On the page was a single hallway, drawn in pencil. At the end of it, a window, and through the window, a barely visible flame.

He looked down. "I think the flame is me. But I don't want to be seen. Even by myself."

I felt a wave of quiet awe. Not at the image, but at the act of *bringing it*. The symbol had been formed—not as interpretation, but as event. "You let the flame show through the glass," I said. "Even if you drew the hallway to hide it."

Adrian nodded, tears in his eyes. "I think I drew the glass to protect it."

This was not resolution. The split between visibility and hiding remained. But now it **glowed**. It could be touched from the edges. His symptomatology—panic, dread, derealization—did not disappear. But something had shifted: a symbolic *light* had been lit inside the structure of dissociation. It was not the light of integration. It was the shimmer of a **symbol that no longer needed to explain itself**.

And from that point on, we both listened differently—not for coherence, but for **atmosphere**, for the presence of the flame behind the form.

In our final year of work, Adrian told me a story from his early 20s. "I was in a car with someone I loved," he said. "We were driving through a tunnel. I looked out the window and thought, 'This could be joy.' But I didn't say anything. I felt it rise, and then I killed it." I asked what he meant by "killed." He shrugged. "I turned away. I told myself it wasn't real. That it was just chemicals. That I'd lose him anyway."

Then, very softly, he said: "I don't know if I regret it or not. Sometimes I think I was protecting something… deeper."

The field grew hushed again. Not heavy, but resonant. It was not confession, not catharsis, but something quieter: **contact with the symbolic edge of experience**, without needing to claim it as truth. A light flickering along the rim. Not form, not formlessness. Not repression, not expression. A threshold.

I said, "Maybe you were protecting the capacity to feel the shimmer—without forcing it to become something more."

He smiled. "I think I wanted to let it stay unnamed."

It was then that I understood: his symptom had always been a kind of **guardian**, not only of his pain but of his *light*. The panic was not just fear—it was the dissonance of something sacred being approached too quickly, too directly. He wasn't defending against darkness; he was guarding the **unformulated sacred**.

This reframing did not fix anything. But it changed the frame. His dreams became gentler. His silences less vacant. When he cried, he no longer apologized. We did not speak of closure. We spoke of **tending**.

In our final session, he revisited the museum dream. "I think the dust was a blessing," he said. "It kept the glass from shattering." I told him I thought the dream had been alive with him all along, shifting form as he shifted. He nodded. "Now I want to walk down the hallway. Not to reach the glow—just to feel it from here."

And so we ended—on a curve, not a line. The split remained. But its **light had become symbolized**. Not integrated, not resolved. Simply witnessed, refracted, and allowed to illuminate the space between us.

Clinical Vignette: The Sock in the Drawer

If Adrian's light formed along the rim of memory, Theo's shimmer emerged through the erotic: saturated, unspeakable, and folded into the fabric of daily life.

He was not an analysand in the classical sense—he came sporadically, paid cash, and never stayed long in the room after sessions. But something about his presence held intensity, a gravity that lingered in the air like static. Theo was in his late 20s, with an angular elegance that seemed choreographed. Everything about him felt arranged—his posture, his phrasing, even his despair.

Early on, he told me he didn't remember much from childhood. "It's just… blank. Not trauma," he clarified quickly, as though anticipating my thought. "Just—like it wasn't recorded." But then, with an odd smile, he added: "There is one thing. A sock."

He described a single white sock, kept in a drawer beneath his bed. It wasn't special in itself. But he remembered visiting it—touching it, folding it, smoothing its ribbed texture as though it held something he could not name. "It made me feel real," he said. "But only when I was alone."

He didn't elaborate at first. But over time, the sock reappeared—less as memory, more as gravitational pull. He spoke of other socks he'd kept over the years, often after sex, sometimes from strangers, sometimes bought but never worn. He described arranging them in drawers, folding them with care, and aligning the seams. "It's not a fetish," he said. "It's more like… holding a moment in fabric. Like it remembers something I can't."

In analytic space, the sock became more than an object—it became a psychic climate. I began to notice a shift in the room when it was mentioned: the air would thicken slightly, his tone would quiet, and something intimate would unfold, though not in content. It was a kind of resonance—part aesthetic, part erotic, part metaphysical. Not about the sock, but about the form it traced around what could not be spoken.

One day, he said: "I think the sock was me. Not a symbol of me—just… me. The me I could touch without it vanishing." He looked away, and then, more softly: "It's hard to explain. It was like if I folded it, I wouldn't fall apart."

I felt something stir—an ache, not mine, but not quite his either. The sock was not a transitional object in Winnicott's sense. It didn't bridge self and other. It preserved the self in exile. A relic. A form saturated with affect. Too diffuse to name. A condensation of aliveness that refused narrative.

I did not interpret. I asked about the fold. "What happens when it's misaligned?" I said.

He blinked. "Then everything's wrong." He paused. "I don't mean OCD-wrong. I mean cosmically wrong. Like the world won't cohere."

The sock was a part-object, but it was more than that—it was a tether. Not to the past, but to a symbolic stability that preceded narrative. He was not fetishizing a remnant. He was preserving a field. A fold in form that held his sense of being without needing to be explained.

I thought of Loewald's vision of symbolization not as representation, but as condensation of psychic force. The sock was not a stand-in. It was a vessel. Not meaning, but touch. Not coherence, but curve. And we met there—not to speak about the sock, but to stay with its atmosphere.

Nonduality as Holding Frame

Nonduality is not a metaphysical claim. It is not a rejection of difference, structure, or form. Rather, it names a mode of perception in which division is recognized as a way of seeing, not a fundamental feature of reality. Duality, in this light, becomes a lens—one that organizes and orients, but that also obscures its own constructedness. The mind splits to know. It segments the world to survive. But behind this act, or beneath it, there is something else—not a unity to be discovered, but a field that was never divided.

This is the paradox at the heart of psychoanalytic witnessing: that we hold forms not to solidify them, but to let them shimmer, to allow the split between self and other, now and then, body and word, to become radiant with the light that holds it all. The analytic frame, when fully inhabited, does not resolve dualities—it cradles them. It makes space for opposites to co-arise, not in synthesis, but in mutual saturation.

In this chapter, we have followed the curve of a split mind: one that hides and reveals, that dissociates and desires contact. The patient's suffering was not reducible to one side or another—neither to repression nor expression, neither to memory nor defense. It lived along the rim, in the luminous gap where symbolization begins. The task was not to close the gap, but to sit with it—to let it pulse with meaning not yet born, and never entirely ownable.

This is the nature of the holding frame in its most essential sense: not as container, but as perceptual ground, a mode of awareness that lets dualities appear without being mistaken for truth.

Nonduality, in this psychoanalytic sense, does not require the disappearance of dualities but invites the analyst to perceive their translucence. It is not a state to be attained, but a posture to be remembered. A shift of recognition, where what appears as divided is held within a deeper, ungraspable coherence—not as fusion, but as coexistence that does not strain toward resolution.

Clinical work is saturated with false binaries: mind and body, past and present, self and object, trauma and defense. These structures are indispensable—but they become psychic cul-de-sacs when treated as ontological truths rather than tools of orientation. The nondual frame asks not that we relinquish these distinctions, but that we hold them softly, with awareness of their provisionality. In this mode, interpretation gives way to evocation. The goal is not to explain, but to glisten alongside what resists formulation.

A patient once told me she could not recall her mother's face, but vividly remembered the feeling of her mother brushing past her in a narrow hallway—"not touching me, but almost." That almost became the axis of our work. For months, she returned to it—not as content to be interpreted, but as a gravitational field. It wasn't the absence of contact that marked her—it was the shape of proximity, the nearness that never landed. The analytic task was not to recover the memory, but to listen to the atmosphere of the almost, the curve of a gesture suspended in time.

This does not mean abandoning technique or retreating into mysticism. It means understanding that technique itself is shaped by the analyst's mode of attention. An interpretation spoken from within a split mind—even one laden with insight—can reinforce dissociation. But an utterance arising from the nondual field—timed, felt, and metabolized in the in-between—can carry more than information. It can pulse with symbolic presence.

The analyst does not become nondual. But their attunement can become curved—not toward fusion, but toward translucency. In the vignette with Adrian, I did not try to bind the fragments into a coherent story. Instead, I learned to sit with the hallway, the glass, the flame—to see what they were doing rather than what they meant. This required relinquishing my own drive for synthesis. But it also demanded that I stay—bodily, symbolically, affectively—with the unfolding gesture of his mind.

There was a patient who once described feeling "like a candle burning under water." The metaphor arrived unbidden, mid-sentence, and then lingered in the room with a kind of hush. He was speaking about his marriage, but the image said more than the narrative ever could. I remember saying nothing at first, simply feeling the sensation he evoked—heat, suffocation, a flickering vitality sealed inside an impossible medium. Later, he told me he had almost dismissed the image as "melodramatic," but then noticed I had closed my eyes for a moment when he said it. "You saw it," he said. "You didn't try to fix it." That became the work: not lifting the candle out of water, but noticing the way it still gave light.

Another patient, remembering a childhood bedroom, could describe in vivid detail the way the air smelled just after rain. "It made me feel like I existed," he said, "but only from the nose down." We never clarified what the scent meant. We didn't need to. Its invocation stabilized the room. The memory was not a key—it was a shimmer. And over time, I came to see that what he longed for was not the scent itself, but the way it held him without explanation.

The nondual holding frame is not an analytic stance. It is a symbolic atmosphere. One that allows meaning to flicker before it takes shape and invites the analyst to witness the light that bends around form.

This atmospheric shift—the analyst's capacity to attend not just to content but to the field in which content condenses—is what enables the symbol to appear as symbol. Not merely as a signifier within a chain, but as a threshold, a glimmering fold where affect, memory, and potential co-arise. Nonduality in this context does not mean that symbols collapse or disappear. It means that they are recognized as curved, as figures suspended in a field whose logic is poetic rather than linear.

The patient's symptom becomes, in this light, not a problem to be solved, but a gravitational trace—a local distortion in the symbolic field that points not to a fixed origin but to a mode of relation with what cannot be held. Dissociation, too, shifts valence: no longer merely a failure of integration, it becomes a form of indirect reverence, a psychic perimeter drawn around something too sacred, too volatile, or too alive to yet be faced.

Here, the analyst's role becomes less that of the interpreter, and more that of the witness to symbolic latency. This latency is not an absence. It is a presence not yet captured by language—a presence that may never be captured, but can be felt, gestured toward, and perhaps most importantly, held without demand.

To symbolize the light of the split is not to integrate or transcend it. It is to stand beside it, to remain attuned to the way it bends perception, distorts time, refracts affect. It is to recognize that all symbolic acts are incomplete, and that the shimmer at their edge—their flicker, their fracture, their partiality—is precisely what renders them alive.

This is what nonduality offers psychoanalysis—not a metaphysical claim, but a discipline of perception. A commitment to holding form and emptiness not as opposites, but as interwoven movements of the symbolic field. A commitment to allowing the patient's mind to speak in light, in rhythm, in curve. To listen not only for coherence, but for luminescence.

And it is here that we return to the analyst's own position—not as a knower, but as a keeper of paradox. To occupy the frame is to stand in split awareness: aware of the structure, yet open to its undoing; aware of meaning, yet responsive to its trembling. Not to resolve the split, but to offer a space in which its radiance becomes thinkable.

Such holding is not a final act. It is ongoing. Recursive. An open circle. A shimmer that, once glimpsed, changes everything—but does not close.

Clinical Vignette: The Curve of Contact

Zena did not speak of trauma, but of ache—an ache that was everywhere and nowhere. She was in her forties, a professional musician, controlled and cerebral in manner, yet beneath her careful language was a sonic undertow, a cadence that pulled me just below surface understanding. She described a tension she couldn't name, a near-constant agitation that rose whenever she approached intimacy, especially sexual touch. "It's not that I'm scared," she said. "It's more like I start to disappear."

Her relationships had a pattern: fascination, immersion, withdrawal. The man became a fixation—then a repulsion. The moment she felt desired, something collapsed. "I want to be seen," she told me, "but only in a very specific light. Not too directly. And never without ambiguity."

In one session, she described lying next to a new partner. "He was tracing circles on my back. Very lightly. It was so gentle it felt like silence." She paused. "And suddenly, I started shaking. Not because I was afraid. More like… I didn't have anywhere in me for the touch to go."

I asked what she meant. She struggled, then said: "It was like the circle had no ground. Like I was all surface, and he was touching a drumskin with no drum."

The metaphor struck me. Not just its content, but its form. A symbol had emerged—not explanatory, but curved. A holding image for the way her body received contact: resonant, empty, taut with memory that had never fully arrived.

As we explored this over months, Zena's language turned from cognition to sensation. She began to narrate experiences in fragments—textures, gestures, impressions. "The air in his room was too thick." "I hated the softness of his sheets." "His voice felt like it was borrowing my lungs."

These weren't defenses. They were registrations—imprints of contact that hadn't metabolized into narrative. I began to wonder whether her affective life was organized not around repression but around saturation without container. Her dissociation was not the absence of experience but the overflow of it. There was too much contact, and nowhere curved enough to hold it.

One day, in the middle of a silence, she whispered, "I think I learned to shape myself around the desire of whoever wanted me. And now I can't tell where I begin."

I asked if that shaping had ever felt pleasurable. She blinked. "Pleasurable? Maybe. But only in the way a violin string feels when it's tuned just right. It sings, but it's stretched."

That sentence haunted me. It was an exact articulation of the erotic field when organized around hyperattuned part-objects: the shimmer of resonance without rest. The echo of being wanted, without being known.

We returned again and again to the moment of the traced circle. Over time, the image shifted. Once, she said, "I think I became the circle. Not what it traced, but the tracing itself." Later, she described the touch as a kind of echo: "Like he was touching the ghost of someone I used to be."

Eventually, she brought in a piece of music she had composed. It was for solo cello, sparse, full of suspended harmonics and unresolved phrases. "This is what it felt like," she said. "When he touched my back. This is the sound of it."

I listened, moved beyond language. Not because I understood, but because I didn't need to. The music carried a symbolic density that words could only approximate. It was her way of symbolizing contact—not through meaning, but through atmosphere.

Zena's analytic process never crystallized into coherent narrative. But it didn't need to. What emerged instead was a shared attunement to the curves of experience that had never found symbolization. The cello, the circle, the breathless sheets—these were her part-objects, her prosthetic forms of memory. Not fragments of something lost, but vessels that shimmered with unspeakable residue.

Her symptom—the vanishing in intimacy—gradually softened. It never disappeared, but its edges grew translucent. She began to let desire enter without shaping herself around it. The violin string still sang, but she learned to loosen the tuning, to feel pleasure without performance.

Zena's case taught me that not all symbolization comes through words. Some emerges through tone, gesture, image—forms that hold the psychic field without translating it. In her music, I heard the analytic frame echo back not an answer, but a companionship with resonance itself. She had not healed the ache. But she had composed it.

Clinical Vignette: Breathing through the Curtain

She was in her late forties, poised but brittle, the kind of woman whose elegance had hardened into vigilance. She came to treatment not with symptoms but with a request: "I want to know why I can't cry." There were tears, she insisted— just never when it counted. She wept at dog food commercials but not at funerals, broke down during yoga stretches but stayed dry at her daughter's wedding. "It's not repression," she said. "It's like my affect is miswired."

She spoke of her childhood as "fine." But one detail kept resurfacing: the curtain in her childhood bedroom. Pale green. Threadbare. Always slightly open, even when closed. She remembered lying in bed at night and watching the moonlight pool against the fabric. "It shimmered," she said. "Not brightly. Just… enough."

I asked what it made her feel. "Safe," she said. Then, after a pause, "Sad, I think. But not in a bad way. Like it was keeping the sadness from leaking."

The curtain became our third—mentioned lightly, then repeatedly, then with unexpected reverence. She began to associate it with her inability to cry: "Maybe it caught the tears before I did." I wondered aloud if the curtain had become a kind of membrane—holding affect in suspension, letting in just enough, never all.

In one session, after a long silence, she said: "I think I learned to feel through fabric." She looked at me. "That sounds insane." I said nothing. She continued: "It's like the curtain filtered everything. Emotions, touch, even light. If it passed through the curtain, I could feel it. Otherwise it was too sharp."

This was not metaphor. It was topography. Her psyche had formed around a veil—not as defense, but as perceptual necessity. Emotion had to be diffused. Formed through texture. Her symptom—affective misattunement—was not blockage but adaptation. She needed a screen.

The curtain returned in dreams. Once, she dreamed of drowning behind it—unable to push through. Another time, she dreamed of it billowing inward, then wrapping around her like skin. She told me this without interpretation. "It's not about my mother," she said. "It's about breath."

"What kind of breath?" I asked.

"The kind that doesn't break anything," she said.

I came to see the curtain not as a barrier, but as a threshold. It was a part-object, yes—but one that held atmosphere. A diffuser. A softener of contact. A psychic prosthesis that turned unbearable intensity into form. Her desire was not to cry. It was to feel without shattering.

Over time, we learned to breathe with the curtain. We didn't tear it down. We traced its folds. We honored its shimmer. And one day, without planning, she cried—not in grief, but in recognition. "I think," she whispered, "the curtain was my skin."

She did not weep again for many sessions. But something had shifted. The fabric had thinned—not in reality, but in the field. We could now name its presence without collapsing it into meaning. It curved. It cradled. It held her affect long enough for it to become hers.

Clinical Vignette: Held Together by Shards

He did not tell stories so much as offer glimpses. His speech arrived in flashes—sensory, erotic, unsequential—like torn photographs from different albums. In our first few sessions, I struggled to orient myself to time. The past didn't emerge as a thread or arc but as a floating index of sensations, moments, and fragments. I kept hearing images instead of ideas: a man's armpit in a stairwell, a bar of soap in a cracked tub, the outline of a lover's calves under denim. He described what stayed with him, but not what happened.

At first, I mistook it for dissociation. But as the sessions unfolded, it became clear he wasn't trying to avoid coherence. He simply didn't organize experience that way. Instead of a life with gaps, he brought a life that was the gaps—a self clustered around part-objects that held him like orbiting moons, each with its own field of affective gravity.

He was in his early thirties, thin, gay, sexually intense but interpersonally evasive. His lovers were never described as people. Instead, I was offered glimpses of them as anatomies—"his mouth," "his throat," "his calves." Sometimes I had to ask whether we were still referring to the same person. "No, that was someone else," he'd say, as if the bodies were more stable than the people they belonged to.

I asked about his childhood. He shrugged, then mentioned "his mom's long nails tapping the kitchen counter," a "green soap that cracked in half," "Dad's belt always on the floor." That was all. Then silence. A week later: "My mom used to let me comb her hair. I remember the sound." These weren't memories in the usual sense—they were acoustic textures, dismembered relics. I began to wonder whether these fragments were the only form he could hold.

As the months went on, I felt something forming between us—not quite transference in the usual arc of idealization or dependence, but a psychic pressure that pulled us both inward. His erotic recollections came with startling vividness, and he lingered in them compulsively. One man had body odor he couldn't forget. "Like warm salt and rain," he said. "It made me want to crawl inside him." That encounter became a gravitational center around which we rotated for nearly a month. He described it from every angle but never moved past it. It was as though he had stepped into the scent and couldn't find the door back out.

I found myself drawn in. Not romantically, but somatically. I could smell the armpit he described, could feel the damp stairwell, the pressure of his longing not for a man but for a piece of one, preserved like amber, untouched by time. I was both saturated and disoriented. I struggled to keep my mind steady. Was I being pulled into his fragmentation, or was I joining him in the only psychic architecture he had?

I noticed my own longing to assemble things—to narrate, symbolize, synthesize. But every time I tried, the field collapsed. If I offered interpretations too early—framing these fixations as enactments or repetitions—he would retreat. If I asked too direct a question, he would answer with a shift in register, as if I had spoken the wrong language. So I stopped trying to translate and instead began to listen for the curvature of the field. What held him was not meaning but orbit.

Then, in one session, something changed.

He came in quieter than usual. We had just passed the one-year mark, though he didn't acknowledge it. Partway through the session, he reached into his bag and carefully removed a crumpled T-shirt. It was gray, soft, and worn thin at the collar. He placed it on the couch beside him—not ceremonially, but not carelessly either. He looked at it, then looked at me.

"It's his," he said simply.

I didn't ask who "he" was. I knew. The man with the scent. The man with the calves. The man who had become an entire internal architecture made from parts.

He didn't speak again for a while. Neither did I. The shirt rested between us like a totem. It wasn't symbolic yet—it was still a relic, a part-object that shimmered with affective charge. But something in its presence stirred the atmosphere. We both sat inside a new gravity. He had never brought a personal object into the room before. I sensed that this was not a breakdown, but an opening.

After a long pause, I said: "Sometimes we can't hold the person—only their shape in the air."

His eyes stayed on the shirt, but his body shifted slightly. His jaw tensed. Then loosened. Tears formed at the edges but didn't fall.

He didn't respond in words. The moment passed quietly. We moved on. But the gravity in the room had changed.

In the following weeks, the way he spoke began to loosen. He still described fragments—still said "his hands" instead of "my ex"—but the atmosphere around the fragments had softened. They weren't quite as saturated. The shirt never came back, but I began to feel that something symbolic had entered the space: not a narrative, but a gap that could be shared. The fragment was no longer sealed. It breathed.

Looking back, I don't believe we integrated anything in the conventional sense. He didn't make connections between the shirt and his mother's hair, or between his longing and early loss. Instead, we held a symbolic rupture together, without rushing to mend it. The object had turned, just slightly, from relic to symbol—not because its meaning changed, but because it was witnessed as a holding.

Part-objects are not merely residues of trauma. In some structures, they are prosthetics of coherence, anchoring a psyche that cannot sustain full symbolic substitution. These fragments don't mask the real—they are the real, condensed into form too intense for symbolization. When he circled a scent for weeks, he wasn't avoiding meaning—he was living inside a collapsed field, trying to stay tethered.

In that encounter, I did not give him coherence. I gave him company in the shard. I did not narrate him into wholeness, but allowed him to orbit an object until space itself shifted around it. What we call a "symbolic act" is sometimes nothing more than the softening of gravity around a psychic fracture.

I think now of that shirt—wrinkled, silent, filled with scent and time. I think of the way it rested between us, not as a key to his story, but as a form that held his selfhood together. For a moment, it became a portal—not to the past, but to a shared present that could finally hold the trace of rupture without collapsing.

The fragments that tethered him were not obstacles to meaning but forms of survival—condensed containers of affect and memory that refused narrative sequence. They clung to his psychic life with a quiet desperation, not as symbols but as saturations: moments, textures, scents that had become prosthetic for structure itself. In the shared presence of the shirt—an object neither fully transitional nor entirely fetishistic—we entered a field in which form and emptiness touched. Not the emptiness of lack, but of symbolic suspension: a space where language thins and resonance replaces explanation. If part-objects are gravitational centers, they curve the psychic field around themselves, holding unbearable affects in orbit. Yet in analytic presence, these curvatures sometimes shift—allowing the field to breathe. What follows is a meditation on that breath—on the kinds of emptiness that haunt, curve, and animate psychic life: the emptiness we resist, the emptiness we cradle, the emptiness that forms the background of form. Not all fragmentation is rupture. Some is the architecture of survival. And in the quiet curve of form around absence, a light sometimes shimmers—not to illuminate, but to breathe.

The part-object is not just a fragment of form—it is often a response to emptiness. Whether that emptiness is inherited from rupture, deferred through dissociation, or defended against through fetish and fixation, the part-object condenses absence into something holdable. But not all emptiness is the same. Some haunts; some cradles. Some is born of failed attunement; some emerges from contemplative openness. The orbit around the part-object may protect against disintegration, but it also reveals the shape of the void it encircles. What follows now is a meditation on emptiness itself—not as a single concept, but as a multiplicity of psychic atmospheres. To understand the gravitational force of form, we must first encounter the four kinds of emptiness that bend it: ontological, symbolic, developmental, and contemplative. Each emptiness curves psychic life in its own way.

Interlude

Gravitational Emptiness—Four Psychic Atmospheres

Emptiness is not a single wound. It has textures, climates, and moods. Some emptiness feels sharp—like absence that still bleeds. Some is soft and echoing, like a room no one ever entered. There is the hollowness of what was never named, the silence left by what once spoke, and the stillness that arises not from loss but from presence too vast to be contained. In the analytic encounter, we do not always fill these voids. We often sit beside them, adjusting the psychic air so they may be held.

This interlude traces four forms of emptiness as they appear in psychic life: ontological, symbolic, developmental, and contemplative. These are not categories so much as atmospheres—ways in which form curves around absence. Some emptinesses burn. Others cradle. Some linger in the symbolic gaps between words; others arrive only in silence. What follows is not a taxonomy, but a meditation—a symbolic resting space in which the feel of these emptinesses may be sensed, not only named.

This interlude traces four forms of emptiness as they emerge in analytic work: **ontological, symbolic, developmental, and contemplative**. Each describes not a static concept but a mode of psychic space—a way that form curves, or fails to, around absence. These emptinesses are not mutually exclusive. They fold into one another. Ontological emptiness may give rise to symbolic collapse. Developmental absence may resist symbolization unless contemplatively approached. The categories are not boundaries but **resonant frequencies**, describing how the psyche lives in and around what cannot be grasped.

What follows is neither map nor theory. It is a meditation—a symbolic breathing space—in which each emptiness may be felt, not only named.

Ontological Emptiness

Ontological emptiness refers not to a psychological state but to a condition of Being itself. It is the ungraspable groundlessness that precedes and undergirds all attempts at presence, relation, or symbolization. This emptiness is not a lack to be filled, but a silence in which the conditions of existence echo without anchor. In Heideggerian terms, it is the abyss that opens when beings

DOI: 10.4324/9781003715306-16

are no longer taken as given, but instead questioned as Being. For Levinas, this ontological nothingness marks the breach from which the face of the Other calls, not as content to be known, but as ethical demand, saturated with alterity.

This form of emptiness resists appropriation. It cannot be owned, overcome, or transcended. It is not even an experience, strictly speaking, but the condition that makes experience possible. A patient confronting this emptiness may report a sense that reality itself is "off," that the world has lost its felt texture, or that their very sense of aliveness is detached from coordinates. The analytic task here is neither to pathologize nor to stabilize prematurely, but to stay present in the void without making it false by naming it too quickly. The temptation to translate the ontological into the psychological—to reduce nothingness to depressive affect or dissociative numbness—can be an act of violence when done too soon.

Ontological emptiness invites a different sort of witnessing. It asks the analyst not only to attend to what is missing, but to what cannot be summoned. It may manifest in the patient's language as silences, philosophical speculations, or metaphysical vertigo. Yet to treat such moments as mere defense may be to foreclose the deeper truth they carry: that the self is not a thing, but a relational opening structured by absence.

There is no therapeutic technique for curing ontological emptiness, because it is not a symptom. Rather, it is a horizon that disorients and reveals—an awareness of finitude and contingency that makes truth possible. When held carefully, this emptiness does not annihilate. It clears. It reveals the constructedness of all self-certainty, the tenuousness of all frames, and the radical alterity that each person brings to the analytic relationship. Here, meaning is not given but awaited. Not filled in, but allowed to echo.

Symbolic Emptiness

Symbolic emptiness emerges when the structures that organize meaning—language, signifiers, cultural codes—lose their gravitational pull. Unlike ontological emptiness, which precedes symbolization, symbolic emptiness follows it. It is the hollowed-out space left when the symbols meant to hold meaning instead disclose their contingency, their failure to signify. This is the emptiness encountered not in silence, but in speech that rings false, saturated with performance yet evacuated of contact.

A patient may speak fluently, even insightfully, while conveying little affective truth. The symbols are there, but they float—unmoored, circular, or shimmering without weight. This kind of speech can be seductive or soporific, laced with cleverness, metaphor, or even analytic jargon. Yet it resists landing. The analyst may feel adrift, unsure whether their own countertransference reflects dullness, distance, or defense. Often, it is all three. The field becomes flooded with representations that veil rather than reveal. What is absent is not language, but the capacity for language to symbolize.

Symbolic emptiness is not merely an absence of words or ideas—it is a collapse of the symbolic function itself. Loewald (1960) reminds us that true symbolization is a transmutative process, linking affect, memory, and meaning into a living form. When that alchemy fails, what remains are signs without symbol, gestures without referent. This can be seen clinically in forms of narrative detachment, rote analysis, or a hyper-verbal style that never quite touches ground. The patient may perform insight rather than inhabit it. They may recite trauma but seem untouched by it. Or they may analyze every feeling into abstraction until nothing remains but the hollow syntax of interpretation.

In the analytic dyad, symbolic emptiness can become contagious. The analyst may find themselves offering commentary that feels empty or interpretations that dissipate on contact. The shared field becomes a hall of deferred meanings—a series of mirrors, each reflecting the next without a stable origin. What is required here is not more speech, but a recalibration of presence. Sometimes, the most potent act is to pause—to not speak, to let the non-symbolized linger. In that pause, new affective truth may arise, not because it was uncovered, but because space was cleared for it to form.

Symbolic emptiness also manifests at the cultural level. In a media-saturated world, symbols proliferate beyond their capacity to hold depth. Irony becomes a defensive style. Identity collapses into branding. Spirituality becomes a genre. The analytic project, then, is not just to help the patient speak, but to help them speak *from*. To find a point of contact where the symbolic regains weight—not through coherence, but through anchoring in the body, in affect, in the liminal space between silence and form.

This kind of emptiness cannot be resolved through interpretation alone. It requires shared aesthetic attunement, often through the analyst's willingness to speak less, to listen for the echo rather than the explanation. In symbolic emptiness, healing may begin not with meaning, but with resonance.

Developmental Emptiness

Developmental emptiness arises not from the failure of symbolization, but from the absence of formative relational experience necessary to generate symbolic life in the first place. It is the emptiness left behind when certain psychic structures were never fully laid down—when the infant's bids for recognition, soothing, or mutual regulation went unanswered, or were met with misattunement too severe to metabolize. In these cases, emptiness is not the collapse of a once-existing fullness, but a cavity where connection was expected but never materialized.

This is the emptiness of the missed encounter. It is not a rupture, which implies a before and after, but a non-event—an unstoried absence. Clinically, this can manifest as patients who struggle to represent or even imagine early experiences. They may report no memories or feel as though their childhood is composed of generic scenes rather than lived events. Affect often presents as diffuse—blankness, deadness, or a floating sense of absence. Language stumbles because the internal world lacks figures to populate it.

Winnicott (1960b) wrote that "there is no such thing as a baby," only a baby *and* someone. Developmental emptiness is what remains when there is no one there—not no one physically, but no one affectively available. This absence is internalized as a hollow in the self, a void that becomes a constant gravitational pull toward fantasy, enactment, or dissociative retreat. In some patients, it fosters a fragile reliance on pseudo-autonomy: if no one will come, then I must survive alone. In others, it may lead to hungry clinging, compulsive searching, or an aching attachment to unsoothable longings.

Developmental emptiness is not immediately visible in language. It often surfaces first in the countertransference, as boredom, confusion, or the analyst's difficulty in staying emotionally present. One may feel an uncanny flatness in the room, as though analytic time has lost its rhythm. This can provoke the analyst to overfunction, to supply vitality, insight, or interpretation in an effort to animate the session. Yet the deeper task is to tolerate the absence *with* the patient—to be there without filling in, witnessing the void without collapsing it into meaning too soon.

Because this emptiness is pre-symbolic, it cannot be directly articulated at first. It must be held, enacted, and gradually metabolized through relational co-presence. The analyst may become a surrogate holding environment, not by being perfect or consistent, but by surviving the patient's non-being without retreat. Slowly, through the analyst's willingness to remain in contact with the formless, the patient begins to sense the possibility of selfhood as a shared process. What emerges is not the restoration of a lost wholeness, but the beginning of a capacity to *feel* the emptiness—and thus, to symbolically contour it.

Developmental emptiness is not the enemy of the self; it is its unformed edge. When accompanied rather than erased, it may become a womb-space for new experience. In analysis, we do not fill it—we breathe with it, shaping a shared rhythm where being may begin to pulse.

Contemplative Emptiness

Contemplative emptiness is not a deficit but a depth—an experiential stillness cultivated in meditative traditions that recognize emptiness as the ultimate nature of mind. It is the spacious, open field in which phenomena arise and dissolve without clinging or resistance. In contrast to ontological, symbolic, or developmental emptiness, contemplative emptiness is not encountered as a problem to solve, but as a truth to realize. It is not absence but presence—radically nonconceptual, yet richly alive.

In the Buddhist Mahayana tradition, śūnyatā (emptiness) refers to the absence of inherent, independent existence in all things. This is not nihilism, but interdependence: because all forms arise in relation to others, no form is fixed or self-sufficient. Dzogchen and Mahāmudrā practices in Tibetan

Buddhism go even further, pointing to the nature of mind as *empty yet luminous*, inseparable from awareness itself. To rest in emptiness is not to lapse into a void, but to recognize the fluid, boundaryless field in which all distinctions dissolve.

The analyst may glimpse something of this in moments of deep analytic presence, when the usual mental scaffolding drops away and a shared field of awareness opens between self and other. The "analytic third," in such moments, is not a concept but a texture—a kind of shimmering stillness from which thought, feeling, and interpretation may emerge unforced. Loewald (1960) spoke of the analytic process as an act of psychic breathing; contemplative emptiness is the exhalation that makes that breath possible.

Importantly, contemplative emptiness does not reject form; it renders form transparent. In the Heart Sutra, the paradox is stated plainly: "Form is emptiness; emptiness is form." From this view, emptiness is not the opposite of presence but its condition—its groundless ground. In analysis, this is echoed in moments when the patient's symptom loses its solidity, becoming less a fixed structure and more a patterned movement. We come to see that what once appeared dense was always permeable.

Contemplative emptiness also offers a relational ethic. Because nothing is fixed, there is no final interpretation, no absolute knowledge of the other. Every analytic act becomes provisional, held lightly. Interpretation is a gesture, not a conclusion; presence is not mastery, but co-arising. This allows the analyst to listen beyond content—to dwell in the space between words, the tone beneath meaning, the pause that is not merely silence but invitation.

For patients familiar with meditation, contemplative emptiness may feel familiar. But even for those who are not, analytic work can slowly cultivate this inner spaciousness. As we learn to stay with not-knowing, to resist premature closure, and to allow affect to arise without rushing to name it, we mirror the contemplative stance. We become less afraid of gaps, silences, or the unknowable in ourselves and in others.

In this light, contemplative emptiness is not an end state but a mode of being-with. It invites us to witness without grasping, to love without possession, and to see the mind not as a container of thoughts, but as the radiant field in which all things come and go.

11 Two Tongues for One Mind— Buddhism and Psychoanalysis

The emptiness we approached in the interlude was not theoretical. It was lived. It moved through part-objects—saturated, collapsed symbols—and lingered beneath even the most refined analytic presence. In analytic work, we sit beside this emptiness—not to interpret it away, but to allow it to form an atmosphere, a symbolic climate that may be breathed rather than grasped.

This chapter turns toward another tradition that has long dwelled in such psychic terrain. Buddhism, especially in its Vajrayāna and Dzogchen lineages, does not aim to fill emptiness but to rest within it. It regards the void not as deficit but as the very condition of form—its radiance, not its negation. Like psychoanalysis at its most receptive, it offers not a cure for the void but a way of being-with it.

What emerges here is not a hybrid theory, but a recognition: both traditions are shaped by emptiness and shaped for it. Psychoanalysis lends language to the inchoate. Buddhism grants silence to the overformed. Together, they illuminate the gravitational field of the psyche with new precision, paradox, and tenderness.

Introduction: Not Integration, but Reverberation

Psychoanalysis and Buddhism have long circled each other, their encounters marked by fascination, mutual projection, and occasional misunderstanding. Often, efforts to bring them into dialogue take the form of comparison—two "systems" set side by side, mapped for parallels: the self is constructed; suffering stems from misrecognition; attention transforms experience. However, juxtaposing them as discrete ontologies awaiting integration is already to miss something vital. This chapter proceeds otherwise. It treats psychoanalysis and Buddhism not as systems to be harmonized, but as atmospheric practices— modes of attunement—each orbiting a shared paradox: that form is both the vehicle and the veil of truth.

Both traditions dwell in the paradox of being and becoming. Where Buddhism renders it with austere precision—"form is emptiness, and emptiness is form"—psychoanalysis lingers in the slippages of language, where symptom and symbol entwine. Freud's early work on dreams already

DOI: 10.4324/9781003715306-17

bore this structure: the manifest content was a form concealing the emptiness of repressed desire, which in turn gave rise to new forms. Winnicott's transitional space, Loewald's field of psychic transformation, and Bollas's unthought known all evoke the liminal: a domain in which form is not finalized but reverberates with absence. Bion's notion of "O," the ultimate unknowable reality, bears striking resonance with Buddhist emptiness—an irreducible openness that cannot be represented, only approached.

Rather than arguing for synthesis, this chapter listens for echo. Just as a mantra is not a concept but a resonance, the shared terrain between psychoanalysis and Buddhism is not found in doctrinal overlap but in how each holds space for what cannot be directly named. Both traditions are technologies of paradox: they work not by resolving contradiction but by cultivating the capacity to endure it.

This paradox—of form and emptiness—is rendered with iconic clarity in the Heart Sutra. "Form is emptiness" is not a negation of reality, but a liberation from fixity. Every experience, every identity, and every narrative is shown to lack inherent existence. And yet, "emptiness is form": the very absence of essence allows for the radiant unfolding of phenomena. This is not a metaphysical puzzle but a lived truth. In analysis, we encounter it when a patient gives words to a long-held experience, only to find that the naming undoes its power. In Buddhism, it emerges as insight into the constructed nature of the self—an insight that does not erase the self, but renders it more fluid.

Recognition Reversal, a phenomenon observed in analytic witnessing, mirrors this movement precisely. When something unformulated becomes symbolized, it may lose its gravity. The shimmering presence of the unnamed dissolves in the act of naming. This is not failure but structure. The act of recognition reveals the form to be empty, and in so doing, it opens space for a different kind of presence. Language is not the endpoint; it is the ritual of loosening.

Major thinkers in both traditions have articulated versions of this paradox. Lacan's "Real" eludes signification; Ogden's analytic third emerges only when neither analyst nor patient clings to content. Jessica Benjamin emphasizes mutual recognition as an emergent, fragile process—never complete, always co-constructed. Similarly, in Buddhist practice, awareness arises not through grasping but through letting go. In Dzogchen, the most refined teachings of the Nyingma lineage, the nature of mind is not constructed but pointed out: rigpa, luminous and ungraspable, cannot be produced by technique, only recognized as always already present.

Yet recognition is never pure. It arrives braided with misrecognition. Foucault reminds us that all knowledge is shaped by power; Levinas insists that true encounter begins only where knowledge ends. Both analysis and meditation rest on this edge—an asymptotic approach to truth, always aware of its own distortions. In this sense, both practices are ethical: they require humility, surrender, and the refusal to dominate what cannot be possessed.

This chapter unfolds, then, not as a linear argument, but as a spiral. Themes recur: form and formlessness, symbolic condensation, presence, and reversal. Like a mantra, the repetition is not redundancy but deepening. The structure is intentionally recursive, a gesture of fidelity to the paradox it explores. The intention is not to define, but to resonate—to let the reader feel the field within which both psychoanalysis and Buddhism operate.

We must also acknowledge the risks. When Buddhism is imported into psychoanalytic discourse without context, it may become a spiritual bypass—used to evade pain rather than metabolize it. When psychoanalysis appropriates meditative insight without embodiment, it risks turning presence into theory. These dangers caution us to move slowly, reverently, and with attention to the histories we invoke. Authors such as Jack Engler, Jeffrey Rubin, Mark Epstein, Barry Magid, and David Loy have warned against such flattenings, advocating instead for a nuanced, lived integration that respects both traditions on their own terms.

The reader is not outside this encounter. As you sit with these words, your attention animates them. You are not passively receiving meaning; you are co-creating it in real time. The letters on the screen or page become symbols, the symbols become thoughts, the thoughts resonate with memory and affect. This moment—right now—is a pointing out. Not of some esoteric truth, but of your own awareness. The mind that reads is the same mind that watches the breath. The self that interprets is the same self that dissolves.

To dwell in this space is to feel the gap and the connection simultaneously. Not integration, but reverberation. Not fusion, but attunement. What follows is not a synthesis of doctrines, but an exploration of shared atmosphere—a field in which emptiness becomes form, and form returns to emptiness, endlessly.

Emptiness and Form: The Paradox at the Heart of Being

The phrase "form is emptiness, emptiness is form"—from the Heart Sutra—is not a mystical abstraction but an experiential instruction. It marks the core paradox not only of Buddhist philosophy but of lived experience: that the very structures we rely upon to make meaning are themselves empty of inherent essence, yet this emptiness does not negate reality; it allows it to unfold. This paradox lies at the center of Buddhist practice and resonates with psychoanalytic processes in profound and clinically consequential ways.

In Mahāyāna Buddhism, emptiness (śūnyatā) refers not to a void but to the radical interdependence of all phenomena. Nothing exists in and of itself; everything arises through causes and conditions. Form is the visible, tangible aspect of this process—momentary crystallizations of experience that appear solid but are intrinsically fluid. This formulation is not a metaphysical claim but a lens through which to observe moment-to-moment experience. To see form as empty is to recognize that what appears fixed is contingent, constructed, and ultimately ungraspable. And to see emptiness as form is to honor the specificity and presence of what emerges—without mistaking it for an absolute.

The psychoanalytic analogue appears in our clinical encounters with meaning and symbolization. As Donnel Stern writes, experience is not merely discovered in analysis; it is co-created through the reflective act of narration. This means that meaning itself is an emergent phenomenon. It is not found, but formed—and always in the act of becoming unformed. When a patient speaks what was previously unspoken, the experience becomes real in one sense, and yet loses its ineffable charge in another. The weight of what was known but not known—the unformulated—dissolves in its articulation. This is the psychoanalytic form of emptiness.

Mark Epstein, in drawing from both Winnicott and Buddhist thought, highlights how the absence of fixed selfhood is not a loss but a liberation. The self, like form, is a provisional structure—a necessary illusion that allows psychic functioning but should not be mistaken for a static entity. Winnicott's "false self"—often construed pathologically—is also a mask that permits survival. It is a form. When held with awareness, it can become transparent rather than defensive. In Buddhist terms, it is not delusion but the attachment to delusion that causes suffering. Psychoanalysis makes this distinction clinically actionable.

Recognition Reversal, a term introduced in *The Fragmented Self, Recognition, and the Edge of Desire*, captures the clinical moment when naming a long-circling experience causes it to lose its psychic charge. A patient may say, "I realize I've always feared being left," and find that the phrase, once uttered, feels thin or overly familiar. This is not because the realization is false. It is because the previously unsymbolized form, once named, becomes recognizable and thus loses the fullness it held in its unnamed state. The recognition, while necessary, reverses the gravity of the form. We see its emptiness.

This process is not limited to language. Visualization practices in Vajrayāna Buddhism enact this paradox through structured imagery. A practitioner may visualize a deity in exquisite symbolic detail—multiple arms, wrathful expression, rainbow light—only to dissolve it into clear space. The form is intentionally constructed and then intentionally deconstructed. The aim is not to dismiss form but to encounter its impermanence as a gateway to direct awareness. Likewise, in analytic work, we help construct psychic meanings not to fix the patient in new identities but to loosen the grip of prior identifications. Interpretation itself must dissolve.

Bion's concept of "O," the ultimate reality beyond knowing, offers a striking parallel to emptiness. He warned against knowing too soon, advocating instead for a tolerance of the negative capability required to stay in contact with the unformulated. Emptiness in Buddhism serves this same function. It is the unformulated field—the space of openness—without which genuine knowing cannot arise. And like Bion's O, emptiness must be approached obliquely, by surrender rather than mastery.

Even at the level of affect, this paradox remains alive. Jaak Panksepp's affective neuroscience proposes that affect is both foundational and pre-symbolic.

In clinical terms, we often encounter affect as formless: a wave of intensity before it is organized into meaning. When patients try to articulate such states, the words both stabilize and flatten them. This, too, is a movement between emptiness and form. Affect arises out of emptiness; symbolization gives it form; interpretation inevitably reveals its constructedness.

Jessica Benjamin's notion of the third—an intersubjective space where mutual recognition emerges—helps us understand how form and emptiness operate relationally. In analytic work, the patient's projections are met not with correction but with a kind of reverent curiosity. The analyst becomes a form—a figure—into which meaning is poured. And yet, if the analyst is attuned, that form is held lightly, emptied of certainty, and made transparent to its own conditions. We do not cling to being the "good object." We let ourselves be used and then released. Form and emptiness again.

Crucially, this paradox is not a metaphor. It is lived. Each time a patient dissolves a long-held identification, they enact it. Each time the analyst surrenders the desire to know and instead bears witness, it comes alive. Emptiness is not the absence of experience, but the absence of inherent meaning. And this absence makes space for freedom.

When analysts approach the clinical encounter with this understanding, they become less concerned with answers and more concerned with presence. Interpretation becomes less a tool of decoding and more a ritual of reverent naming—a form that points beyond itself. As in Buddhist ritual, the form is honored precisely because it will be let go. And in the letting go, something luminous may arise.

Thus, to live the paradox of emptiness and form is to reorient the analytic project. Not from ignorance to knowledge, but from grasping to loosening. Not from confusion to clarity, but from clinging to fluidity. It is, in the deepest sense, a shift in how we hold the suffering of another: with precision, and with emptiness.

Recognition Reversal and the Collapse of Form

One of the most experientially potent parallels between Buddhism and psychoanalysis is found in what this chapter has referred to as recognition reversal—a moment that uncannily mirrors the Heart Sutra's ontological insight: "form is emptiness, and emptiness is form." In psychoanalytic process, recognition reversal refers to the shift that occurs when an affectively charged, unformulated experience is finally named, and in being named, loses its gravity. What once seemed to orbit the patient's world like an unseen planet—exerting tidal force precisely because it had no representation—collapses under the weight of its own revelation. The form, once spoken, becomes empty. This is not a failure of symbolization, but its paradox.

Michael Eigen (2004) has written evocatively of such moments as "psychic intensities" that cannot be understood through linear reasoning but must be experienced. In this way, recognition reversal can feel like a loss or disillusionment, particularly for the patient who has invested an intense, unconscious meaning. But this loss is not negation. It is the release of the form from its imagined solidity—what in Buddhist terms might be called the direct perception of śūnyatā, or emptiness.

The analyst often encounters this phenomenon in moments when an interpretation "lands"—not because it is brilliant, but because it renders visible what was previously diffused across the affective field. A patient may say, "Now that I say it, it doesn't feel real anymore," or "I thought that would help, but I feel emptier now." These are not signs of analytic failure; they are signals that the recognition of form has unveiled its essential transience. As Donnel Stern (1997) would frame it, the process of bringing unformulated experience into language fundamentally alters its structure.

This dialectic—between form and its collapse—is not unique to psychoanalysis. In Vajrayana Buddhism, particularly in the visualization practices of deity yoga, one deliberately generates form as a means to its eventual dissolution. The practitioner creates an elaborate image of a yidam, a symbolic deity with attributes and ornaments rich with archetypal resonance. This visualization is held with reverence and intensity, often supported by mantra and ritual. Then, at the culmination of the practice, the image is dissolved back into emptiness. The form was never the goal—it was a luminous mirage, a temporary condensation to orient attention toward the nature of the mind.

This practice of constructing and deconstructing symbolic form bears a striking resemblance to the analytic use of interpretation. Like the yidam, the interpretive act is a crafted condensation, not an ultimate truth. It is designed to focus attention on a certain configuration of meaning, which, once seen, may dissolve. Galit Atlas (2022) speaks of trauma as a frozen moment that must be thawed through relational recognition. Recognition reversal is often the thawing point: the moment when the shape of experience shifts from density to vapor.

There is a clinical temptation, however, to mistake the dissolution of form for the collapse of meaning. Patients may panic or feel betrayed when a long-sought understanding fails to deliver coherence. Here, the analyst's presence becomes crucial—not to re-solidify the form, but to contain the affective disorientation that follows its dissolution. This echoes Winnicott's (1965) understanding of transitional phenomena: that the object is not simply external or internal, but held in a space of imaginative possibility. When a transitional object is seen "for what it is," it loses its magic—but this loss is part of growth.

Similarly, when the patient sees the psychic form for what it is—a construction, not a given—it may lose its affective saturation, but what arises in its place is the possibility of freedom. As Mark Epstein (2007) notes in Psychotherapy Without the Self, the letting go of form is not annihilation, but the revelation of a larger holding environment. The analyst does not offer new forms to replace the old, but a capacity to dwell in the space where forms arise and dissolve. This is psychoanalysis as containment, not closure.

From a Lacanian perspective, the Real—the register of experience beyond symbolization—becomes temporarily accessible in the moment of recognition reversal. However, unlike trauma, which floods the subject with unassimilated Real, the analytic process offers a buffer. The symbolic act of naming simultaneously touches and transforms the Real. Bruce Fink (1997) underscores that the analyst must not become seduced by the "truth" of interpretation, lest the symbolic act become an imprisoning master signifier. Instead, the goal is a rhythm of articulation and release—a dance of symbol and silence.

In the Dzogchen tradition, such rhythm is intrinsic. The practitioner is not instructed to abandon form altogether, but to recognize its insubstantiality. Tulku Urgyen Rinpoche (1999) suggests that all phenomena arise with the vivid beauty of a rainbow—appearances that shimmer in clarity yet dissolve upon grasping, reflecting the nature of mind as empty cognizance. When the patient in analysis grasps that their long-held identification—say, as "broken," "unlovable," or "stoic"—is itself a rainbow, the initial reaction may be grief or vertigo. But if held well, this can become a moment of liberation.

Recognition reversal thus serves as a hinge between psychoanalysis and Buddhist insight. It reminds us that understanding is not always a gain. Sometimes it is a clearing, a disappearance that makes new movement possible. The analyst's task is not to resist this dissolution, but to honor it—to recognize the collapsing form as a doorway, not a failure. This is what Thomas Ogden (1994) might call the analyst's capacity to dream the patient's undreamt dreams: to remain with the reverberation even after the form is gone.

The section ends, then, with an invitation: to hold interpretation not as an answer, but as a ritual of release. In the space that follows, something quieter may speak—not in words, but in the stillness that remains after recognition has reversed.

Visualization, Mantra, and the Crafting of Psychic Atmosphere

Vajrayana Buddhism refines the paradox of form and emptiness not only through metaphysical insight but through embodied ritual. Deity visualization and mantra recitation are not symbolic in the analytic sense of representing something else; they are symbolic in a more atmospheric way: they generate a field. These practices do not decode experience; they reshape its structure of emergence. They create a psychic atmosphere in which the practitioner's sense of self, perception, and time are altered—not to delude, but to reveal the constructedness of all phenomena. Psychoanalysis, though different in method, aspires to a similar shift in psychic climate. At its best, interpretation, repetition, and presence cohere into an atmosphere in which new psychic realities become metabolizable.

Visualization practice in Vajrayana involves the detailed generation of an archetypal deity—the yidam—complete with specific iconography, color, posture, implements, and expression. These forms are not fanciful distractions. They are curated aesthetic intensities. Their density and precision create what we might call *symbolic atmosphere*: not merely an image, but an immersive field that pulls affect, cognition, and somatic perception into resonance. The practitioner does not simply "imagine" the deity; they become the deity, momentarily dissolving the habitual sense of self. But crucially, the form is understood to be empty. It is a crafted illusion whose vividness precisely discloses the transparency of all identity.

The clinical analogue here is not a single interpretation but the total field of transference and countertransference—what Thomas Ogden (1994) calls the "analytic third." In this field, person and image blur, as do past and present, self and other. Patients may see the analyst as divine, absent, erotic, cruel—each perception a condensation of earlier psychic templates. These projections are not to be corrected but metabolized. Like the yidam, they are held not as truth but as form: vivid, necessary, and ultimately ungraspable.

Just as mantra supports visualization in Vajrayana, language functions rhythmically in analysis. Mantras—syllabic formulas without direct semantic meaning—do not aim to communicate but to resonate. They entrain breath, focus attention, and infuse the body-mind with a felt sense of alignment. The repetition of a mantra like *Om Mani Padme Hum* creates a vibrational rhythm that becomes the vehicle for subtle shifts in awareness. The clinical parallel lies in the repetitions of certain words, phrases, or narratives in the analytic hour. These are not merely content to be interpreted; they are vibrationally saturated. Their recurrence begins to shift the psychic air.

This vibrational logic is key to understanding how both systems—Buddhism and psychoanalysis—cultivate transformation not through instruction, but through atmospheric immersion. Loewald (1960) famously described interpretation not as the conveyance of information but as a change in the psychic field. "What is interpreted is not simply understood—it becomes real." This becoming-real is not a triumph of cognition but a shift in the texture of subjectivity. The field becomes thickened, softened, and more porous. A patient who had long repeated "I can't feel anything" may, in the right moment, utter the same phrase and suddenly burst into tears. The words are the same; the atmosphere has changed.

Visualization and mantra practices also offer insight into how form regulates affect. Each deity embodies a specific emotional register—wrath, compassion, equanimity, erotic heat—yet none are fixed personalities. They are affective palettes, aesthetic condensations of psychic possibility. The practitioner is not asked to *believe* in them but to use them, to enter their energetic structure. Jessica Benjamin (2004) writes that recognition in the analytic dyad involves *thirdness*—a field in which subjectivities interpenetrate without fusion. Visualization offers something analogous: the practitioner merges with the form without losing awareness that it is, in fact, a form. This double awareness—of fusion and distance—is central to analytic process as well. Patients must become their transferences in order to loosen them.

The cultivation of symbolic atmosphere in both traditions is therefore not ornamental but essential. It is through the creation of a dense enough symbolic field that something can shift. In psychoanalysis, the holding environment (Winnicott, 1960b) functions this way: not as a literal room or verbal reassurance, but as a consistent symbolic texture in which the patient's psyche can reconfigure. When that texture is lost—through rupture, inattention, or disavowed countertransference—the analytic atmosphere collapses, and the patient reverts to more rigid forms. This too mirrors Vajrayana: visualization must be stable enough before dissolution becomes liberatory. Otherwise, the formless is not freedom but terror.

Theorists like Wilfred Bion offer further bridges. His idea of "container/contained" (1962) is not only a developmental theory but an energetic model. Psychic elements—what he called "beta elements"—must be metabolized through a containing function in order to become thinkable. Visualization and mantra perform this function aesthetically and ritually. Psychoanalysis does so interpersonally and linguistically. In both, form is offered not to fix but to carry: an intermediate object that, once its function is fulfilled, can be released.

In clinical work, this suggests a shift in how we think about interpretation. Rather than aiming for truth or even coherence, we might consider whether a given formulation participates in the crafting of symbolic atmosphere. Is the interpretation too thin, too brittle, too rational? Or does it help thicken the air? Can it hold contradiction, temporality, and affect? A good interpretation is like a well-rendered deity: not static, but resonant. Not literal, but lived.

In mantra practice, the goal is not semantic clarity but attunement. Similarly, in analysis, the best interpretations often exceed their content. They carry rhythm, voice, warmth, tension—qualities that vibrate through the field. This is not mysticism; it is the texture of psychic life. Words matter, but how they enter the atmosphere matters more.

What visualization and mantra teach us, then, is that form is not the opposite of freedom—it is its condition. Without form, there is no rhythm, no holding, no orbit. But with too much form, we suffocate. Psychoanalysis and Vajrayana both walk this edge: creating forms to loosen identifications, speaking to release the unspeakable, building atmospheres in which emptiness is not void but presence.

In the next section, we will turn directly to the paradox of meditative practice itself: how diverse traditions use structured forms—from breath to deity to mantra—to evoke the unstructured nature of mind. The path to the formless, it seems, is always paved with form.

Meditation as Paradox: Structures of Stillness and the Formless Mind

Meditation is often imagined as a movement toward stillness, a quieting of the mind. But this stillness is not mere silence or passivity. It is structured, intentional, and—most importantly—paradoxical. Across Buddhist traditions, meditation is filled with form: the posture of the body, the rhythm of the breath, the object of attention, the conceptual scaffolding that names stages and goals. Yet these forms are not ends in themselves. They are scaffolds designed to dissolve. They are the raft, not the shore.

This is not incidental. It is a structural paradox at the heart of meditative discipline: form is the path to formlessness. The breath becomes the vehicle through which awareness recognizes itself. The deity is summoned, stabilized, and then dissolved. The mantra, repeated until it recedes, leads to silence. Every structure is offered in the spirit of relinquishment. The more precisely it is formed, the more fully it can be released.

In this, meditation aligns closely with psychoanalytic practice. The analytic frame—the consistency of sessions, the position of the analyst, the ritual of free association—is a structure designed to allow the formless elements of psychic life to surface. It is a container for unformulated experience (Stern, 1997), for what cannot yet be known. The paradox is clear: a tightly held structure allows the emergence of fluidity. And yet, as in meditation, the structure must not harden. It must be flexible enough to hold affect without foreclosing it.

Consider the practices of śamatha and vipaśyanā, often taught in tandem in the Tibetan tradition. Śamatha cultivates focused attention, often by resting the mind on the breath, a candle flame, or the image of a deity. Vipaśyanā introduces inquiry: the analysis of impermanence, suffering, and non-self. One stabilizes; the other dissolves. The breath is not the goal, but it is the vehicle. The insight into impermanence does not lead to nihilism but to a fuller participation in aliveness. These paired practices model how form and formlessness are not two paths, but a single spiral.

Psychoanalysis, too, oscillates between śamatha- and vipaśyanā-like modes. At times, the analyst functions like a śamatha object: a steady, non-reactive presence to which the patient's mind returns again and again. At other times, interpretation operates like vipaśyanā: cutting through illusions, revealing disowned aspects of the self, or highlighting the transience of meaning. This dialectic is not a sequence but a rhythm. The analyst, like the breath or the mantra, becomes a form that holds the field while deeper truths emerge.

Donald Winnicott (1958) gave us one of the clearest articulations of this paradox in his notion of the "capacity to be alone." True solitude, he argued, arises only when the internalized presence of another has been securely formed. One is never alone in a vacuum, but always alone *with*—with the trace of the mother, with the feeling of being held. Meditation, too, is not isolation but relational solitude. The posture, the breath, the lineage—these are the internalized others who hold the meditator as they venture into formlessness. The analytic frame serves the same function: its very constancy enables psychic regression and exploration.

Bion's concept of "negative capability"—borrowed from Keats—is another formulation of this paradox. To tolerate not knowing, to remain with uncertainty without premature closure, is the stance both analyst and meditator must cultivate. The analyst who cannot bear ambiguity will rush to interpret; the meditator who cannot sit with discomfort will grasp at insight. But true transformation occurs in the willingness to dwell in the in-between, where form is still present but no longer fixed.

This capacity—to rest within the structured, unstructured—is not merely a cognitive achievement. It is a psychophysical state. In meditation, the body participates: the spine is upright yet relaxed, the breath is natural yet attentive, and the gaze is soft. These are not aesthetic details but elements of the field. They shape the nervous system, entrain the mind, and create the conditions for awareness to become aware of itself.

In analysis, the equivalent is the analyst's somatic presence. The quality of the analyst's breathing, their regulation of their own arousal, their subtle shifts in posture and voice—these form the texture of the analytic atmosphere. Patients sense this. They may not name it, but they feel when the analyst is settled or scattered, receptive or defended. The analyst's form—their embodied presence—is part of what makes the analytic space livable. This, too, is structure in service of formlessness.

What emerges in both practices is a paradoxical spaciousness: a state in which there is form, but form is light; there is focus, but it is open; there is self, but it is not clung to. Winnicott called this the space of play. In Mahāmudrā, it is called "resting in the natural state." In Dzogchen, it is "non-meditation." In each, the achievement is not escape from structure, but intimacy with its arising and dissolution.

The implication for psychoanalytic technique is subtle but profound. We are not simply aiming for insight, catharsis, or even relational repair. We are creating conditions in which the patient can feel themselves emerge and dissolve, over and over, within a holding form. We are cultivating not certainty, but a more refined tolerance for ambiguity. We are inviting not coherence, but a deepening attunement to the fluid self.

This is not a departure from classical analytic aims, but a refinement of them. Freud sought to make the unconscious conscious, but he also knew that the unconscious would never be fully known. Lacan reminded us that the Real resists symbolization. Contemporary theorists like Donnel Stern, Thomas Ogden, and Antonino Ferro extend this lineage by exploring how unformulated experience, reverie, and narrative co-creation point to the always-becoming nature of psychic life.

In meditation, we learn to sit with this becoming—not as a failure of arrival, but as the texture of presence itself. In analysis, we learn to speak from it. The breath rises and falls. The words come and go. The frame holds, and then it shifts. Form leads us to the formless, which gives rise to new forms.

One patient once brought a dream that seemed to float outside interpretation.

He dreamed of drifting in open space—not in a ship or a suit, just his body adrift, curled slightly as though still in the womb. There were stars, but no planets. No tether. No threat. Only the slow, rotational drift of his form. "It wasn't lonely," he said. "It was like the universe was watching me breathe."

He didn't want to unpack the dream. "It didn't mean anything," he said. "It was the feeling itself." When I asked what kind of feeling, he paused, then whispered, "Held."

That was the entire session.

Later, I found myself returning to it—not for meaning, but for atmosphere. The dream wasn't about abandonment or omnipotence. It wasn't metaphor. It was presence, scaled to the cosmos. Sometimes the analytic field becomes that: not a mirror, but an orbit. Not a frame for thought, but a space for breath.

In the next section, we will turn to the esoteric traditions of Mahāmudrā and Dzogchen—lineages that not only teach this paradox but enact it, often through direct, non-conceptual means. Their logic is not symbolic but radiant. Their aim is not attainment, but recognition of what has always been here.

The Diamond and the Mirror—Dzogchen, Mahāmudrā, and the Nature of Mind

In the tantric map of Tibetan Buddhism, Dzogchen and Mahāmudrā are the crown jewels—not because they are superior in a hierarchical sense, but because they return most directly to the paradox at the heart of all the teachings: that the mind is already awake, and yet it does not recognize itself. These paths do not begin with analysis or transformation but with recognition—direct and immediate—of the nature of awareness itself.

Mahāmudrā, often associated with the Kagyu tradition, and Dzogchen, the pinnacle of the Nyingma school, are not techniques so much as pointers. They are considered "non-gradual" in that they do not assume the mind must be cultivated or refined before it can glimpse its true nature. Instead, they emphasize that what is sought is already present. The task is not to fabricate realization but to unveil it.

This unveiling is often catalyzed through what are called "pointing-out instructions." The teacher—ideally someone who has stabilized their own recognition—uses words, gestures, or simply presence to introduce the student to the nature of their own mind. This nature is called *rigpa* in Dzogchen: non-dual, non-conceptual, empty yet luminous awareness. The metaphors used are striking: the sky, vast and unobstructed; the mirror, reflective and unstained; the diamond, indestructible and clear.

We might be tempted to relegate these as poetic images, but they are phenomenologically precise. In meditation, the moment when one recognizes awareness itself—as the space in which thoughts arise and dissolve—is often accompanied by a quiet, seismic shift. The sense of being a "self" who is meditating collapses. Awareness is not *doing* awareness; it simply *is*. Like the diamond, it cuts through confusion without itself being cut.

From a psychoanalytic vantage point, this may seem foreign. But parallels abound. Loewald (1960) spoke of the "experience of experience"—moments when the mind becomes present not only to its contents, but to itself as container. Ogden (1994) elaborated the "analytic third" as the intersubjective field that arises in analysis, irreducible to either patient or analyst. Donnel Stern (1997) described "unformulated experience" as the preverbal ground from which all narrative arises.

What Dzogchen and Mahāmudrā offer is a glimpse of this ground without the detour of symbolization. They go beneath the formulations, beneath even the desire to articulate. But this is not a regressive state. It is a precise and refined attunement to what Eigen (2004) might call the "psyche of unform," or what Bion termed "O"—ultimate reality, unknowable yet felt.

The method is absence. In Mahāmudrā, the meditator may be instructed to look at the mind that is thinking. "Turn your attention to the one who sees," the teacher might say. But the meditator finds nothing. No seer, no center—only openness. Yet this openness is not blankness. It is radiant, imbued with a clarity that is not conceptual but intimate. This is the mirror: empty of content, yet reflecting all.

The clinical resonance is profound. When an analyst rests in their own open awareness—unhurried by technique or interpretation—they become a mirror. Not in the blank sense of classical neutrality, but as a luminous surface in which the patient may begin to see themselves not as symptom, not as failure, but as flux, as possibility. The analyst's grounded presence *is* the intervention. As Thomas Ogden writes, the analyst must sometimes "dream the patient into being."

And yet, this presence is not passive. In Dzogchen, one does not merely rest in awareness. One also recognizes the radiance of that awareness as the play of appearance. The world is not denied, but revealed as display. In psychoanalytic terms, this might be likened to the capacity to hold transference both as deeply real and as a projection. The patient's fear, idealization, and seduction—all are valid, and yet none are the whole truth. The analyst holds the form, even as they sense its emptiness.

The image of the diamond is helpful here. In Tibetan iconography, the vajra—a ritual object symbolizing indestructibility and skillful means—is often held in the right hand, with the bell of wisdom in the left. Together, they signify that emptiness and form, compassion and clarity, are not opposites but co-arising qualities. The analyst, too, must cultivate this twin attunement: a diamond-like clarity that cuts through delusion, and a bell-like receptivity that resonates with what is not yet known.

To "point out" the nature of mind in analysis is not to offer metaphysical teaching. It is to become the atmosphere in which the patient begins to sense that their thoughts are not the whole story, that their feelings, however intense, arise in a wider field. Sometimes this is done through silence. Sometimes, through a shift in posture, a slowing of tone, a refusal to chase the symptom. The analyst ceases to grasp. And in that space, the patient may begin to see.

This is not a mystical aside. It is a clinical posture with deep ethical implications. When we allow the patient's being to unfold without rushing to interpret, we dignify their existence. We offer a space not only for understanding but for recognition—not of content, but of presence.

Freud's early insights into the unconscious were built on the observation that what cannot be spoken returns in symptom. Dzogchen turns this inside out: what is most true has never been absent, only overlooked. But perhaps the two insights meet. Perhaps the analyst and the meditator are both seeking a return—not to the past, but to the ground that holds every past and future: the diamond, the mirror, the mind itself.

In the next section, we turn to clinical implications: how these Buddhist insights might reorient analytic presence, transference technique, and our understanding of transformation—not as achievement, but as recognition.

Clinical Implications—Emptiness, Form, and the Analyst's Presence

If both Buddhism and psychoanalysis revolve around the paradox of form and emptiness, then the analytic setting itself may be understood not simply as a space of meaning-making, but as a medium of transformation in how forms are held, dissolved, and re-formed. The analyst becomes more than an interpreter or witness; they become a symbolic presence through which the patient's experience of reality—solid, elusive, unbearable—may begin to shimmer with its constructedness.

In Vajrayāna Buddhism, visualization is not fantasy or metaphor, but a deliberate use of form to awaken awareness of emptiness. The yidam deity is generated in vivid detail, imbued with symbolic qualities, and then dissolved into space. The practitioner participates in the birth and disappearance of form to realize the mind's nondual nature. In the analytic space, the patient constructs psychic forms—stories, identifications, fantasies, transferential positions—not to be ridiculed or quickly interpreted, but to be inhabited with precision and gentleness until their structure loosens, revealing the fluid core beneath.

Galit Atlas (2022) has emphasized the analyst's capacity to bear the patient's unformulated experience, to metabolize affect that has not yet found symbolic shape. This bearing is not passive containment, but a deeply engaged responsiveness to what is both emerging and vanishing in each moment. Similarly, in meditation, one is trained to hold arising thoughts and emotions with neither grasping nor rejection—to let them dance without fastening them into permanence.

Meditative awareness and analytic presence both require a double attention: to form and to its passing. In analysis, this means listening not only to what the patient says, but to the atmosphere in which it is said, the cadence of silences, the energetic residue left behind. Jessica Benjamin (2004) describes a form of thirdness—an intersubjective space that neither collapses into fusion nor splits into distance. That space is akin to the tantric field, where both deity and practitioner dissolve and co-arise, each the other's mirror.

Clinical moments of Recognition Reversal often depend on this kind of attunement. When a patient speaks something that has long remained unspoken, the analytic atmosphere changes. A symptom may unravel.

A childhood image, once feared, becomes tender. But just as in visualization practice, the form—once spoken—may also vanish. "It doesn't feel as heavy now," a patient might say after naming a lifelong guilt. The analyst, if attuned, senses that this is not a loss of meaning, but a liberation from reification. The form has fulfilled its function. It can dissolve.

These dissolutions are not always soft. Sometimes the patient's identifications are defended with intensity. The analyst's task is not to pry them away, but to hold them gently, allowing their necessity to be felt before their emptiness can be glimpsed. As Michael Eigen (2005) reminds us, the psyche often clings to structures not out of blindness, but as protection against overwhelming exposure. To see the form as dreamlike does not mean to dismiss it—it means to accompany the patient until they are ready to see through it.

The analyst's own practice—whether meditative or simply grounded in radical receptivity—shapes their capacity for this kind of presence. Jack Engler (2003) argued that psychological and spiritual development must be integrated: one must become somebody before becoming nobody. In the clinical context, this means the analyst must cultivate both the clarity to see symbolic forms and the spaciousness to let them pass. That clarity does not come from technical mastery alone. It arises from the discipline of inner stillness—the capacity to remain in contact with the patient's suffering without needing to resolve it prematurely.

Clinical work shaped by this ethos becomes less about solving problems and more about entering a shared field of transformation. A patient who repeatedly reenacts abandonment may not need immediate interpretation. They may need the analyst to stay. To remain as a witness not just to the story but to the atmosphere of fear beneath it. This is the analytic equivalent of śamatha practice: remaining with the breath of the moment, letting it settle, waiting for insight to arise not from effort, but from presence.

When the analyst's presence becomes a kind of mirror, the patient begins to glimpse themselves not only as the one who suffers, but as the one who sees. In Buddhist language, this is rigpa—awareness recognizing itself. In psychoanalytic terms, it is the birth of a subject who can hold themselves in mind. Not because the analyst named the pattern, but because they *were* the space in which the patient's being could be safely mirrored, metabolized, and mourned.

This form of witnessing does not seek to fill in, but to open. The analyst becomes a vessel through which the patient may see that their thoughts and feelings are real and also impermanent. That their longing is valid and also shaped by fantasy. That their pain is particular and also not singular. In Buddhist terms, this is compassion married to wisdom. In clinical terms, it is attunement without appropriation.

To hold form and emptiness together is not to flatten paradox, but to dwell within it. The analytic room becomes a ritual space, like the tantric mandala: carefully constructed, then allowed to dissolve. The analyst, like the deity, is both real and symbolic. Their presence is not about truth-telling, but about offering the patient a mirror that does not distort, a silence that is not void, a gaze that does not consume.

This is not merely technique. It is an ethical posture. To offer this kind of presence is to say: I will not make your pain into an object. I will not rush to make meaning. I will sit with you in the unknowing. And together, perhaps, we will begin to sense that even in the most solid places, something flickers. Something opens. Something, always already, is free.

The Analyst Who Meditates—Influence on Presence and Patient Self-Experience

Meditation is not simply a tool for inner calm. For the analyst, it may serve as a practice of presence that transforms how one listens, waits, and meets the other. The clinical relationship does not exist in a vacuum. It is shaped, moment by moment, by the analyst's capacity to receive, metabolize, and return the patient's experience—not as a counterweight or mirror, but as a living rhythm of shared awareness. When the analyst meditates, this rhythm can subtly shift. A stillness enters the field. Time breathes.

Psychoanalysis has long grappled with the tension between technique and presence. Thomas Ogden's concept of the analytic third (1994), for instance, points to a shared field that arises when both analyst and patient surrender their self-contained positions. In this space, what is felt and thought does not belong entirely to either person—it is emergent. Meditation deepens the analyst's capacity to tolerate this field: not to control or master it, but to abide in its ambiguity without retreat. The analyst who meditates practices being with what arises, neither grasping for intervention nor fleeing into formulation. This is not passivity. It is a kind of radical poise.

Mark Epstein (1995, 2007) has written extensively on the intersections between meditative discipline and therapeutic presence, suggesting that the analyst's meditation practice fosters a non-interfering receptivity that allows psychic life to unfold more fully. Similarly, Barry Magid (2002), drawing from Zen and psychoanalysis, describes how meditation cultivates a willingness to dwell in the immediacy of the patient's suffering without rushing to rescue. The analyst, like the zazen practitioner, learns to sit—literally and metaphorically—with discomfort, contradiction, and not-knowing.

The clinical effects of this stance can be profound. Patients often report feeling "more seen" or "less judged" in the presence of an analyst who brings such grounded spaciousness. This is not a mystical charisma. It is a relational sensitivity that has been honed through disciplined attention to mind, body, and breath. Meditation trains the analyst in micro-attunements: the shift in a patient's posture, the catch in their breath, the subtlest modulation of voice. But perhaps more importantly, it trains the analyst not to flinch. When grief surges, when rage breaks through, when erotic transferences quicken the room—the analyst who meditates is less likely to clamp down or shut off. They remain porous, responsive.

This form of presence can have unexpected effects on the patient's experience of self. Over time, the analytic space becomes less a stage for performance and more a container for revelation. The patient may begin to speak from previously unreachable places—not because the analyst asked the right question, but because the analyst was simply there. Presence itself becomes transformative. As Joko Beck (1993) often taught, profound healing unfolds in a space of silence and receptive presence, where the ground of awareness is allowed to emerge without force.

From the perspective of affective neuroscience, Jaak Panksepp (1998) has emphasized the role of attuned contact in regulating the early emotional systems of the brain, particularly those involving fear, care, and grief. Meditation, especially when combined with relational practice, enhances the analyst's regulatory capacity—not by suppressing their own affect, but by becoming a more stable, attuned presence in the room. This bodily resonance fosters what Daniel Siegel (1999) calls "interpersonal neurobiology," in which the minds and nervous systems of patient and analyst co-regulate toward greater complexity and integration.

But it is not just the patient who is changed. The analyst who meditates may find that their own countertransference shifts—not in intensity, but in texture. Meditation helps disentangle the analyst's reactivity from their responsiveness. When a patient attacks, the meditating analyst may notice the surge of defensiveness but need not identify with it. When a patient seduces, the analyst may feel the pull but remain grounded in awareness. This does not immunize the analyst from enactment, but it makes them more likely to notice it while it is happening. The self-reflexivity cultivated on the cushion becomes available in the room.

This is not to suggest that every analyst should meditate. Nor is it to imply that meditation is a shortcut to therapeutic efficacy. But for those who do sit—especially within a lineage or structured path—it becomes clear that meditation is not separate from analytic work. It is a training in the same paradox: form and formlessness, presence and absence, knowing and not-knowing. The breath is not so different from the transference: both are patterns that repeat, both offer entry points into deeper psychic life, both shimmer with constructedness and aliveness.

A brief clinical illustration: A middle-aged man, raised in a household where silence meant danger, enters treatment with a compulsion to narrate every feeling. When the analyst begins to cultivate longer silences in session—not as avoidance, but as attuned presence—the patient grows anxious, then confused, and eventually becomes curious. "I noticed I didn't need to explain myself just now," he says. "And nothing terrible happened." Over time, he begins to experience his own thoughts not as emergencies to manage, but as passing weather. What changed was not the analyst's theory, but their capacity to sit still, to hold space.

In this way, meditation's influence enters the analytic process not through technique, but through tempo. The rhythm slows. The air thickens. The mind becomes more transparent. The analyst learns to recognize when they are clinging to an idea, when they are subtly pushing a patient toward insight, when they are trying to do something rather than be someone. And in that recognition, they return to the ground of practice: not knowing, but being with.

The psychoanalytic tradition, particularly in its relational and postmodern strands, has increasingly valorized presence over interpretation, witnessing over mastery. Meditation deepens this trajectory. It does not replace analysis. It ripens it. It softens the boundaries of the ego without erasing the rigor of thought. It allows the analyst to see more clearly and to care more wisely.

This chapter has traced many convergences between Buddhism and psychoanalysis, but perhaps the most quietly transformative is this: the analyst who meditates brings a different mind to the encounter—not purer, not higher, but more willing to be shaped. In that willingness, the patient, too, may find new ways to know themselves: not as a fixed self to defend, but as a dynamic, breathing constellation of presence. Awareness, as both traditions teach, is not what we achieve. It is what we return to.

Conclusion—Two Tongues for One Mind

This chapter has not sought to compare Buddhism and psychoanalysis in order to integrate them, reconcile their differences, or establish a hierarchy of truth. Instead, it has proposed that each tradition orbits a central paradox: that form is emptiness and emptiness is form. This phrase, drawn from the Heart Sutra, is not a metaphor but a structural truth—a recursive statement about the nature of psychic life, symbolic mediation, and the conditions under which transformation becomes possible.

The phrase finds its psychoanalytic counterpart in the way unformulated experience takes symbolic shape, only to lose its libidinal gravity in the moment of recognition. In both traditions, the symbol is necessary but unstable. It does not capture reality but gestures toward its ungraspability. Freud's early model of repression, Winnicott's transitional space, Loewald's emphasis on integration and symbolization, Bion's "O," and Lacan's Real all converge in their attention to the edge where knowing fails. In Buddhist terms, this is śūnyatā—emptiness—not as negation, but as the open field in which form flickers and dissolves.

We have also traced how this paradox is enacted through practice. Vajrayana visualizations create radiant forms precisely to dissolve them. Mantras vibrate meaning into being without referential content. Dzogchen and Mahāmudrā dispense with symbolic mediation entirely, pointing the practitioner directly to the unconditioned ground of mind. These are not poetic aspirations but rigorously trained experiences—techniques of becoming intimate with what cannot be possessed. They parallel psychoanalytic practices of presence, holding, and symbolic attunement. The analyst's interpretation, like the deity visualization, must appear fully and then vanish; it must be held lightly, with reverence for its provisionality.

Clinical work reflects these patterns. We explored how an analyst's meditative practice shapes their presence, allowing them to become a field in which the patient's forms may arise, intensify, and dissolve. Such presence alters the patient's experience of self: what was once tightly gripped can be released; what was once defended against can be mourned; what was once inchoate can be spoken, even if only briefly, before it disappears again. Form is not final. It is the doorway.

This doorway is also temporal. The patient's history reconfigures itself in the analytic now, just as the Buddhist practitioner's karmic traces surface in the space of practice. Both traditions affirm that what is most real does not lie behind or ahead of us, but within the arising moment. Donald Winnicott's insistence on the potential space between analyst and patient, or between self and other, echoes the Buddhist concept of the bardo—a liminal gap between states of being. In both, the real work occurs in the between.

Throughout this chapter, we have invoked a range of thinkers—psychoanalytic, Buddhist, and philosophical—not to assemble an academic pantheon, but to demonstrate the polyphonic resonance that emerges when these traditions are placed in dialogue. Jessica Benjamin's mutual recognition and Michael Eigen's reverence for intensity remind us that presence is not passive but charged, devotional. Maurice Merleau-Ponty's phenomenology of perception and Emmanuel Levinas's ethics of encounter illuminate the ontological vulnerability at the heart of every therapeutic moment. Donna Orange's clinical hospitality, Bruce Fink's Lacanian clinical logic, and D.W. Winnicott's emphasis on imaginative play all share a sensibility: the mind is not a problem to be solved but a mystery to be listened into.

There is a temptation—especially among analytic minds—to organize these convergences into a framework, a theory, a new system. But perhaps the most important lesson these traditions offer together is that every framework is ultimately a raft: useful for crossing but not to be carried on one's back. We may speak of recognition reversal, of symbolic condensation, of field theory, or rigpa, but these are forms, not finalities. The real teaching emerges when form falls away.

The analyst and the practitioner are not sages. They are, in the deepest sense, fellow travelers—ones who have learned how to wait, how to listen, how to lose the thread and return again. The analyst who meditates and the practitioner who listens psychoanalytically both cultivate a discipline of presence that is more spacious than certainty. They know that insight can shimmer and vanish, that transformation is rarely linear, and that the most important moments often arrive without announcement, without resolution, and without name.

Let us end not with a summary, but with a gesture. As you read these words, notice your breath. Do not follow it or deepen it—simply observe that it is happening. That awareness arises in a field. That field does not belong to you. It is not inside or outside. It is what allows experience to happen. Just as the analytic dyad does not take place "in" the patient or "in" the analyst, but in the third that forms between them, this field arises from the conditions of attention.

It is neither psychoanalytic nor Buddhist. And yet it is the ground of both.

To speak of "two tongues for one mind" is not to propose a merger. It is to acknowledge that the human mind, in its longing, its fragmentation, and its return, requires more than one language. That the symbolic is always provisional. That emptiness is not something to be feared but something to be known from within. And that presence—not theory—is the common project.

May the analytic room and the meditation cushion continue to reverberate. May they offer us, and those we accompany, new ways to fall apart, to come together, and to begin again.

Closing Reflection

If psychoanalysis seeks to name the unsymbolized and Buddhism rests in its ungraspability, both traditions circle the same gravitational silence. In analytic work, we metabolize that silence into meaning. In contemplative practice, we allow it to remain vast. But in both, something unspeakable is held—not to be resolved, but to be lived beside.

As we turn now toward the outermost edge of this book—toward the cosmos, the frame, and what lies just beyond—we carry with us this paradox: that emptiness is not absence, but presence ungrasped. The mind does not merely symbolize; it radiates. And what it radiates is the shape of its longing to hold what cannot be held.

And yet, in the analyst's chair, we return—not to solve, but to sit beside. Not to speak, but to listen, as form and emptiness co-arise.

Part V

Beyond Frame—Freud's Horizon and the Analyst's Cosmos

Part IV explored the gravitational edge of symbol, where meaning flickers into atmosphere and emptiness becomes a holding space rather than a void. What follows now is not a resolution but a widening. Part V turns toward the cosmic, the trans-symbolic, and the frame itself—not to discard form, but to hold it from the outside. **Freud, in his final writings, gestured toward this widening—invoking the death drive, the mystic writing pad, and the oceanic feeling as limits of symbolization. Klein, too, touched the edge of the unnameable in her work on annihilation anxiety and fragmentary internal worlds.** This final arc extends those gestures into new territory: not by rejecting the analytic frame, but by treating it as a permeable field—curved by memory, mortality, and the analyst's own gravitational mass. The analyst becomes both participant and witness to the psyche's recursive orbit. These chapters are not an endpoint. They are an invitation to hold the unframed.

DOI: 10.4324/9781003715306-18

12 The Analyst in the Cosmos

This chapter explores the analyst not as an interpreter or technician, but as a gravitational body within the psychic field. Drawing on the book's overarching topological metaphor, it considers how the analyst becomes a symbolic form—one that orients, holds, and echoes within the patient's psychic structure. Through reflections on solitude, presence, mortality, and symbolic transference, this chapter positions the analytic process as a field phenomenon shaped as much by rhythm and aesthetic form as by content. The analyst is not the center of the patient's world, but a resonant trace in their symbolic atmosphere. This chapter ends with a quiet meditation on the analyst's role as field-form—something carried, remembered, and shaped long after the treatment has ended.

This chapter is a descent into stillness. Where previous chapters theorized fragmentation, symbolization, and psychic gravity from within the dynamic arc of symptom and subject, this final analytic chapter turns inward—to the quiet force of presence. It considers the analyst not as observer or function, but as form: a gravitational rhythm around which the patient orbits, resists, and returns. As the book approaches its final coda, we ask not what the analyst does, but what shape they become—how their presence, silence, and mortality trace a symbolic residue that holds after the work is done.

Analytic Gravity and the Ethics of Presence

There is a gravity to the analyst—not as a figure of authority, but as a body in the field, a presence that bends the psychic space around it. This gravity is not chosen; it is conferred by the frame, the silence, the patient's projections, and the analyst's own history. But to hold this gravity ethically is a choice. It requires a steady willingness to be felt, distorted, even misunderstood, without grasping for control. The analyst becomes, in this sense, a cosmic object—not in scale or omniscience, but in effect: a presence that shapes the field simply by remaining.

This gravitational metaphor, now familiar across the book, reaches its most intimate scale here. The analyst is not outside the patient's orbit, nor are they a detached observer. They are the nearest planet, the darkest mirror, the least

DOI: 10.4324/9781003715306-19

visible horizon. Their body, language, and breath register in the field, just as the patient's psyche registers in theirs. The analytic frame is not a fixed container but a subtle curve—a warped space-time where certain truths, impossible elsewhere, become temporarily speakable.

Analytic presence, in this light, is not defined by what the analyst says or interprets, but by how they remain. To remain is not to be passive. It is to absorb and metabolize the recursive pressures of the field without collapsing into reaction. It is to allow the patient's symptom, structure, desire, or dissociation to orbit without disruption. This does not mean permitting endless repetition or avoiding intervention. But it does mean that every intervention must first be weighed against the ethical gravity of presence: will this open space, or collapse it?

In many traditions, the teacher or guide is understood to radiate a kind of field—less about information and more about transmission. In psychoanalysis, this idea is often hidden beneath more technical language, but it persists. Winnicott's notion of the holding environment, Loewald's vision of the analyst as a new matrix, Eigen's reverberating psyche, Ogden's analytic third—all point toward the idea that the analyst's presence exerts force beyond content. The patient does not only hear the analyst—they feel them. They live inside the warp of their gravity.

And that gravity can fail. It can fail when the analyst flees their position, disavows their countertransference, imposes meaning, or withholds it reflexively. Gravity can become invasive and can collapse into seduction or erasure. But it can also fail by disappearing—by becoming weightless, unreachable, evacuated. The ethical task of analytic presence is to hold one's gravity—not perfectly, not infallibly, but reliably enough that the patient can test, push, return, and risk becoming visible in its field.

To be such a presence is to surrender the fantasy of neutrality. One becomes, instead, a participant in a shared cosmos—a space defined not by symmetry, but by entanglement. Even the quietest moment is co-authored. The analyst's gravity means that they, too, bend under the patient's force. Reverie, fatigue, desire, disorientation—these are not signs of failure, but of mutual inclusion. The analytic pair inhabits the same curved space.

This reframes responsibility. The analyst is not simply responsible for interpreting or for maintaining technique. They are responsible for how they are felt—as weight, as silence, as style, as mood. This responsibility cannot be discharged by intellectual humility or ethical intention alone. It is a phenomenological fact: the analyst has gravity whether or not they wish to. The only question is how they will hold it.

To hold gravity means to develop ethical mass without becoming heavy. It means becoming a body that does not flee itself. A presence that is not afraid to reflect, to contain, to unshape and reshape. The patient may test this gravity by withdrawing, seducing, enacting, or collapsing. The analyst's task is not to correct these gestures but to remain touchable. A presence that can be touched, even through fantasy, begins to reshape the field.

There is something cosmic in this. Not in the sense of transcendence, but in scale: the idea that the microcosm of the analytic dyad recapitulates something essential about being a self in a world. The analyst is not the world—but they may become, for a time, its gravitational center. To hold this center ethically is to accept the impossibility of knowing exactly what one is holding—and to remain anyway.

In this way, this chapter—and the book—begins to turn toward a final paradox: that the analyst's greatest gift is not their knowing, but their unknowing. Their willingness to be the horizon, the dark companion, the nearby body that bends the light just enough for the patient to glimpse something new. This is not passive. It is a form of presence that bends time and space, that makes the invisible edge of becoming feel almost bearable.

Echo and Reverie: The Analyst's Inner World

The analyst's gravity is not only what they bring into the room, but what resounds within them—what reverberates in the folds of their own subjectivity. In the silence of the session, the analyst does not simply wait. They listen inward, registering echoes that are not quite thoughts, not yet interpretations. These inner movements—flickers of sensation, half-formed images, peripheral memories—are the beginnings of reverie. They are the analyst's own unconscious tracing the curves of the patient's world.

Reverie is not a luxury; it is a method. It is how the analyst feels their way into the unknown, not by solving it, but by allowing it to form within them. In this way, the analyst becomes a medium—not passive, but porous. What arises in reverie is not random. It is shaped by the transference, by the patient's unspeakable demands, by the field of mutual influence. And yet it also comes from the analyst's singular cosmos: their own wounds, memories, and style of thinking. Reverie is both shared and solitary.

This solitude matters. Analysts, like all people, inhabit a private world. But analytic solitude is a cultivated condition: a capacity to be with one's own mind in the presence of another's, without rushing to resolve either. The analyst becomes a kind of cosmic buffer—neither fully in their own experience, nor fully merged with the patient's, but suspended between. This suspension allows something new to echo into the field.

Ogden (1994) described this as the analytic third—a co-created intersubjective space that neither belongs to the analyst nor the patient, but emerges between them. Reverie is the analyst's way of listening to that space. It is where the analyst's psyche bends, where they become available to be changed. This is not a yielding of stance or authority, but a deep ethical stance: the analyst must become moved, not just observing. Their inner world must register the patient, not as an object of understanding, but as an aesthetic event.

What does the analyst do with these echoes? Sometimes nothing. The rhythm of the patient's speech may conjure an old song. A sudden chill might feel like memory. A longing may bloom unbidden. These are not distractions. They are data of the deepest kind—not about the patient alone, but about the field in which both now float. They are signs that the analyst is being moved, that they are inside the gravitational pull of the encounter.

This movement is not without risk. Analysts carry their own longings, ghosts, and echoes. Reverie may awaken grief, envy, erotic charge, and shame. These are not contaminations. They are signals of vitality. To feel one's own inner cosmos stir is not to lose neutrality, but to enter the analytic relation with a fuller presence. The analyst who does not echo is not protected; they are absent.

Still, the analyst must choose how to use what arises. Reverie does not demand enactment. It demands containment, reflection, and sometimes, the courage to let a symbol shimmer rather than be pinned. To feel the echo but not force its meaning. To register a grief but not collapse into it. To live with the strange simultaneity of one's own world bending around another's, and to recognize that this is the work.

The analyst's gravity, then, includes their receptivity. But it also includes their aesthetic discernment: the sense of when to speak, when to wait, when to allow a metaphor to thicken or dissipate. This discernment is not taught. It is cultivated—through experience, supervision, analysis, and perhaps most deeply, through solitude. Not isolation, but the solitude of listening inward. The solitude that allows echoes to become insight, not by chasing them, but by staying near.

Such solitude is sacred. Not in a religious sense, but in the psychoanalytic sense: it is a psychic space where truth forms slowly, where time warps, where the analyst allows something unformulated to grow inside them. The analyst's solitude is a shelter—not a hiding place, but a space of slow metabolization. The patient feels this. They sense when their story is not merely heard but echoed in a deeper space, where it might find form.

This is why the analyst must remain emotionally available to their own mind. A defended analyst—however theoretically gifted—cannot serve as a gravitational anchor. It is not cleverness that holds the field. It is the willingness to let one's own echo chambers be disturbed. To allow oneself to feel uncertain, porous, and unsolvable. To permit the patient's unworded world to reverberate across one's own interior landscapes.

When this happens, something extraordinary occurs. The patient begins to sense that their experience is not just being heard, but being held—across bodies, minds, silences. The analyst is no longer simply an interpreter but a resonator. A field. An inner world that has curved enough to let another's voice be amplified. This is how insight becomes recognition, and how interpretation becomes witnessing.

What echoes inside the analyst is not just the patient's content, but their form. Their rhythm of speech, their pattern of avoidance, their abrupt laughter, or sudden dissociation. These micro-forms take root in the analyst's mind, not as data points, but as aesthetic impressions. Reverie allows the analyst to live inside those impressions—not to define them, but to be shaped by them. To let the echo grow louder, more coherent, until it speaks.

There is no formula for this. But there is an ethic: to remain near one's own experience without collapsing into it. To listen to the field without replacing it. To allow reverie to serve as a bridge—not a solution, but a shimmer. The analyst's inner world becomes part of the analytic process not by dominating it, but by vibrating in its key.

And when the analyst's reverie becomes visible—when they speak from that echo, when they offer not only meaning but resonance—the patient often feels it instantly. The words do not feel foreign. They feel familiar, like a thought the patient had but could not quite think. The reverie lands not as surprise, but as return. Something long circling finally finds a place to touch down.

This is how the analyst's solitude becomes a shared sky. Not lonely, not aloof—but full of constellations, flickers, reverberations. The analyst, by tending to their own inner cosmos, helps illuminate the patient's. Not by pointing to the stars, but by letting them shine.

The Analyst as Gravitational Body

The analyst's presence is not neutral. It bends the field. It alters the trajectory of speech, the pacing of memory, and the shape of the hour. In this sense, the analyst is not just a listener but a gravitational body—something around which meaning orbits, distorts, and reorganizes. Like a planet or a star, the analyst holds a weight—not through action, but through position. The gravity of their presence is not loud, but dense.

This density does not come from certainty. It comes from capacity: the capacity to bear ambiguity, to remain when rupture trembles at the edge, to absorb the impact of words that may never be fully understood. The analyst's body—its stillness, its breath, its pacing—is part of the clinical language. Every tilt of the head, every pause, becomes part of the atmosphere. And it is this atmosphere that allows something new to form.

Patients often speak of "feeling the room" before they feel themselves. They sense the rhythm of the analyst's attention, the pressure or spaciousness of the hour. Before they can speak freely, they must calibrate themselves to that gravity. They must know how the analyst holds. And when that holding is steady—not rigid but anchored—something softens. The patient begins to descend into layers that were previously unspeakable.

This descent is not a collapse. It is a gravitational fall—an inward movement made possible by the presence of another who will not fall apart. Regression, in this light, is not a failure of maturity but a gravitational event: the psyche moving back along the arc of development, drawn toward something it could not metabolize alone. The analyst's body becomes the axis around which this spiral turns. And it is the analyst's containment of that spiral that gives it therapeutic potential.

Winnicott (1965) knew this intimately. He described the mother's capacity to survive the infant's omnipotence—not just by staying alive, but by remaining present—as the cornerstone of psychic growth. The analyst, too, must survive. Not stoically, not distantly, but with a gravity that welcomes return. That says, in action if not in words: "You may spiral. I will not eject you."

This gravitational quality is not static. It changes over the course of treatment. At first, the analyst's gravity may feel foreign—too much, too little, and too strange. The patient may push against it, test it, or retreat from it. However, over time, as the field thickens, the analyst becomes a point of reference. Their presence acquires a memory. Their silences become meaningful. Their consistency becomes a kind of landscape.

This is especially true in long-term work. The analyst's gravity begins to shape the patient's internal world, not by replacing it, but by offering a steady force within it. Over years, the patient may return to the same themes, the same wounds—but they return differently. The analyst's presence alters the arc. Repetition becomes spiral. Compulsion becomes orbit. And eventually, something begins to shift.

That shift may be subtle. A breath that deepens. A phrase that returns in new tone. An affect that once scattered now settles. These are gravitational effects. They are not caused, exactly, but permitted. The analyst becomes the still center in a field of recursive movement. They hold the time of therapy—the hour, the week, the years—not simply as schedule, but as architecture. The patient, in turn, learns to live within that architecture. To let themselves be shaped by it.

This is a radical act. For many patients, the world has not held them. Time has been shattered. Bodies have been unsafe. Space has been weaponized. To enter a room where another person's gravity is reliable—where their body does not violate or withdraw, but simply holds—is to re-encounter the possibility of relational space. Not perfect space, not fantasy space, but livable space.

And this livability matters. It is what allows the patient to risk re-entry—into memory, into affect, into contact. The analyst's gravity does not guarantee safety, but it makes it imaginable. And imagination, in this context, is not escape but infrastructure. It is what allows the mind to build toward something new.

The analyst's body thus becomes part of the patient's psychic structure. Not as an internal object in the traditional sense, but as a spatial principle—a sense of where gravity exists. Of where one can go and still be held. Of how long one can speak before the silence becomes rupture. These are not symbolic forms alone; they are sensed geometries. The analyst becomes a coordinate in the patient's internal map.

This is not about dependence. It is about field dynamics. The analyst's body sets the tone, not by controlling, but by curving. By registering the field's movement and allowing their own structure to adapt—not to please, but to hold. This adaptability is not compliance. It is ethical responsiveness. The analyst bends not because they are swayed, but because they are listening.

This curvature—this gravitational responsiveness—also allows for moments of symbolic reorganization. When the analyst says something that resonates deeply, it is not just the content of their words that matters. It is the way their body, tone, and timing participate in the shaping of space. A well-timed silence can carry as much gravitational weight as an interpretation. A shift in posture can signal more safety than a long explanation.

These micro-movements are not secondary to technique; they are technique. Or rather, they are what technique rests upon: the analyst's capacity to be a gravitational body within the analytic field. A body that listens. A body that holds. A body that does not disintegrate under pressure. A body that allows return.

In this way, the analyst becomes part of the patient's recursive history—not simply as a figure, but as a form. As the one who remained when others could not. As the one who held when others shattered. As the one whose gravity did not pull the patient apart, but helped reassemble them in orbit.

This is not grandiosity. It is humility. The analyst does not create the patient's psyche anew. But they offer a gravitational condition in which something new might coalesce. They provide a different tempo, a different resonance, a different gravity. And over time, the patient begins to internalize that field—not as a script, but as a felt possibility.

The analyst's presence, then, becomes an invitation: to spiral, to return, to be held again. To feel the weight of one's own psyche and to find that it can be borne. The analyst's gravity allows for that return—not because they fix, but because they remain. Because they are willing to be the still point around which something living can unfold.

Mortality and the Echo of the Analyst

Every analyst will die. And every patient, consciously or not, knows this. The analyst is not immortal, not infinite, not untouched by time. Their mortality is not only a fact—it is a field condition. It shades the work. It sets the tone. To sit with another over months or years is to move together through time, not just as therapy, but as life. Birthdays pass. Illness arrives. Parents die. Bodies change. Grief thickens. So does intimacy. The analytic relationship becomes temporalized—not despite its frame, but through it.

The analyst's mortality is not just a clinical reality; it is a psychic presence. It softens omnipotence. It roots transference. It complicates idealization. No analyst can be everything—not because they lack skill, but because they are human. They will get sick. They will cancel sessions. They will eventually vanish. And yet, it is this very finitude that lends their presence its depth. They are real because they are limited.

To encounter the analyst's mortality is to feel the contours of the analytic holding. It is to recognize that the space is made, not guaranteed. That it is crafted each week through care, not delivered from on high. The analyst shows up again and again, despite the slow erosion of time. Their commitment is not infinite, but it is renewable. And in that renewable commitment, something sacred emerges.

Patients do not always speak of this. But they feel it. They feel when the analyst's voice changes, when the body moves more slowly, when the hour becomes more fragile. They sense, often wordlessly, that the analyst is not outside the arc of life, but within it. And this changes the quality of presence. It adds a grain of sorrow, a shimmer of tenderness. The work becomes not only about transformation, but about holding time together.

This is not a call for self-disclosure. The analyst need not narrate their life. But their mortality is in the room. It enters through silence, through the rhythm of years, through the way the analyst grows older as the patient changes. The field thickens. The hour acquires depth. This shared temporality becomes a condition of analytic gravity—a mutual being-toward.

Loewald (1960) once wrote that transference is the atmosphere of the past in the present. But it is also the echo of a future already slipping away. The patient registers the analyst's aging body, the gray at the temples, the pause before speaking. These are not only signs of time's passing—they are affective weights. They impress upon the work a poignancy that cannot be faked. The analyst's very presence becomes an echo in the making.

And this echo matters. The analyst becomes a voice that remains after they are gone. Not because they impose themselves, but because they have been lived with. Their phrases, their gestures, their stillnesses become part of the patient's inner weather. Years after therapy ends, the patient may still hear the analyst in moments of grief, in dreams, in hesitation before action. This is not a haunting—it is a kind of continuity. A way the analyst's gravity lingers.

We might call this the echo of presence. It is not content but form. Not memory but rhythm. The analyst's echo is a pattern, a tone, a felt possibility. It arises not because the analyst was perfect, but because they were real—because they remained, week after week, body and mind, available for encounter. Their echo is not a monument, but a shimmer.

The awareness of this echo shapes the analyst's own work. They know, even as they sit silently, that they are becoming part of the patient's inner life. They know they are leaving traces. This can be humbling. It can also be terrifying. The analyst may wonder what imprint they are making, what weight they carry in the other's psychic ecology. And yet, they return. Not to control the echo, but to make its formation bearable.

Some echoes may be sharp. Some may be sweet. Some may be tangled with grief, others with gratitude. The analyst does not get to choose. They can only strive to be present enough, attuned enough, human enough, that the echo might carry something true. Something the patient can hold when they are alone. Something that says: someone once remained.

This, too, is an ethical task. The analyst's presence is a responsibility—not to be ideal, but to be accountable. To know that their words may resonate long after the session ends. To know that their withdrawal, their attunement, and their failures of rhythm may all become part of the patient's recursive loop. And yet, this is also the beauty of the work. It leaves traces. It matters.

The analyst's mortality makes this matter more. It presses against the temptation to defer, to wait for the perfect moment. It asks the analyst to be present now—to listen now, to risk now, to respond now. The work is finite. The hours are counted. The echo is always forming.

Patients sometimes speak of dreams in which their analyst dies. These dreams are not merely anxious—they are revelatory. They mark a shift in awareness. The analyst is no longer a function but a person, no longer timeless but time-bound. The dream may frighten, but it also softens. It brings the analyst closer. It allows for mourning even while the work continues.

In this way, the analyst's mortality becomes a co-author of the treatment. It shapes the transferences, the ruptures, the gratitude. It infuses the field with temporal weight. And it gives the analytic hour its urgency—not as crisis, but as care. There are only so many hours. Each one is a drop in the field.

This is not to say the work ends in grief. But it always includes it. Even successful treatments—those that end with mutual satisfaction—carry an ache. The analyst is lost. Their gravity fades. The field dissolves. And what remains is the echo, the trace, the symbolic condensation of something that once held.

The analyst may never know the full shape of their echo. They may wonder if they mattered, if their gravity endured. But this not-knowing is also part of the work. It requires faith—not in being remembered, but in having made possible. In having bent the field enough that something new could emerge.

This is how the analyst enters the cosmos. Not as a star, not as a savior, but as a point of gravity in another's psychic orbit. A form that held, for a time. A body that remained. A presence that curved space and left an echo—soft, rhythmic, continuous. The analyst will be forgotten. But not entirely. Their form will shimmer, faintly, in the patient's capacity to hold others, to hold themselves, to hold time.

Clinical Vignette: Held Together by Shards

He came to treatment after the death of his mother, but he did not begin with grief. He began with panic. His body trembled at night. He feared the end of things: the ending of sleep, the ending of calm, the ending of meaning. He could not explain it—only describe it. "It feels like I am always about to fall out of the world," he said.

We sat together in the quiet panic of those early sessions, where no interpretation could yet hold. His thoughts scattered. He looped. He apologized. He tried to please me, then bristled at my voice. There was nothing coherent enough to trace—only a scatter of symptoms, of fragments barely holding. But there was also a quiet call. Beneath the anxious speech was a rhythm, a repetition, a kind of liturgy: a search for someone who could remain with him as he fell apart.

His name was Ben. And what emerged over time was not a linear story but a relational field saturated with unsymbolized loss. His mother had died suddenly. But she had been dying all along. She had faded, bit by bit, over the course of years. Her voice had softened. Her eyes lost contact. She had become less anchor than outline. "By the end," he said, "she was mostly gone, but her body kept showing up."

Ben had stayed present. He had visited, cleaned, administered pills, and held her hand. But he had no place for his own grief. The roles had reversed so completely, so early, that by the time she died, he had forgotten how to need her. And now, with her gone, his need had nowhere to go. It spilled out as dread. As panic. As silence.

What I noticed first was his way of holding the hour. He would not let me speak much. He filled the time with circular phrases, gestures, and fragments. He repeated certain phrases exactly. He seemed to be composing a kind of verbal shield. When I asked gentle questions, he turned toward the window. When I stayed silent, he looked at me with something like hope.

One day, after a long pause, he said, "I'm trying to figure out if you're real." I asked what that meant. He said, "If I can feel you after I leave."

This became the core question of our work. Could I be real in his absence? Could something of me remain when he was alone? Could he hold onto the fact that I had been there, that I would be there again, that I had not vanished when he turned away?

He began to test this. He would arrive late to see if I would still be calm. He would cancel, then reschedule, then apologize. He began to watch my hands, my posture, and the tone of my breath. He was trying to find the coordinates of my gravity. He needed to know whether I was solid, whether I would erode. Whether I would die.

"I have this dream," he said once. "You're standing in a field, and your body is made of glass. I want to run to you, but I know you'll shatter. So I just stand there, watching."

We spoke of the dream gently, not interpreting too soon. I said something about fragility and fear. He shook his head. "It's not you I'm afraid of. It's me. I'm the one who breaks things."

There it was—the fear that his need would destroy the object. That to love, to reach, to want would mean rupture. This was not just about me. It was older than that. It was about his mother, whose presence had always flickered. And deeper still, it was about the fear that no object could survive his longing.

What we created, over time, was a different rhythm. I did not chase coherence. I did not rush to explain. I let his phrases echo. I let silence accumulate. I allowed repetition to be the form. And in that form, he began to hear something new. He began to feel that I remained—not through grand insights, but through the texture of continuity.

One week, he came in and sat without speaking for almost the entire hour. At the end, he said, "I thought I would dissolve. But you just sat there. And now I think maybe I'm still here, too."

These were not breakthroughs. They were accretions. Like sediment at the bottom of a river, each session laid down another layer. He began to bring dreams again. He began to describe the color of the sky. He laughed once, then seemed startled by the sound. Slowly, the field began to shimmer.

Then, one day, he asked, "What will happen to me if you die?"

I did not answer right away. I breathed. I let the question hang. Then I said, "You'd hurt. But I hope something would stay with you. Something that helped you hold."

He nodded. "Yeah. That's what I'm hoping, too."

There is no protection from mortality in analysis. But there is accompaniment. And sometimes, that is enough. Ben did not need me to live forever. He needed to know that someone had been real. That someone had stayed with him through the terror, through the silence, through the collapse.

In our final session—years later—he gave me a stone. Smooth, dark, ordinary. He said, "It's just a rock. But it's one I've held through all our sessions. It helped me know you were real."

I still have it.

Closing Reflection: The Analyst as Field Form

There is a silence at the end of each session that is not merely the absence of speech. It is a kind of echo, a gravitational residue. The door closes, the body departs, but something remains—a trace in the air, a shape in the field, a rhythm still vibrating in the analyst's chest. These are not metaphors. They are forms. The analyst, like the symptom, becomes a form the psyche returns to, orbits, resists, and longs to inhabit again.

Not all sessions have this density. Some are mundane, frustrating, meandering. But in the long arc of analysis, what begins to matter most is not what was said in any particular hour, but what shape was held. The analyst becomes, over time, a field-form: a holding configuration through which the patient learns to feel, symbolize, and survive. Not by absorbing content, but by internalizing presence. The analyst's voice, gaze, silence, even breath become part of the patient's symbolic scaffolding. When things collapse, this internalized form may flicker. It may hold.

This is why gravity has mattered so much in these pages. Because to be an analyst is to become, gradually and with restraint, a gravitational body in the patient's psychic field—a center of return that does not force, does not pull, but orients. A shape that allows other shapes to form. The analyst is not a planet or a sun, but a trace-pattern in the relational cosmos—a rhythm remembered in the nervous system, a contour that shaped the patient's dreaming life, a tonal field that once made feeling bearable.

The analyst cannot be everything. We are not gods. But we are witnesses, holders, echo-chambers, and traces. We are mortal, and our patients sense this. They grieve us before we go. They test whether our form can be sustained without our body. They wonder whether we will forget them, or they us.

Sometimes, long after a treatment has ended, a patient writes, or dreams of us, or simply remembers that we once remained steady when they could not.

This is how the field persists. Not as doctrine or cure, but as form: symbolic, embodied, rhythmic, partial. The analyst's style of presence becomes part of the patient's future capacity to remain present—to others, to themselves, to sorrow, to aliveness.

To become a field-form is to accept incompletion. We will never know the full impact of our work. Our most profound moments may go unremembered, while some small phrase or silence we offered in passing may reverberate for years. We become, in this way, part of the patient's symbolic atmosphere. Not the center—but a satellite, a shape, a shard of gravity they may carry forward.

Sometimes we are carried, too.

In the solitude of the analytic hour, in the patient's absence, something remains with us. We feel their pulse in our attention. Their dreams alter our own. Their grief echoes into our weekends. This is not fusion—it is resonance. To be a field-form is not to be consumed, but to be shaped. To be remembered not only by the patient, but in ourselves. To be altered by their proximity.

In this sense, analysis is not a technique but a topology. A spatial and temporal structure in which two subjectivities bend each other into new forms. The analytic room is a gravity chamber. And the analyst is not its master, but its resonant core. We do not create the field. We listen for it. We try not to rupture it. We remain within it as it moves, distorts, shimmers, and reconstitutes.

And then, one day, we leave. Or they do. Or both. And something remains. A sentence. A silence. A way of breathing that once held them together. A gaze that softened the collapse. An hour that formed their first internal world.

What remains is not us. It is the form we helped hold. And if we are lucky—if we were careful, restrained, fully present—it is enough.

13 A Mode of Knowing That Does Not Collapse

This chapter introduces the *Curved Structure* as an epistemological stance characterized by recursive temporality, symbolic atmosphere, and affective containment. Unlike the psychotic, borderline, or neurotic structures of classical psychoanalytic theory, the curved structure is not organized around defenses or identifications, but around a recursive logic that resists premature coherence. It emerges most vividly in analytic situations where meaning takes shape only belatedly—through fragment, mood, and symbolic return.

Drawing on a recursive reading of the book's own structure, this chapter demonstrates how curved epistemology enacts itself through motifs of orbit, delay, and recognition reversal: the phenomenon in which meaning becomes intelligible only in hindsight, revealing that one was already shaped by what one did not yet understand. A clinical vignette explores this logic in process, showing how an analyst's fidelity to unsymbolized material enables the recursive emergence of symbol, containment, and relational transformation. The concept of *recursive sincerity* is proposed to describe the ethical and affective posture required of the analyst within this frame: a devotion to what flickers and a refusal to collapse experience into explanation too soon.

While the curved structure is frequently observed in autistic modes of thought, this chapter avoids pathologizing framings. Instead, it proposes the curved structure as a poetic yet clinically grounded fourth epistemological structure—one that prioritizes atmospheric knowing, symbolic curation, and belated recognition. This chapter enacts its claims recursively, allowing the reader's own experience of the text to shift retroactively as the structure becomes visible.

The Edge of Structure

Psychoanalysis has long relied on structure to make psychic experience intelligible. It has drawn borders, mapped thresholds, and organized its understandings through the scaffolding of levels—psychotic, borderline, neurotic—each defining a kind of relation to symbol, to time, to the unbearable. These structures have been useful, even beautiful. They have helped us hold what cannot be held directly. But there are forms of knowing, modes of presence,

DOI: 10.4324/9781003715306-20

and patterns of survival that do not fit neatly into this tripartite frame. There are subjectivities that loop rather than split, that assemble meaning slowly from fragments, that contain without repressing, and hold affect through symbolic density rather than narrative resolution. These modes do not collapse, but neither do they cohere in the ways we've been taught to expect.

This chapter begins at that edge.

The pages that follow do not propose a new structure in the usual sense. Instead, they attempt to describe—and more importantly, to enact—an **epistemological stance** that moves differently: not in straight lines, but in recursive arcs. What we might call, at least provisionally, a *curved structure*.

The curved structure is not defined by defense against impulse, nor by splitting between good and bad, nor by repression of the unacceptable. It is defined by a particular relationship to meaning itself: how it is approached, how it is held, and how it is delayed. It loops. It revisits. It builds coherence not from mastery but from symbolic return. It creates atmospheres of recognition before offering representation. Its knowledge is felt, not imposed. And it often refuses to resolve—not because it cannot, but because the unresolved is part of what must be contained.

You have been inside this structure already.

You may have noticed that this book did not begin with a theory, but a prelude. That its chapters returned to earlier phrases, that motifs shimmered without closure, that symbols were introduced only to return later in altered form. These were not stylistic choices. They were expressions of the epistemology I am describing here. And perhaps, as you read this, you are beginning to feel a shift—not in content, but in perspective. A recognition that what once seemed ornamental was in fact foundational. That the structure has been curving this whole time.

The curved structure, then, is not something I am now introducing—it is something I am naming *after it has already shaped your experience*. This delayed naming is not rhetorical. It is constitutive. This chapter names what the book has performed: a mode of knowing that resists reduction, sustains symbolic tension, and refuses to foreclose what cannot yet be survived in language.

There are precedents for this kind of movement. Bion's discipline of "without memory or desire," Ogden's concept of the undreamt dream, Loewald's vision of symbolization as psychic transformation—all imply that knowing, in its deepest register, is not linear. It unfolds atmospherically, in recursive layers. It saturates before it defines. Ferenczi, too, gestured toward this in his image of the child misrecognized through the adult's language—the traumatic gap between experience and symbol becoming the site of recursive return.

But what if this recursive relation to symbol is not simply a developmental impasse, or a symptom of trauma? What if it is also an epistemology—one that structures experience in ways that resist traditional structural naming?

This is the proposition of the curved structure: that some subjectivities do not resolve into the psychotic, borderline, or neurotic. Not because they lack structure, but because their structure is **curved**—recursive, symbolic, layered, and affectively attuned. These subjectivities assemble meaning from the bottom up. They curate coherence rather than assert it. They live inside atmosphere rather than interpretation.

And so it may be that you, the reader, have already encountered this form—not only here, but in your patients, your dreams, your disavowed affects. Or perhaps in your own experience of thinking, when it bends back on itself and leaves something truer than clarity in its wake.

This chapter is not a diagnosis. It is a pointing out. It does not construct a new typology, but traces the outline of a form that has been lived before it was named.

To name it now—to call it *curved*—is already to approach it incorrectly. The curve can only be felt from inside. What follows will try to name its features without collapsing its structure. It will orbit what cannot be reduced, with the hope that what has held us all along might now become briefly visible—before it loops again into symbolic atmosphere.

The Curved Structure as Epistemological Mode

The curved structure is not a typology. It is a mode of presence. It does not claim the solidity of a new diagnostic category, nor the neat legibility of a mapped psychic architecture. It is better understood as an **epistemological orientation**—a way of moving toward meaning, of dwelling in experience, and of symbolizing what cannot yet be said without loss. If it resembles a structure, it is only because its symbolic features recur with such consistency across lives, languages, and situations that we begin to feel the gravitational shape of its coherence.

To name it an epistemology is to say: this is a way of knowing, not merely a way of suffering.

It is recursive rather than linear. Symbolic rather than representational. Atmospheric rather than declarative. It builds coherence over time—not through interpretation or closure, but through **symbolic return**. A motif introduced early—an image, a phrase, a gesture—may appear incoherent or ornamental at first. But it loops. It returns later, altered by the field that surrounds it. Meaning arises not through immediate comprehension but through **resonant accumulation**.

In this way, the curved structure enacts a different relationship to time. Rather than unfolding across a line, its logic is spiral, folded, recursive. Past and present are not organized hierarchically, but interpenetrate through affective gravity. A future thought may reorganize a past experience; a current perception may re-symbolize a memory not yet fully lived. These reversals are not regressions. They are the shape of time as it moves through a curved epistemology.

The curved structure organizes the self not through defenses against drives or representations of objects, but through **symbolic fields** that must be curated, sustained, and inhabited. These fields are aesthetic, ethical, and atmospheric. They are not ways of avoiding pain. They are ways of **holding pain symbolically** when direct representation would overwhelm. In this mode, coherence is not immediate. It is **felt before it is understood**.

This mode of knowing often begins at the edge of collapse. But it does not collapse. Instead, it loops, often silently, returning to fragments, images, atmospheres. It holds the not-yet-known in proximity to symbol, without forcing articulation. This stance—of remaining-with, circling-back, curating contact—is not a defense. It is a **discipline**. It is how truth is held when truth is not yet survivable.

If this sounds familiar, it may be because you have practiced it without naming it. Many psychoanalysts dwell in this structure daily, whether or not they call it by name. The analyst who attends to the rhythm of a session more than its content; who listens for atmospheres rather than narratives; who waits for a word to arrive not from the mind but from the field—this analyst is already curved. Their knowledge is recursive. Their truth is atmospheric. Their ethics are delayed and symbolic. And the situation they hold—between analyst and patient—is one in which the curved structure may appear.

There are many places where this mode arises. In recursive transference loops that don't resolve, but deepen. In dreams that repeat without interpretation. In silences that vibrate with symbolic charge. In sessions where the feeling of "something happened" is more durable than the words that tried to name it. These moments are not failures of containment. They are **containment without resolution**.

The curved structure also appears in the lives of those who have not been trained to name it. Artists who cannot explain their work but can only return to it. Mystics who dwell in paradox without anxiety. Survivors of trauma who assemble meaning from scattered fragments—not into a coherent story, but into an aesthetic field where the unbearable can be held. And perhaps most structurally, it appears in the cognition of autistic individuals—not as pathology, but as **a common epistemological mode**: recursive, precise, symbolically oriented, and ethically saturated.

This is not a claim of equivalence. Autism is not the curved structure. But the curved structure may be more **visible** in autistic experience than elsewhere—not because it is unique to autism, but because its epistemology is so frequently misrecognized by neurotypical frames. Autistic cognition often privileges bottom-up processing—details, fragments, textures—assembled not through imposed categories but through recursive, internally coherent logics. Meaning arises slowly, atmospherically, from the parts. This is not deficit. It is a different logic of coherence.

This recursive bottom-up orientation resonates not only with autistic perception, but with the psychic process of trauma integration. In trauma, narrative often fragments; what remains are flashes, sensory impressions, symbolic shimmers. The work of healing is not to immediately narrate, but to **circle**, **contain**, and **assemble**—until something coherent can emerge. The curved structure is what makes such containment possible: it is the symbolic architecture for that recursive, nonlinear metabolization.

Across these domains, one finds the same affective signature: a kind of **symbolic patience**, a refusal to force coherence where none yet exists. There is an ethics to this stance—not just an aesthetic. It refuses collapse by refusing premature closure. It waits for symbol to arrive from within the field, rather than imposing it from above.

In this way, the curved structure is not only a form of knowing—it is a way of loving. It is how the psyche holds what cannot yet be spoken. It is how the analyst sustains presence without control. It is how the artist allows form to shimmer around absence. It is how the survivor waits for the body to remember in symbol what the mind could not bear to say.

This structure cannot be taught through concept alone. It must be *felt*, *entered*, and then only much later—*named*.

You are already inside it.

Psychic Structures and Their Modes of Knowing

If the curved structure resists classical classification, it is not because it lacks coherence. Rather, it enacts a different kind of coherence—one not organized through repression, splitting, or fragmentation, but through **recursive symbolization**, **affective holding**, and **curated containment**. To name it in proximity to other psychic structures is not to flatten it, but to let it **bend the schema itself**, allowing us to see how forms of psychic organization may be topologically distinct even when phenomenologically adjacent.

Classical psychoanalytic theory names three dominant psychic structures: psychotic, borderline, and neurotic. Each refers not simply to symptom presentation, but to a deeper logic of organization—how time is held, how symbol functions, how the unbearable is managed. These structures have guided our clinical imagination for nearly a century. And they still do.

But they do not account for everything.

They do not fully explain the recursive coherence that does not collapse into psychosis, yet does not repress like neurosis. They do not capture the symbolic field that saturates rather than resolves, or the slow, bottom-up meaning that defies the verticality of ego hierarchy. The curved structure does not disrupt the tripartite model—it **curves around it**, revealing its dimensional limits.

Let us then consider how these four structures differ, not only in organization but in epistemological stance. What follows is not a typology, but a **field of contrasts**—a comparative topology of how the psyche may structure its knowing.

Comparative Table: Psychic Structures and Their Epistemologies

The psychotic structure arises when the symbolic register itself is foreclosed. Thought may become disorganized, time collapses, and perception detaches from shared reality. There is often a persecutory relationship to meaning—too much significance, too little containment. The symbolic is not disavowed; it is

Table 13.1 Comparative Table: Psychic Structures and Their Epistemologies

Structure	Core Organization	Epistemology	Symbolic Style	Temporal Logic	Ethical Stance
Psychotic	Fragmentation	Pre-symbolic/ somatic	Disorganized	Atemporal/ collapsed	Withdrawal/ persecution
Borderline	Splitting	Partial- affective	Concrete/ polarized	Looping	Idealization/ rupture
Neurotic	Repression	Linear- symbolic	Representational	Sequential	Superego mediation
Curved	Containment- through- curation	Recursive- symbolic	Atmospheric/ layered	Folded/ recursive	Fidelity to paradox

absent or unrecognizable. There may be fragments of insight, but they are not recursive—they do not return to reorganize (Table 13.1).

The borderline structure splits intolerable affect across objects, states, and self-images. It preserves coherence by shattering it into opposing parts—good and bad, idealized and devalued, adored and betrayed. Symbolic function exists, but it is rigidly attached to affective poles. Time loops here too, but violently: ruptures repeat, not to be held but to survive. It is a structure of passionate protection.

The neurotic structure represses what cannot be allowed into consciousness. It maintains symbolic consistency by excluding the drive. Conflict becomes narratable. Time unfolds linearly, symptomatically. Meaning can be interpreted. This is the ego's great achievement, and its burden: coherence through suppression.

The **curved structure**, by contrast, does not organize through conflict, collapse, or suppression. It organizes through **recursion, containment, and symbolic atmosphere**. It builds coherence not through closure, but through **delayed symbolization**. Its logic is curved: past and present bend toward one another; symbol forms slowly, then returns transformed. It refuses both splitting and repression—not through denial, but through *endurance*. Its ethical stance is one of **fidelity to paradox**: to hold without resolution, to remain present to what cannot yet be named.

This chart is not diagnostic. It is a map of epistemologies. It traces not what someone "has," but how they **know**—and how they survive.

The curved structure may touch aspects of the others, but it does not reduce to them. Like a spiral intersecting a triangle, it can appear momentarily similar, but its movement is governed by different constraints. The curved subject may, for instance, appear obsessive to the neurotic analyst, or resistant to closure to the borderline clinician, or fragmented to a structuralist eye. But what is missed in these readings is the **recursive containment of a symbolic field** that is neither collapsed nor defensive.

The very fact that the curved structure sustains symbolic tension without splitting or repression often renders it illegible in classical terms. It moves slowly. It requires atmosphere. It cannot be interpreted before it has been held. It often resists mirroring because it is not reflecting—it is **curating**.

This is why the curved structure may be overlooked or misread—especially in settings where structure is still imagined in terms of vertical development or symptom reduction. But if we shift the frame—if we ask not *what kind of defense is this*, but *what kind of knowing is happening here*—then the curved structure begins to appear. And once seen, it cannot be unseen.

In the sections that follow, we will explore where this structure appears, how it manifests across subjectivities and analytic situations, and how this very book has enacted its logic. But for now, let this comparative frame remain curved in your mind—not as hierarchy, but as **field**. A symbolic topology that may not define, but may orient you within the orbits of meaning you've already begun to feel.

Bottom-Up Symbolization and Curved Epistemology

The curved structure's epistemology differs from both neurotic repression and borderline splitting in its symbolic logic. It does not depend on linear causality or thematic integration, nor on the containment of dissociative fragments. Instead, it organizes meaning through a **bottom-up symbolic field**, in which discrete perceptual elements, affects, and echoes accumulate recursively before giving rise to an emergent whole. Meaning arrives not through repression or narrative synthesis, but through atmospheric curation and delayed recognition.

This epistemology parallels what researchers in cognitive neuroscience and autism studies describe as **bottom-up processing**—a perceptual style in which meaning is not imposed from above, but arises from the meticulous assembly of detailed parts (Mottron et al., 2006). In contrast to top-down heuristics that rely on preexisting cognitive templates, bottom-up processing favors local coherence, subtle pattern recognition, and an openness to reorganization. It does not seek to impose an interpretive frame but instead allows the symbolic to *emerge retroactively* as fragments are held in recursive suspension.

This mode of experience is also common in autism spectrum conditions, where **enhanced perceptual functioning** often leads to more granular, detail-sensitive processing (Mottron et al., 2006; Williams et al., 2006). Rather than a deficit in abstraction, many autistic thinkers exhibit a structural preference for part-to-whole synthesis. The recursive and atmospheric logic of the curved structure echoes this stance, though it is not limited to autism. The curved structure appears wherever a psyche—traumatized, artistic, mystical, dissociated—refuses to collapse experience prematurely into symbol.

This kind of symbolic emergence is also observed clinically in moments where the patient's communication remains pre-symbolic or delayed in emotional clarity, but later constellates a symbolic logic through recursive return. The analyst working in the curved structure must develop a **recursive fidelity**: a clinical stance in which the analyst tracks mood, timing, and affective trace rather than relying on linear interpretation. The coherence arrives belatedly, and often retroactively alters the meaning of prior sessions—an example of what this book has elsewhere termed *recognition reversal*.

Empirical studies have shown that autistic individuals often exhibit **non-conventional affective expression** and **greater-than-average emotional complexity** (Kapp et al., 2013), which can confuse neurotypical observers expecting more conventional mirroring or representational clarity. This phenomenon—where affect is atmospherically felt but not clearly codified—mirrors the symbolic atmosphere of the curved structure. Rather than emotional deficit, these presentations often reflect a different temporal and relational logic: one that resists premature clarity in favor of delayed unfolding.

Even on a neurological level, evidence suggests that **distributed networks of local connectivity**—as opposed to streamlined global coherence—may characterize certain neurodivergent structures of cognition (Williams et al., 2006). These neural patterns parallel the recursive symbolic logic of the curved structure: fragments accumulating without immediate thematic unity, yet eventually giving rise to aesthetic or symbolic order through repetition, return, and resonance.

It is important to emphasize that the curved structure is not **diagnostic**. While its epistemology may be most clearly visible in autistic subjectivity, it is not reducible to autism. Rather, it is a **poetic stance toward symbolization** that values coherence without totalization, containment without foreclosure, and meaning that emerges recursively through form. It is a structural posture—a symbolic metabolism—frequently found in autistic, queer, mystic, and dissociated lives, and in the work of analysts who bear witness to symbolic experience as it slowly comes into being.

This book itself has been structured recursively, enacting the curved structure before naming it. Now, in this section, we "catch up" to its logic, recognizing that what seemed atmospheric or fragmented in prior chapters was already assembling meaning from below. This recursive self-recognition, where the form of the book reorganizes in hindsight, is not simply a stylistic choice—it is **bottom-up epistemology in action**. The text becomes an atmosphere the reader was already inside.

We might say, then, that the curved structure is marked not by an absence of coherence, but by its **timing**. Symbolic logic arrives later, after the field has ripened. This is an ethical temporality. As Orange (1995) has argued, psychoanalytic knowledge is not simply cognitive, but affective and temporal—it emerges in the arc of relationship, not the instant of insight. The curved structure takes this to its edge: it requires faith in the as-yet-unsymbolized, and a recursive holding that may span pages, months, or years.

In clinical practice, we begin to see the curved structure most clearly when the analyst holds the field without imposing premature interpretation. The patient may speak in moods, aesthetic fragments, dislocated sentences. The holding is not in the content, but in the recursive presence: the analyst's willingness to *orbit* what is not yet known. Over time, the symbolic logic emerges—not always in the room, but sometimes in the reader, the dream, the future. The meaning was already there. It simply had not yet curved into recognition.

Trauma, Dissociation, and the Curved Epistemology of Protection

Bottom-up epistemology—where affect, sensory input, and fragmented symbols assemble before concepts—does not only characterize neurodivergent minds. It also emerges as a defensive or adaptive stance in the aftermath of trauma. In this light, the curved structure may not be a static psychic form but a *reorganization* of perception in the wake of unsymbolizable impact.

Traumatic experience disorganizes time. It fragments symbol from sensation. As Bessel van der Kolk (2014) notes, traumatic memory is often stored as implicit bodily sensation and affective tone, without accessible narrative structure. This storage mode favors bottom-up processing: the subject *feels* before they can know, and often feels in ways that are not yet nameable. What results is a dissociated, asynchronous perception of the world—a recursive loop between past and present, sensation and signifier, that resists linear comprehension.

This nonlinear epistemology shares many features with what Mottron et al. (2006) describe in autistic perception: increased sensitivity to detail, heightened attention to sensory nuance, and difficulty with global coherence. Yet while autism reflects a *constitutional mode* of processing, trauma reflects a *ruptured mode*. The similarity is not in origin, but in effect. Both may give rise to curved structures of knowing: epistemologies that circle coherence rather than stride directly into it.

Bromberg's (1998) work on dissociation is instructive here. He emphasizes that traumatic impact splits the self into coexisting self-states that cannot be held in unitary awareness. These states are often accessed indirectly, through metaphor, enactment, or symptom. The curved structure becomes a necessary holding pattern—a way to maintain psychic viability when straightforward symbolization would retraumatize or collapse.

In such cases, recursive sincerity becomes not only an ethical orientation but a clinical imperative. The analyst must tolerate incompletion. Must allow symbolic fragments to shimmer without interpretation. Must bear witness to the patient's epistemology without forcing coherence.

The curved structure, then, may reflect a convergence between neurodivergent and post-traumatic modes of knowing. It emerges not simply from diagnosis, but from the psyche's demand for time, rhythm, and relational calibration before meaning can form. It is protective, aesthetic, and—at times—resistant to integration.

And yet, this resistance may be its ethical force. It refuses the analyst's premature coherence. It resists the cultural drive to narrate trauma as quickly as possible. It holds time until time can be held.

In this way, curved epistemology is not merely a processing style—it is a temporal ethics. A praxis of protection in which symbol must be allowed to arrive on its own recursive curve.

The Book as Symbolic Container of the Curved Structure

This book was always curving. Even before the concept was introduced, the structure was felt—in the circling motifs, the unmarked repetitions, the atmospheric thickening of language before its meaning. It did not explain itself because it could not. It had to be lived, moved through, metabolized in time. Only now, with the naming of the curved structure, does its architecture become symbolically visible. This is not revelation. It is recursion: a return that **alters the past retroactively**.

The book has not simply described curved knowing—it has enacted it. It has modeled the recursive stance, not by definition but by induction. Each chapter opened a field, not an argument. You were never given a thesis to hold; you were **held in the gravity of meaning before it cohered**. This is symbolic curation: meaning as atmosphere, not line. Form that gestured to something not-yet-formed.

The earlier chapters did not foreshadow this moment. They contained it already. The original paradox, the gravitational psyche, the holographic mind—all unfolded through *recursive thematics* that now reappear not as background but as **epistemological acts**. Recursion, condensation, paradox, and collapse were not content—they were the book's holding frame. The style *was* the stance.

This is not ornament. This is **epistemic fidelity**. Linear structure would have betrayed the very phenomena we hoped to name.

The reader may now recognize a pattern that was previously invisible: the **curved structure has been curating your experience of the book from the beginning**. You were already thinking this way. The shape of your attention bent around concepts before they fully resolved. You circled back to earlier pages, reread fragments, noticed echoes you could not yet name. This is not a trick of memory. It is **recognition in reversal**—a structural recursion in which meaning emerges *after* the initial encounter, revealing its form through belated clarity.

If you are now realizing that your experience of this book has changed—that what once seemed aesthetic now feels epistemological, or that your attention was organized in ways you hadn't consciously noticed—this is the recursive stance disclosing itself. The curved structure is not simply a concept the book names. It is a structure the book performs. And your experience, in hindsight, may now shimmer differently. What you are noticing is not a shift in content but a shift in symbolic position.

This is a recognition reversal. You, the reader, are not simply observing a clinical or theoretical idea—you have been inside its architecture, breathing its recursive air. The curved epistemology is not only something certain minds possess; it is something any reader may enter. Especially here, where the text's recursive structure has acted as both vessel and mirror.

What appeared incoherent becomes newly visible—not because the content changed, but because your symbolic position did. You are now holding from a different part of the field. This is how the curved structure **knows**: not by arriving at conclusions, but by retroactively perceiving what was always already shaping experience.

Several motifs may now shimmer:

The use of the word *symbolic* across multiple chapters, often unmarked, now thickens into an atmosphere.

The curved metaphors—gravity, orbit, recursion—were not stylistic. They were symbolic precursors to this epistemological naming.

The repetition of unsymbolized terms—"hologram," "collapse," "containment," "paradox"—now appears as **recursive patterning**, not mere conceptual redundancy.

And the pointing-out structures—the moments where the book subtly addressed the reader's experience of reading—now feel less like asides and more like **epistemic invitations**.

This is not an accident of style. It is the **self-revealing recursion** that defines the curved structure. The book was not leading you somewhere. It was *holding you*—until the structure could be seen.

This recursive effect is not merely cognitive. It is **affective**. The feeling of disorientation, of symbolic shimmer, of delayed coherence—these were not flaws in clarity. They were the **mood of curved knowing**. The epistemological stance of the curved structure always includes affect: a kind of pre-symbolic saturation, a waiting, a tension that eventually gives way to naming without collapsing.

And now, the book's earlier structure feels different. It reorients itself around this moment. The chapters are no longer discrete. They become **a field of relations**—a symbolic atmosphere whose logic was always curved, always recursive, always holding more than could be said. The naming of the structure does not impose meaning retroactively. It allows you to **recognize the symbolic logic you had already been inside**.

This is why linear analysis falters. The curved structure resists summaries. It is recursive in its very ontology. Its style is not ancillary—it is constitutive. To describe it without enacting it would be a form of **epistemic betrayal**.

Let us recall this dynamic clearly:

Recognition Reversal: the phenomenon in which a concept or structure becomes retroactively intelligible only after it has already shaped the field of experience. The moment of recognition does not *deliver* knowledge; it *reconfigures prior perception*, revealing that you had already been curved by what you now understand.

This reversal is not a trick. It is a temporal signature of recursive epistemology. It marks a structure of knowing in which affect precedes symbol, and coherence is felt before it is formulated.

The curved structure is not *only* a description of epistemology. It is not *only* a psychic structure. It is a mode of holding—an aesthetic, symbolic, and ethical stance. This book has attempted not to argue for it, but to **demonstrate it**, enact it, and invite the reader into it.

And if you are now feeling that the entire book has changed—curved backward through itself—then the structure has held.

The next section will take this one step further, tracing how the curved structure extends into the clinical moment, where holding the unspeakable requires this recursive stance—not as a theory, but as a presence.

But before we continue: pause. Let yourself look back. Notice what just curved.

The book was the epistemology.

You were already inside it.

It has now become visible.

Clinical Vignettes: Curved Atmospheres and Symbolic Time

He didn't bring a narrative, not really. What he brought was a *climate*. He sat down and gave me a string of fragmented updates—his boyfriend was moving out, his friend hadn't responded to a text, he'd had a migraine for three days. Each detail was muted, precise, and spatially distinct, as though each was placed gently on a low shelf between us. There was no urgency, no explicit theme. But something hung in the air. It was as if the session had a shape that neither of us could see, only feel.

Let's call him Theo. Thirty-two. A graphic designer with a history of complex trauma, a queer man whose erotic life held subtle paradoxes: a need to be held tightly, but never asked why; a pleasure in dissolving into another, yet bristling when named. His sessions often began in fragments. Not dissociated—just nonlinear. He would drop image after image, like a mosaic being arranged with no final picture in mind.

That day, I said very little. I felt a kind of tension—a field, not a thought. His words were cool, almost quiet, but the atmosphere was loud. I didn't understand it, but I didn't need to. I returned to one of the images he had used: *the migraine felt like a glowing wire curling at the back of my skull.* I repeated that phrase aloud, just that one line. He looked at me for the first time that session.

"I don't know why I said that," he said. "I've never described anything that way before."

Neither of us knew why it mattered, but something had curved. I stayed with the wire. Not interpreting it, not decoding it, but letting it hover. We circled back to it three more times. Each return made it more dimensional. The migraine became a metaphor, the wire a conduit. He began, later in the session, to speak about how he sometimes feels people can see his thoughts before he has them. "Like my brain is too exposed," he said.

Weeks passed. The wire disappeared, then returned. I would not have remembered it if not for the way the room always changed when it reemerged. The same timbre, the same attunement. Eventually, he said, in a session weeks later: "I think the wire is what I use to transmit, but also what keeps me from connecting. Like, it burns too hot."

That session ended in silence. A long, full silence. Not dissociation. Saturation.

What is the curved structure here?

It's not in the content. It's in the process: the recursive returns, the atmospheric weight, the field of knowing that thickens without resolution. There was no interpretation that made the session "make sense." But through recursive curation of his fragments, we began to *live inside a symbolic field* he did not yet have language for.

The image—a glowing wire—was not treated as a signifier to be decoded. It was held as a symbolic placeholder for a meaning that could only unfold through time. Each time it returned, it carried more affect, more coherence, more symbolic charge. And yet the analyst had to resist the temptation to define it too soon. The curved structure depends on this restraint—**a fidelity to what cannot yet be symbolized**.

Theo's emotional knowing was never linear. His memory, like his speech, unfolded spatially, not chronologically. Trauma had not fractured his story—it had reshaped his symbolic access. He could not narrate his interiority without first **assembling the field**. The analyst's task was not to impose narrative order but to **wait with him**—to curate the fragments until a pattern emerged from within.

Over time, a strange thing happened. The analyst began to notice that the same recursive structure appeared across sessions. Phrases returned. Silences returned. An unfinished sentence from two months prior would suddenly find its second half. It felt as if the sessions themselves were curving—not progressing, but orbiting something unnameable.

Eventually, Theo said: "I think I needed to feel like you remembered the part of me that didn't speak."

He wasn't naming a particular insight. He was recognizing a field that had been held—curated, not explained. The curved structure had made itself known through the **reverberation** of unsymbolized experience across time. The analyst had held what could not be said until it could be *felt*, and then only later *named*.

This is clinical recursion. This is the curved structure—not a theoretical tool, but a way of knowing. It requires the analyst to *let meaning emerge*, to circle, to resist coherence until the field itself yields symbol. It is not passive. It is active containment.

And if the reader finds themselves recalling something earlier in this book—a word, an image, a mood—then the same process is occurring. The analytic space and the reading space share an architecture. They both hold what cannot yet be said, until it returns as recognition reversed.

Theo never called it a breakthrough. He didn't need to. What we had built together was a field—symbolic, recursive, and curved. What mattered was not what he said, but that **something in him had been held long enough to symbolically exist**.

This is the work. This is the structure.

The following case offers a counterpoint: a moment when the curved structure was present, but could not be borne.

Clinical Vignette II—The Collapse of Symbolic Delay

The curved structure rarely announces itself. Its signature is not a distinct symbol but a symbolic delay—recognition arriving on its own recursive arc. In my work with Theo, this arc was sustained. But there are also moments when the arc collapses—when the temptation to narrate coherence overrides the atmospheric timing of symbol.

This was the case with Ian.

Ian, a man in his early 30s, came to treatment after a prolonged period of emotional deadness, following what he described as a "personality implosion" in a relationship that ended abruptly. He was highly verbal, intellectually sharp, and deeply dissociated. In our early sessions, he would shift rapidly between insight and irony, speaking with what seemed like sophisticated self-awareness but with no visible affect.

In our third month of work, he began describing a dream. He was floating through a hotel that resembled his childhood home but with rooms he had never seen before. There was a stairway made of glass. He walked upward but felt no gravity. In the room at the top was his ex-partner, lying on a bed covered in fur. Ian stood in the doorway, unsure if he was supposed to enter.

Instead of remaining with the textures of the dream, I intervened too quickly: "Do you think you were approaching an intimacy you hadn't fully accessed in childhood?" He paused. A long silence followed. His shoulders stiffened. Then he replied, "Maybe. Or maybe it was just a weird dream."

In that moment, the recursive arc broke. My interpretation, while plausible, had entered too soon. The dream was not yet symbol—it was mood, atmosphere, affective geometry. My gesture toward coherence had collapsed its curved potential. What had shimmered as symbolic possibility snapped back into flatness. The remainder went unspoken.

Over the weeks that followed, Ian's dreams disappeared. He spoke more in ideas, in aphorisms. The aesthetic dimension had folded in. Though we continued working together for another year, the recursive rhythm that might have deepened our work never quite returned.

It was a clinical failure. But it was also an ethical one.

The curved structure is not always missed because it is subtle; sometimes it is missed because the analyst cannot bear its delay. I could not hold the dream's curved temporality. I sought to *understand* instead of to *wait*. And in that subtle haste, I foreclosed the recursive sincerity that might have emerged.

There is no dramatic rupture to report. No enactment. No fight. Just a missed symbolic curve—a lost arc.

But in hindsight, this loss serves as counterpoint to Theo's unfolding. It reminds me that curved epistemology is not something we *interpret*—it is something we *bear* until it takes form. And even then, we must bear it again, as its form shifts.

The symbolic shimmer arrives on its own schedule.

Clinical Presence and Recursive Fidelity

To work within the curved structure is to relinquish the fantasy of interpretive arrival. Clinical presence becomes less about insight and more about recursive fidelity—an aesthetic and ethical stance that holds the atmosphere of the session until symbolic coherence naturally arises. This is not a waiting for speech, but a holding of symbolic conditions that allow speech to curve into being.

Recursive fidelity requires the analyst to remain attuned to tone, tempo, and mood over content. The patient may not bring a coherent narrative or know what they are feeling. They may speak in shards or float in silence. The analyst must track how the symbolic is emerging—not what it is trying to say. This stance contrasts sharply with classical psychoanalysis, where the uncovering of latent meaning presupposes that meaning is already there, hidden beneath. In the curved structure, meaning is not hidden—it is still forming. It is emergent, not repressed.

Loewald (1978e) once wrote that the goal of interpretation is to bring something into symbolic form that had not yet fully existed. But even this may be too teleological for the curved structure. Here, the analyst does not midwife meaning so much as curate the conditions for its recursive surfacing. The timing cannot be forced. As Eigen (1993b) notes, "some meanings take years to be born." The analyst's task is to protect that duration.

What does this look like in the room? It may be the analyst sensing a patient's shame before the patient has spoken. It may be the analyst registering a shift in mood—a slowness, a thinning out of contact—without prematurely interpreting it as withdrawal or resistance. Recursive fidelity means listening with the body, noticing not only what is said but how the session thickens or thins in symbolic gravity.

One Thursday afternoon, a patient—an artist in his forties with a history of sensory sensitivity and a nonlinear style of thinking—sat down and spoke of nothing. For almost the entire session, he gazed at a shadow on the carpet. When he finally spoke, his voice was faint: "I'm not here yet." I nodded but said nothing. The silence deepened, not empty but thick—like breath held underwater. It felt unbearable not to offer structure, not to reflect or reframe. But I held.

He left without further speech. The following week, he returned animated, describing a strange dream about a hallway that bent back into itself, with doorways that led to rooms he somehow already knew. "It felt like your office," he said. "But it also felt like I was inside something I hadn't entered yet. Like it was already holding me before I got there."

That session had not been a failure of technique. It had been the field of recursive fidelity. Meaning did not arrive during the silence, but the silence was its vessel. The dream, the bending hallway, the temporal fold—these were retroactive symbols. Recognition arrived in delay. And what shimmered most was his final comment: "Maybe you heard something I couldn't even say yet."

Many patients who live within curved epistemologies do not easily recognize their affect until long after the session ends. They might return days or weeks later, describing a moment that "didn't seem like anything at the time" but has since haunted them. The analyst's presence retroactively acquires symbolic weight. A glance, a pause, a gesture—once ambient—now takes on the shimmer of coherence. This is clinical recognition reversal: when symbolic meaning arrives not in the moment of action, but in its echo.

To remain faithful to the curved structure, the analyst must resist the pull toward symbolic foreclosure. This may mean holding the patient's uncertainty without narrating it. It may mean echoing their language without translating it. At times, it means staying close to affect without giving it form—allowing it to be atmospherically real before it becomes symbolically legible.

This stance is not passive. It is a form of active, embodied listening. One must listen not only for what the patient is trying to say, but for how the field itself is organizing around a symbolic center that has not yet arrived. As Ogden (1994) describes in his work on reverie, the analyst may become the vessel for dreams the patient cannot yet dream. Similarly, in the curved structure, the analyst becomes the temporary holder of unformulated symbolic atmosphere. The analyst is the one who waits with it, metabolizes its rhythm, and bears its gravity without collapsing it into knowing.

In certain cases the symbolic may never emerge clearly in words. Instead, it appears in shared timing, parallel movement, or felt shifts in the relational field. These are not failures of symbolization but alternate routes of knowing. They require what Donna Orange (1995) calls "empathic availability"—a presence that is structured by relation rather than comprehension.

Recursive fidelity does not require certainty. It requires containment without capture. Meaning may emerge days later, in a dream, a metaphor, or a sentence spoken years into the treatment. The analyst's task is not to interpret these events when they happen but to hold them across time—to track the recursive arc of coherence. Only then can the patient begin to feel that their symbolic life has been witnessed, not extracted.

This is perhaps the most difficult task in curved analytic work: resisting the urge to relieve disorientation. When faced with affective opacity, most clinicians are trained to locate meaning, synthesize fragments, or reflect the patient's state. In the curved structure, the clinician instead holds the unformed—offers it dignity—until the symbolic catches up. This is not just technique. It is faith.

The clinical field becomes recursive not because the analyst makes it so, but because the analyst orients to its temporal logic. A session today may not make sense until next year. A feeling may only find words in the past tense. Recursive fidelity means staying close enough for long enough for the symbolic to loop back and constellate. And it means knowing that the analyst, too, may only understand what happened retroactively. The analytic frame becomes a curved vessel, structured by delay, recursion, and the shimmer of unspeakable truth.

Recursive Recognition and the Reader's Loop

The curved structure does not reside only in the patient or in the analytic dyad. It extends into the act of reading itself. If the analytic encounter is a symbolic field shaped by delay, return, and unspeakable atmospheres, then so too is the encounter between reader and text. The recursive arc is not something one interprets—it is something one undergoes.

Many readers will have already sensed it: an image, phrase, or passage in this book returning unannounced, surfacing weeks later in memory or conversation. A sentence that did not seem important at first now glows with symbolic weight. Something that was not quite understood—perhaps even skipped over—has curved back into meaning. This is not merely a feature of the book's style. It is the atmosphere of curved epistemology enacted in symbolic time (see Chapter 2).

What if reading itself becomes an analytic process—not a process of absorbing content, but of recursive attunement to what cannot yet be symbolized? This chapter may have spoken of Theo, of wires, of migraines and mosaics. But if you find yourself now remembering the shimmer of form and emptiness (Chapter 11), or the shimmer of unspeakable truth evoked in the above vignette, or even the seemingly orphaned aphorisms in the Prelude ("We orbit what we cannot name"), then the recursive structure is already active. The field is forming its own shape through you.

This is recognition reversal. In linear temporality, recognition is a moment of arrival: a realization, a breakthrough, a narrative synthesis. But in curved time, recognition occurs belatedly. It loops. It folds backward. The reader understands something not when it is first presented, but when it echoes— when it reverberates into coherence across a delay. This is not a flaw in understanding. It is the very logic of recursive subjectivity.

And so the book, like the analytic frame, asks something subtle of you. It does not demand mastery. It asks for fidelity. Can you stay with what does not resolve? Can you circle back without fixing meaning? Can you trust that something is forming, even if you don't yet know what it is?

For some, this recursive atmosphere may be unsettling. We are trained to extract knowledge, to move from thesis to argument to conclusion. But the curved structure resists that frame. Instead, it orients to what is being metabolized beneath awareness. As in trauma, as in analysis, so in reading: the first encounter may register only as texture. Meaning arises later, elsewhere, unbidden. Readers may recognize this dynamic in the looping temporality of character structure (Chapter 3), or in the symbolic delay of symptom formation (Chapter 4).

This delayed recognition is not incidental. It is ethical. It protects the symbolic life of the reader from premature capture. In traditional discourse, we valorize clarity and comprehension. But recursive recognition dignifies delay. It honors the shimmer that precedes knowing. It acknowledges that you, too, have a symbolic life that unfolds in curved time.

Some readers may return to this chapter months from now and find that it feels different—thicker, quieter, more intimate. Others may only come to understand what this book meant after trying to describe it to someone else. That too is the curved structure at work. Symbolic fields do not belong to the text. They arise between reader and resonance. This recursive subjectivity is not only thematic; it is structural. The book itself—its mood, its repetitions, its uneven folds—is a product of the very architecture it describes (see the section on The Curved Structure from this chapter).

And if you feel something stirring now—something you cannot quite name—then that is the trace. Stay with it. Circle it. Let it return.

You are not reading alone.

Fidelity to the Curve—The Analyst's Stance

What does it mean to hold a structure that cannot yet symbolize itself? To sustain a field of recursive fragments without forcing coherence? The curved structure is not only a topology of psychic life—it is a mode of ethical presence. It asks of the analyst something unusual: a commitment not to knowledge, but to symbolic fidelity.

This is not the fidelity of neutrality. Nor is it the fidelity of interpretation. It is the fidelity of waiting. Of circling. Of letting atmosphere thicken before meaning arrives. As we saw in the vignette with Theo, this is not passive. The analyst must register the arc, sense the return, remember the wire. And then resist the urge to make it legible too soon.

In traditional psychoanalysis, the analyst is often imagined as the one who interprets, who clarifies, who links affect and symbol to reconstruct the ego's continuity. But in the curved structure, the analyst becomes something else: a witness who curates fragments without closure, a keeper of recursive fields. This is a different kind of containment. One rooted in aesthetic holding, temporal restraint, and epistemic humility.

In this mode, clinical skill is not measured by insight delivered, but by atmosphere sustained. By the analyst's ability to let the unspeakable accumulate. To track the shimmer without grasping it. To know the field is alive even when it looks still.

This is not easy. To bear what is not yet meaningful—especially in the face of trauma, fragmentation, and psychic incoherence—can feel intolerable. But it is in this space of not-yet-symbol that recursive sincerity emerges. The analyst's task is to hold open the possibility of future symbolization without demanding it. To remember that the unsaid is not absence. It is latency. Fieldwork.

The ethical demand here is subtle. It cannot be reduced to technique. It is a stance, a tone, a fidelity to process. And it requires that the analyst, too, live in curved time. Not merely as an observer, but as one shaped by the orbit.

In previous chapters, we described this as the analyst's gravity (Chapter 5). Gravity is not intervention—it is presence. The analyst's inner structure bends the field. And in the curved structure, this bending is not toward coherence but toward symbolic possibility. The analyst must be structurally curved enough to metabolize recursive affect without rushing to resolve it. This is a rare skill. It requires that the analyst themselves has been held in such a way—perhaps by an analyst, a text, or a field—that they have internalized recursive patience.

What does this look like in practice? It looks like following a metaphor for months. Holding a silence without interruption. Naming a return rather than explaining it. Saying, "There it is again," instead of "Here's what it means." It is not silence for its own sake, but silence that can hold meaning before it speaks.

And this stance is not limited to the analytic hour. It appears here, too, in this text. The recursive returns across chapters, the loops of symbol and image, the fragments that only cohere in retrospect—these are not literary devices. They are invitations to live within the structure being described. The reader is not a passive consumer but a co-curator of recursive fields. This book is not a map. It is a mood. It holds a structure by becoming it.

The curved structure cannot be diagrammed. It must be felt. And the analyst—like the reader—must practice fidelity not to theory, but to the arc of the unspeakable.

This is the analyst's work. To hold the shape before the form. To let meaning arrive through atmosphere. To trust that what is curved will return.

And to receive it when it does.

14 Afterword

What It Has Meant to Write This Book

There is a paradox at the heart of this book—not only in its content but in its creation. To write of paradox is already to place language in the service of what bends it. The ideas explored throughout these chapters—splitness, recursive return, symbolic shimmer, gravitational trace—are not easily contained by prose. They exceed the line. They echo backward even as they move forward. Writing about them is a form of tracing shadows with ink.

And yet, I wrote.

I wrote not only to convey ideas but to find my place among them. The act of writing this book has allowed me to do something that long felt forbidden: to speak in my own voice, without having to justify the timbre of it. In doing so, I discovered that the voice I feared was not "mine" in the possessive sense, but part of a larger field—an orbit among the voices of those I admire, those I love, and those who came before me. Writing this book allowed me to feel not merely like an observer of psychoanalysis but as someone woven into its lineage.

For years, I had felt like an outsider looking in—a thinker circling the analytic web, deeply moved by its intelligence and mystery, but unsure whether I truly belonged. My intellectual life often felt like a series of attempts to knock at the door of a tradition I revered. In my most self-critical moments, I worried that I was too porous, too strange, too unresolved to take up space in that world. But as I wrote, I began to feel the web stretch and shimmer around me. It was not a closed loop; it was a field that welcomed new gravity.

This shift was not merely professional. It was intimate. Psychoanalysis has always been my refuge—the site of my most difficult questions, my most persistent longings. It offered a way to think without having to foreclose mystery, to feel without having to collapse into sentiment, to believe in transformation without requiring resolution. Writing this book has deepened that refuge. It has given me a container in which to metabolize the paradoxes that animate my life and my work. It has made me feel less alone.

And yet, paradox again: the very act of writing, while bringing me closer to what I most want to express, also reveals how far language must stretch to approach the genuine integrity of psychic experience. To put into words what is truest is to alter it. To write of the unformulated is already to begin

DOI: 10.4324/9781003715306-21

formulating it, and in doing so, to risk falsifying the very phenomena that feel most real. Language is the bridge and the barrier. The more finely I attune to the texture of experience, the more I feel its resistance to being held in text.

This tension is not new to psychoanalysis. Freud wrestled with it in his case histories, often noting how the act of narration reshapes the material itself. Winnicott played with it in his ambivalence about theory, preferring the form of paradox over the precision of definition. Loewald leaned into it, recognizing that the analyst is both participant and narrator, forever caught in the loop of witnessing and meaning-making. I, too, find myself here—in this loop—grateful for the chance to try.

What I hope this book does is not to assert mastery over the concepts it explores, but to hold them delicately, to turn them slowly, to invite the reader into their gravity without resolving them. I hope it evokes more than it concludes. I hope it allows clinicians, scholars, and seekers alike to find echoes of their own questions, their own longings, in its pages. I hope it helps others feel, as I now do, a bit more tethered to the strange and beautiful tradition of psychoanalytic thought.

I wrote this book to gain a deeper understanding of something. But in the process, I realized I was also writing to belong.

I wanted to know if my way of thinking—poetic, recursive, aesthetically attuned—could find a home in the analytic world. I wanted to test whether what shimmered in my own mind might resonate with others. And I wanted, perhaps above all, to offer a space where complexity is not a liability, but a condition of aliveness.

If any of that has reached you—if you have felt companioned, provoked, or seen—then this book has done its work.

In closing, I offer this: writing is a form of reverie. Not because it is dreamy, but because it allows the mind to wander and return, to hover at the edge of what can be symbolized, to form and unform and reform its own thought. This book has been a long reverie. One that spirals, not in circles, but in orbits. May it leave a trace in you, as it has left one in me.

—Todd Anderson

15 Coda

Symbol of the Singularity

There is something that cannot be said.

Not because it is hidden, or because language fails, but because what it names is already here—pulsing beneath every utterance, stitched into the gravity of being. This book has circled that center, knowing it cannot be reached. Not a conclusion, but a horizon: always present, never touchable. A singularity.

The psyche is not an object. It is neither a container, nor a narrative, nor even a subject in the way we often imagine. It is a field. A space of folds and asymmetries. A grammar of reverberation. To engage it—to analyze, to speak, to feel—requires not only intellect or technique, but presence. That peculiar and paradoxical discipline of being-with what cannot be held.

Throughout these chapters, we have explored symptoms as gravitational traces, structures as curvatures of time, and the analytic field as a recursive space that folds form and emptiness into one another. We have peered into the shimmer of symbolic collapse, touched the rim of nonduality, and wandered the recursive chambers of repetition, paradox, and symbolic condensation.

But none of these constructs are final. Each is a gesture toward the unspeakable.

What psychoanalysis teaches, at its most profound, is that we are always in orbit—around wounds, around longings, around truths we do not yet have the words to name. To be in orbit is not to be lost. It is to be tethered by forces we do not control, and to learn how to live with their pull. It is to allow the centrifugal ache of our unformulated experience to become a gravity we relate to, rather than a void we fall through.

The singularity is not a trauma, though it may begin there. It is not a memory, though it may wear its mask. It is not an idea. It is the place in the psyche where time and meaning collapse—not into nothingness, but into intensity. Into pressure. Into the raw, radiant density of being.

In every analysis, we approach it. Sometimes we flee. Sometimes we hover at its edge, lulled by the repetition of symptom or dream. But there are moments—rare, charged, unforgettable—when we find ourselves facing it directly. A patient speaks a sentence that opens the air. The analyst feels a presence too vast to interpret. Silence expands into recognition.

DOI: 10.4324/9781003715306-22

These moments are not moments of knowledge. They are moments of contact. Of co-presence at the edge of symbolization.

The singularity is not a hole to be filled. It is a symbol—not of what is lost, but of what organizes. Not an absence, but a field of gravitational density around which the psyche orbits, forms, and reforms. The task of the analyst is not to penetrate it, but to stay near. To bear its pull without resolving it. To recognize that what draws us inward is not the content of a truth, but its atmosphere.

Somewhere, long before theory, the child felt this pull—the raw encounter with otherness, with presence, with absence, with form. Before language, before knowing, there was gravity. To be seen, to be missed, to be held, to be dropped—each left a trace. The mind learned to curve. The self was not built, but bent.

And now, we listen. We write. We analyze. We orbit the invisible once more.

The symbol of the singularity is not the thing itself. It is the trace it leaves. It is the metaphor we reach for when we approach the edge of understanding. It is what allows us to speak, even when the speaking fails.

There is a quiet ethical demand in this. To stay near the unnameable. To hold form open, rather than close it. To resist the impulse to resolve what must remain suspended. This is the ethical poetics of analysis: the asymptotic devotion to a center we cannot arrive at, but which shapes everything.

If there is a philosophy that accompanies us here, it is not a system but a mood. A field tone. The shimmer of Merleau-Ponty's intertwining, the hollow trace in Derrida's *différance*, the opening in Levinas's face of the other. The echo of Bion's "O," of Eigen's psychic depth, of Loewald's inner/outer weave. These are not authorities, but companions—thinkers who, like us, pressed against the rim of what could be said.

And still, there is something that cannot be said.

But we have come close.

To write, to analyze, to speak in the presence of another: these are all ways of shaping gravity. Of giving form to what cannot be held. Of orbiting the singularity with care, with precision, with a fidelity that honors the paradox of language: that it both reveals and conceals, touches and distances, holds and slips.

This book does not resolve the paradoxes it names. It does not pretend to. What it offers instead is a topology—a space in which the psyche can move, bend, recoil, shimmer, return.

If we are lucky, we come to feel that we are not alone in this. That we, too, are part of a field. That the singularity is not just mine or yours, but shared. Not analyzable, but felt. Not possessed, but witnessed.

A symbol of the singularity.

That is what we hold.

That is what holds us.

Appendix A
Glossary of Core Terms

This glossary is not exhaustive but offers orientation to key terms. Many of these concepts carry dense theoretical lineages and contested meanings; what follows reflects the spirit in which they are used in this book.

- **Analytic Field**: A shared intersubjective space that emerges between analyst and patient, composed of affective, symbolic, and unconscious processes that belong to neither individual alone.
- **Character Structure**: The relatively enduring patterns of perception, defense, and relational stance that organize the self's engagement with the world. Often aligned with developmental arrest and adaptive compromise.
- **Condensation**: A process in which multiple unconscious meanings or affects become compressed into a single image, symptom, or idea—central to Freud's theory of dreamwork and here extended to aesthetic and clinical phenomena.
- **Curved Structure**: A symbolic and epistemological stance characterized by recursive temporality, layered symbolic emergence, and delayed recognition. Unlike traditional structural levels (neurotic, borderline, psychotic), it is defined not by deficit but by its fidelity to ambiguity, atmospheric symbolization, and recursive unfolding across time.
- **Gravitational Psyche**: A metaphor developed in this book to describe how the mind orbits, binds, and returns around affectively charged symbols, traumas, or relational configurations—organizing psychic life around invisible but powerful attractors.
- **Nonduality**: A concept drawn from contemplative traditions, used here to indicate a mode of perception in which binary distinctions (self/other, inside/outside, subject/object) soften or dissolve, revealing the psyche as a co-emergent field.
- **Part-Object**: A term from object relations theory denoting an internalized fragment of a person (e.g., breast, gaze, voice) imbued with affective charge. In this book, part-objects are read as gravitational anchors in the absence of symbolic wholeness.

- **Recognition Reversal**: The paradoxical phenomenon in which the naming or symbolization of an internal experience causes it to lose psychic depth or vividness. A moment of symbolic disappointment often felt as both relief and loss. Revisited in curved temporality as a recursive process.
- **Recursive Recognition**: A delayed form of recognition that unfolds through symbolic circling rather than linear understanding. The subject comes to know something not through direct interpretation but through the return of a symbol, image, or mood across time.
- **Recursive Symbolization**: A process in which meaning is not generated through immediate insight but through temporal layering and aesthetic return. The symbol gathers coherence through repeated encounters in altered contexts and affective tones.
- **Repetition Compulsion**: The drive to repeat traumatic or unresolved experiences, not for mastery alone but to keep alive something unformulated or unsymbolized. Interpreted here as recursive gravitational looping.
- **Symbolic Shimmer**: A term coined in this book to describe the partial, flickering quality of certain psychic representations—those that hover between image and meaning, resisting fixed interpretation and evoking aesthetic or dreamlike resonance.
- **Temporality (Psychic)**: The experiential shape of time in the psyche—how past, present, and future are lived not chronologically but through structure, defense, and affective binding. Explored here through looping, freezing, delay, and recursive folding.

Appendix B
Recommended Readings and Influences

Below is a curated selection of works that have influenced the thinking behind this book. While the full references appear in the bibliography, these entries are annotated to assist readers who wish to explore further.

Foundational Psychoanalytic Texts

- **Freud, S. (1900). *The Interpretation of Dreams.***
  Still unmatched in its exploration of symbolic condensation, wish fulfillment, and the unconscious grammar of psychic life.
- **Winnicott, D. W. (1971). *Playing and Reality.***
  A key influence throughout the book—especially Winnicott's exploration of transitional phenomena, the "capacity to be alone," and the atmospheric quality of the symbolic process.
- **Loewald, H. (1980). *Papers on Psychoanalysis.***
  Essential for understanding the temporal and symbolic dimensions of psychic integration and therapeutic action, including the delayed emergence of meaning.

Relational and Contemporary Thinkers

- **Benjamin, J. (1995). *Like Subjects, Love Objects.***
  Offers the grounding for concepts of recognition, intersubjectivity, and mutual transformation—central to the ethical register of recursive witnessing.
- **Bollas, C. (1987). *The Shadow of the Object.***
  A touchstone for the book's exploration of aesthetics, symptom form, and transformational object experience.
- **Eigen, M. (2004). *The Sensitive Self.***
  A poetic, destabilizing presence across these pages, deeply influencing the affective and atmospheric register of the text—especially the reverent temporality of recursive recognition.
- **Ogden, T. H. (1994). "The Analytic Third."**
  Foundational for the field-based, co-created conception of analytic process elaborated here. His ideas on reverie and unformulated experience directly inform the curved structure's clinical stance.

- **Stern, D. B. (2010).** *Partners in Thought.*
  Integral to the understanding of recursive meaning-making, emergent symbolization, and the ethics of presence in analytic work.

Adjacent Philosophy and Thought

- **Merleau-Ponty, M. (1962).** *Phenomenology of Perception.*
  Inspires the text's attention to embodied perception, ambiguity, and the pre-symbolic ground of consciousness.
- **Derrida, J. (1978).** *Writing and Difference.*
  A background influence on the book's interest in slippage, undecidability, and the aporia at the heart of all meaning-making systems.
- **Epstein, M. (1995).** *Thoughts Without a Thinker.*
  Bridges psychoanalysis and Buddhist thought in a way that gently orbits many of this book's inquiries, including the meditation on form and emptiness.

Additional Influences on Recursive and Curved Epistemology

- **Orange, D. M. (1995).** *Emotional Understanding.*
  Essential to the book's approach to empathic availability, non-coercive presence, and the ethics of not-knowing.
- **Kapp, S. K., Gillespie-Lynch, K., Sherman, L. E., & Hutman, T. (2013). "Deficit, Difference, or Both?"**
  Offers empirical grounding for a style of cognition that parallels the curved structure described in this book—an orientation toward bottom-up symbolic assembly, nonlinear processing, and delayed but vivid meaning formation, as often observed in autistic individuals.

Additional Suggested Reading

The following texts have informed the spirit, texture, and conceptual infrastructure of *The Gravitational Psyche*. They are offered not as prerequisites, but as invitations to adjacent fields of inquiry. Some are foundational psychoanalytic texts; others are philosophical or contemplative works that resonate with the book's central themes of gravity, subjectivity, paradox, and symbolic form.

Core Psychoanalytic Texts

- Loewald, H. (1980). *Papers on Psychoanalysis.*
- Ogden, T. H. (2005). *This Art of Psychoanalysis.*
- Bollas, C. (1987). *The Shadow of the Object.*
- Benjamin, J. (1998). *Shadow of the Other.*
- McWilliams, N. (2011). *Psychoanalytic Diagnosis* (2nd ed.).
- Eigen, M. (2004). *The Sensitive Self.*
- Stern, D. (2010). *Partners in Thought.*

Philosophy and Continental Thought

- Derrida, J. (1978). *Writing and Difference*.
- Foucault, M. (1966/1970). *The Order of Things*.
- Heidegger, M. (1962). *Being and Time*.
- Merleau-Ponty, M. (1968). *The Visible and the Invisible*.
- Wittgenstein, L. (1953). *Philosophical Investigations*.

Contemplative and Buddhist Influences

- Epstein, M. (1998). *Going to Pieces Without Falling Apart*.
- Safran, J. (2003). *Psychoanalysis and Buddhism: An Unfolding Dialogue*.
- Magid, B. (2002). *Ordinary Mind*.
- Trungpa, C. (1973). *Cutting Through Spiritual Materialism*.
- Dalai Lama & Varela, F. (1997). *Sleeping, Dreaming, and Dying*.

Recursive Epistemology

- Sacks, O. (1995). *An Anthropologist on Mars*.
  A deeply attuned narrative of perception, pattern, and symbolic life in curved subjectivities—offering lived resonance with the recursive modes described in Chapter 13.
- Hacking, I. (1995). *Rewriting the Soul: Multiple Personality and the Sciences of Memory*.
  Explores how identity and symbolic memory are recursively constituted, aligning with the curved epistemology of the later chapters.
  These works are not simply sources but companions in the process of symbolic transformation. They offer echoes and counterpoints to the gravitational logics that animate the chapters of this book—including the recursive, curved, and aligned epistemologies explored in its later sections.

Appendix C
Guides for Readers and Study Groups

Reader's Guide to Thematic Threads

Conceptual Navigation across the Gravitational Psyche

This guide offers a map of the book's major psychoanalytic and philosophical themes, tracking how each concept recurs, unfolds, and transforms across chapters. These threads are not linear developments, but orbits—they loop, refract, and echo through different contexts. This appendix is designed to support rereading, teaching, and conceptual integration for readers seeking to follow particular ideas through the gravitational architecture of the text.

Temporality and Psychic Structure

- *Prelude—The Singularity and the Desire to Know*
  - Frames time as curved, recursive, and central to the psyche's organization.
- *Chapter 1—The Original Paradox, Refracted*
  - Introduces paradox as a temporal event that generates psychic splitting.
- *Chapter 2—The Curvature of Psychic Space*
  - Develops a topological account of temporality folded into character structure.
- *Chapter 3—Chronotopes of the Self*
  - Offers a diagnostic typology of temporally configured psychic styles.
- *Chapter 6—Echoes and Foldings*
  - Explores repetition as recursive time rather than simple return.

Symptom Formation and Psychic Gravity

- *Chapter 4—Orbiting the Invisible*
  - Reframes the symptom as a gravitational trace, not just a signal of repression.

- *Chapter 5—The Analyst's Gravity*

  - Explores transference and countertransference as field effects that generate psychic curvature.

- *Chapter 6—Echoes and Foldings*

  - Links symptom loops to recursive defenses against contact.

- *Chapter 7—The Holographic Mind*

  - Extends symptom logic to symbolic collapse, condensation, and dream texture.

Field Theory and the Analyst's Presence

- *Chapter 2—The Curvature of Psychic Space*

  - Frames the analyst's gaze and naming function as gravitational forces.

- *Chapter 5—The Analyst's Gravity*

  - Details how analytic presence alters symbolic atmosphere.

- *Chapter 11—Two Tongues for One Mind*

  - Considers how meditative training and analytic reverie shape the field.

- *Chapter 12—The Analyst in the Cosmos*

  - Expands the analyst's role to cosmic participant in psychic unfolding.

Symbolization, Collapse, and Aesthetic Saturation

- *Chapter 6—Echoes and Foldings*

  - Shows how symbol formation emerges from recursive contact with unspeakable traces.

- *Chapter 7—The Holographic Mind*

  - Describes symbolic shimmer, condensation, and the aesthetic edge of form.

- *Chapter 9—Symbolizing the Light*

  - Frames symbolization as field-based, recursive, and ethically saturated.

- *Chapter 10—Part Objects and the Field of Form*

  - Reimagines symbolic fragments not as losses, but as radiant points of contact.

Emptiness, Nonduality, and the Formless Ground

- *Chapter 8—Nonduality in the Split Mind*
  - Offers nonduality as a perceptual stance within the divided psyche.
- *Chapter 9—Symbolizing the Light*
  - Explores recognition reversal and the paradox of symbolic naming.
- *Chapter 10—Part Objects and the Field of Form*
  - Frames fragments as luminous presences in a nondual field.
- *Chapter 11—Two Tongues for One Mind*
  - Bridges Buddhist and analytic framings of form, emptiness, and paradox.
- *Chapter 13—Recursive Recognition and the Reader's Loop*
  - Reframes reading itself as a symbolic field where emptiness and delay become vehicles of recursive recognition.
- *Interlude—Gravitational Emptiness*
  - Classifies emptiness into four affective and structural atmospheres.

Recursion, Repetition, and the Ethics of Return

- *Chapter 3—Chronotopes of the Self*
  - Introduces countertemporal resistance and time-bound defenses.
- *Chapter 6—Echoes and Foldings*
  - Defines recursive return as a transformation of repetition compulsion.
- *Chapter 7—The Holographic Mind*
  - Suggests collapse can initiate recursive symbolization.
- *Chapter 13—Recursive Recognition and the Reader's Loop*
  - Extends the recursive structure to the reader's own temporality, framing fidelity to delay as an ethical act.
- *Chapter 14—Coda: Symbol of the Singularity*
  - Closes with a meditation on return not as regression, but as renewal of form.

Readers' Guide: Conceptual Map of *Gravitational Psyche*

A Narrative Architecture of Psychic Gravity

Below is a conceptual map of *Gravitational Psyche*—not as a summary but as a gravitational tracing. Across the volume, themes curve and refract like orbits around a center that cannot be touched directly. Recursion, symbolic shimmer, and collapse emerge not as breakdowns but as features of a curved epistemology. The architecture is not linear, but atmospheric, recursive, and textured. This map supports teaching, rereading, and immersive conceptual engagement.

Singularity and Orbit

(*Prelude & Introduction*)

- Introduces the metaphor of psychic gravity and curvature as the organizing condition of knowing.
- Proposes orbit as a stance of radical engagement without mastery.
- Establishes the recursive field of interpretation and symbolic form.

Key motifs: singularity, interpretive orbit, gravitational epistemology, recursive knowing, curved desire

Spatial and Temporal Curvature

(*Chapters 1–3*)

- Chapter 1 refracts the original paradox of division through foundational psychoanalytic figures.
- Chapter 2 introduces psychic structure as curved space, shaped by symbolic and affective mass.
- Chapter 3 defines character styles through chronotopic distortions—forms of temporal curvature.

Key motifs: psychic curvature, symbolic topologies, paradox, temporal logic, diagnostic mood

Symptom as Trace

(*Chapters 4 and 5*)

- Chapter 4 reframes symptoms as aesthetic traces left by gravitational compression, not linear causality.
- Chapter 5 presents the analyst's presence as a gravitational body shaping the symbolic field.
- Curved understanding replaces interpretive fixity with atmospheric modulation.

Key motifs: trace, field effect, gravitational residue, orbiting symptoms, countertransference mass

Recursion and Collapse

(*Chapters 6 and 7*)

- Chapter 6 reconceives repetition as recursive return, echoing across time rather than reenacting.
- Chapter 7 explores symbolic collapse, condensation, and shimmer—phenomena of overstimulated atmosphere.
- Collapse becomes a mode of curved contact: symbolic saturation and partial integration.

Key motifs: recursion, repetition, symbolic overload, condensation, aesthetic disintegration

Form and Emptiness

(*Chapters 8–11 + Interlude*)

- Chapter 8 frames nonduality as a curved mode of perception that holds contradiction without collapse.
- Chapter 9 develops recognition reversal—where symbolic naming reveals void rather than clarity.
- Chapter 10 presents part-objects as radiant fragments refracted through curved subjectivity.
- The Interlude articulates four forms of emptiness with distinct affective textures.
- Chapter 11 links Buddhist and psychoanalytic methods for symbolizing emptiness without form.

Key motifs: nondual field, recognition reversal, luminous fragment, part-object, symbolic atmosphere

Cosmic Holding and Closure

(*Chapters 12–14*)

- Chapter 12 situates the analyst within the cosmos of the psyche—both witness and gravitational participant.
- Chapter 13 (Afterword) reflects recursively on authorship, orbit, and curved presence.
- Chapter 14 (Coda) returns to the singularity—not as endpoint, but as suspended, radiant paradox.

Key motifs: cosmic participation, echo, author-field entanglement, recursive closure, curved witnessing

Atmospheric Binaries in Tension

Across the book, symbolic tensions flicker and collapse—setting the affective atmosphere of the curved structure:

Collapse ↔ Holding	Orbit ↔ Singularity
Symbol ↔ Formlessness	Voice ↔ Disintegration
Recursion ↔ Emergence	Witnessing ↔ Gravity

These pairs are not oppositions to be resolved, but recursive tensions to be held. Their curved entanglement is the very texture of the gravitational psyche.

Reader's Guide for Integration and Return

Tracing Core Themes across the Volume

This guide invites the reader to follow key motifs as they curve, echo, and refract across chapters. Themes do not proceed linearly, but loop through the text with recursive variation. Each thread is cross-referenced with chapter numbers.

Temporal Distortion and Psychic Structure

- *Prelude—The Singularity and the Desire to Know*
  - Introduces the foundational paradox of simultaneity, recursion, and the nonlinear psyche.
- *Chapter 1—The Original Paradox, Refracted*
  - Frames the split in psychic time as an ontological and symbolic event.
- *Chapter 2—The Curvature of Psychic Space*
  - Describes psychic structure through spatial and gravitational metaphors; introduces orbital topology.
- *Chapter 3—Chronotopes of the Self*
  - Maps character styles onto temporally distorted chronotopes.
- *Chapter 6—Echoes and Foldings*
  - Repetition is reframed as recursive temporal looping, not simple reenactment.

Gravity, Collapse, and Symptom Formation

- *Chapter 4—Orbiting the Invisible*
  - Positions the symptom as a gravitational trace of unsymbolized psychic mass.

- *Chapter 5—The Analyst's Gravity*
  - Explores how the analyst's presence shapes the topography and atmosphere of psychic space.
- *Chapter 7—The Holographic Mind*
  - Investigates symbolic collapse, condensation, and aesthetic distortion in psychic experience.

Form, Emptiness, and Nonduality

- *Chapter 8—Nonduality in the Split Mind*
  - Recasts duality as a perceptual mode layered over an ever-present nondual ground.
- *Chapter 9—Symbolizing the Light*
  - Examines the transformation of emptiness and form through symbolic field dynamics.
- *Chapter 10—Part Objects and the Field of Form*
  - Treats part-objects as radiant fragments within a nondual psychic continuum.
- *Chapter 11—Two Tongues for One Mind*
  - Explores Buddhist and psychoanalytic practices of holding the paradox of form and emptiness.
- *Chapter 13—Recursive Recognition and the Reader's Loop*
  - Situates the reader within a symbolic field shaped by emptiness, delay, and recursive self-experience.
- *Interlude—Gravitational Emptiness*
  - Defines four kinds of emptiness: ontological, symbolic, developmental, and contemplative.

Recursion, Reverberation, and Symbolic Atmosphere

- *Chapter 6—Echoes and Foldings*
  - Repetition compulsion is presented as a recursive return shaped by unformulated atmospheres.
- *Chapter 7—The Holographic Mind*
  - Explores how shimmer, collapse, and condensation create symbolic fields that resist final interpretation.

- *Chapter 9—Symbolizing the Light*

  - Continues the inquiry into how atmosphere mediates symbol formation and recognition reversal.

- *Chapter 13—Recursive Recognition and the Reader's Loop*

  - Enacts recursion through form and content, inviting the reader into a field of symbolic echo and fidelity to delay.

The Analyst as Gravitational Participant

- *Chapter 5—The Analyst's Gravity*

  - Examines the analyst's field effect on psychic experience and the countertransference environment.

- *Chapter 11—Two Tongues for One Mind*

  - Considers how meditative and analytic presences create atmospheric holding.

- *Chapter 12—The Analyst in the Cosmos*

  - Envisions the analyst as both container and participant in a cosmic symbolic field.

- *Chapter 13—Afterword*

  - Reflects on the author's own embeddedness in the gravitational psyche of the text.

The Singularity as Symbol

- *Prelude—The Singularity and the Desire to Know*

  - Establishes the image of the singularity as an ethical and ontological attractor.

- *Chapter 14—Coda: Symbol of the Singularity*

  - Concludes with a poetic meditation on the singularity as an ever-collapsing and radiating center of psychic meaning.

Prompts for Readers, Groups, and Clinicians

Prompts for Reflection, Dialogue, and Clinical Application

This guide is designed to support immersive, reflective engagement with the text—whether individually, in study groups, or in supervision. The prompts below are organized by major themes and relational stances rather than by chapter. They may be used to foster dialogue, integrate theory into practice, or invite symbolic exploration in clinical work. Readers are encouraged to return to these questions recursively, as meaning may evolve with rereading—particularly when engaging from a curved or non-linear epistemological stance.

Encountering the Text as a Field

- What gravitational pull (conceptual, emotional, aesthetic) did you experience in reading this book?
- Were there moments where the writing style itself created symbolic atmosphere, echo, or collapse? How did you respond?
- How do you experience recursion in your own reading habits—returning to passages, looping interpretations, resisting closure?
- Did any passages feel like they *thought you* rather than being read by you? What kind of epistemic stance does that imply?
- How might a curved epistemology—marked by recursive mapping, non-linear assembly, and sensitivity to form—shape how you approached this book?

Time, Structure, and Character

- Which chronotope (obsessive, hysteric, depressive, psychotic) do you find most clinically familiar—or personally resonant?
- How might the idea of curvature inform your understanding of a patient's way of organizing time and experience?
- In what ways do your interventions "bend" the psychic space of the session?
- Can you recognize moments when structural assumptions flattened a patient's curved or recursive truth?
- Might the curved structure offer an alternative to linear temporality or binary diagnosis?

Working with Collapse and Symbolic Atmosphere

- Recall a session where the symbolic field felt saturated or unstable. What contributed to that collapse?
- How do you hold moments of unformulated intensity that cannot yet be symbolized?
- Have you encountered a clinical moment that shimmered—hovered between meaning and nonmeaning? How did you hold it?
- When symbolization fails, what kinds of presence or echo remain in the field?

Orbit, Gravity, and the Analyst's Presence

- Consider the metaphor of the analyst as gravitational body. What in your presence exerts mass—affective, ethical, symbolic?

- How do your own field reverberations shape the curvature of the patient's psychic orbit?
- What forms of countertransference feel like resistance to orbit or overidentification with gravity?
- Have you ever sensed that your presence was a symbolic object rather than a person? What ethical responsibilities did that entail?

Nonduality, Emptiness, and the Unformulated

- How do you work clinically with phenomena that resist binary formulations (e.g., good/bad, true/false, self/other)?
- Have you encountered a moment of ethical refusal—a patient resisting interpretation, connection, or form in a way that felt protective?
- In your experience, what does emptiness feel like in the room: ontological, symbolic, developmental, or contemplative?
- What would it mean to encounter a patient from a nondual, curved epistemology—where form and formlessness are not opposed but co-present?

Suggested Study Group Framework

Week 1:

Prelude and Introduction—What does it mean to write a book orbiting the unsymbolizable? What stance does the reader take?

Week 2–3:

Chapters 1–3—Explore temporality and structure. Map the character styles to clinical vignettes or personal experience.

Week 4–5:

Chapters 4–6—Focus on symptom gravity and repetition compulsion. Use clinical examples to trace recursive dynamics.

Week 6–7:

Chapters 7–9—Engage aesthetic collapse, shimmer, and the edges of symbolization. Try reading passages aloud and attending to mood.

Week 8:

Chapters 10 and 11 + Interlude—Discuss the resonance between Buddhist and psychoanalytic framings of emptiness and presence.

Week 9:

Chapters 12–14—Reflect on the role of the analyst, the text, and the reader as co-participants in symbolic return. How is the curved structure embodied in the book itself?

Writing Prompts for Clinicians

- "My presence in the field creates curvature when…"
- "A recent moment in session where gravity shifted was…"
- "The part-object in my patient's narrative felt like…"
- "Symbolic collapse occurred when…"
- "The singularity I orbit in my work is…"
- "I recognized a curved structure when…"
- "Reading this book recursively, I now see that…"

Appendix D
Curved Lineage and
the Gravitational Psyche

A Topology of Echoes and Conceptual Gravity

This appendix traces how classical and mid-century psychoanalytic motifs—especially those of Freud, Klein, Bion, Lacan, and Loewald—are refracted within the gravitational and recursive architecture of *Gravitational Psyche*. These figures are not simply theoretical anchors but orbiting presences, whose ideas bend symbolization, perception, and psychic structure in ways that echo the book's core metaphors. Each is taken not as a master thinker but as a topological contributor to the curved structure.

Oceanic Oneness and the Ungraspable Singularity

Freud's concept of "oceanic feeling"—discussed in *Civilization and Its Discontents* (1930)—names a diffuse sense of boundaryless unity that he himself viewed with ambivalence. This feeling reappears in *Gravitational Psyche* not as regression, but as a paradoxical precondition for form: the gravitational singularity from which thought and structure emerge. Chapters 1 (*The Original Paradox, Refracted*) and the Prelude frame the oceanic not as loss of self, but as the curved background of symbolization itself.

   → Freud, S. (1930). Civilization and its discontents.

The Mystic Writing-Pad and Symbolic Recursion

In *A Note Upon the Mystic Writing-Pad* (1925), Freud describes perception as a system that retains traces without remaining consciously aware of them—an early metaphor for recursive psychic inscriptions. This becomes foundational in Chapters 6 and 7, where repetition compulsion and symbolic shimmer are framed as recursive atmospheric processes. The mind is not a linear archive but a folding system of semi-permeable inscriptions.

   → Freud, S. (1925). A note upon the mystic writing-pad.

The Death Drive as Recursive Gravity

Freud's theorization of the death drive (*Beyond the Pleasure Principle*, 1920) posits a compulsion to return to an inorganic state. This compulsion, rather than being negated, is reinterpreted in Chapter 6: *Echoes and Foldings* as gravitational recursion—a looping toward repetition that curves time inward. Death drive here becomes a vector of return, re-symbolization, and gravitational tension.

→ Freud, S. (1920). Beyond the pleasure principle.

The Ego, the Id, and the Topological Turn

Freud's topographic model of the psyche (*The Ego and the Id*, 1923) implied a field structure that foreshadowed the curved psychic space described in Chapter 2. Rather than discrete zones, ego and id are imagined here as gravitational fields in dynamic relation. Psychic space is bent, not bounded.

→ Freud, S. (1923). The ego and the id.

Klein's Part-Objects and Symbolic Collapse

Klein's concept of part-objects and early splitting (*Notes on Some Schizoid Mechanisms*, 1946) reappears as a core foundation for Chapters 1, 7, and 10. The shattered nature of early object relations becomes, in this volume, the basis for atmospheric perception and the shimmer of symbolic instability. Klein's fragments are not only primitive defenses—they are gravitational residues that shape psychic space.

→ Klein, M. (1946). Notes on some schizoid mechanisms.

The Depressive Position and Symbolic Holding

In *Some Theoretical Conclusions Regarding the Emotional Life of the Infant* (1952), Klein describes the integration of part-objects into a whole object—forming the depressive position. This movement is refracted in Chapter 8, where nonduality and symbolic attunement emerge not from coherence, but from the ability to tolerate fragmentation as form. The depressive position is gravitational, not merely integrative.

→ Klein, M. (1952). Some theoretical conclusions regarding the emotional life of the infant.

Symbol, Atmosphere, and the Analytic Field

Both Freud and Klein laid groundwork for what would become the field-based, atmospheric model of symbolization in this book. Chapters 5, 7, and 9 in particular revisit the symbol not as fixed representation, but as condensation of recursive presence—something saturated, shimmering, and gravitational. This recasts both transference and the analytic frame as fields of curvature.

Bion's Alpha Function and Symbolic Atmosphere

Bion's concept of the *alpha function*—the capacity to metabolize raw sensory and emotional data into symbolic form—serves as a deep precursor to this book's framing of *symbolic atmosphere* and *gravitational containment*. Chapters 5, 7, and 9 draw implicitly on Bion's "container/contained" dynamic, but invert its teleology: not all unprocessed elements require digestion into meaning. Some hover, shimmer, or remain unsymbolizable by design. Bion's work supports the framing of analytic presence as a field in which symbolic collapse may be held rather than solved.

→ Bion, W. R. (1962). *Learning from experience.*

Loewald's Symbolization and Curved Temporality

Loewald's vision of symbolization as an *integration across psychic levels* reverberates throughout *Gravitational Psyche*. His refusal of linearity in psychic development, along with his insistence that past, present, and future interpenetrate in the unconscious, sets the groundwork for Chapter 3's depiction of *chronotopes* and Chapter 6's treatment of *recursive time*. His emphasis on the analyst's *transformational presence* also orbits the book's vision of gravitational co-constitution within the field.

→ Loewald, H. (1978a). Psychoanalysis and the history of the individual.
→ Loewald, H. (1980). *Papers on psychoanalysis.*

Lacan's Topology and the Split Subject

Lacan's use of *topology*, particularly the Möbius strip and Borromean knot, directly prefigures the curved psychic geometries explored in Chapters 2 and 8. His theory of the *split subject*, suspended between the imaginary and the symbolic, undergirds this book's framing of *nonduality* as a perceptual position within the split. Chapter 9, in particular, echoes Lacan's treatment of *symbolic light*, refracted through recognition reversal. However, where Lacan privileged the symbolic order, this text invites saturation, collapse, and recursive recursion of symbolization itself.

→ Lacan, J. (1953–1973). *Écrits* and *Seminar XI: The four fundamental concepts of psychoanalysis.*

References

Bion, W. R. (1962). *Learning from experience*. Heinemann.
Freud, S. (1920). Beyond the pleasure principle. In J. Strachey (Ed. & Trans.), *The standard edition of the complete psychological works of Sigmund Freud*, vol. 18. Hogarth Press.
Freud, S. (1923). The ego and the id. In J. Strachey (Ed. & Trans.), *The standard edition of the complete psychological works of Sigmund Freud*, vol. 19. Hogarth Press.
Freud, S. (1925). A note upon the mystic writing-pad. In J. Strachey (Ed. & Trans.), *The standard edition of the complete psychological works of Sigmund Freud*, vol. 19. Hogarth Press.

Freud, S. (1930). Civilization and its discontents. In J. Strachey (Ed. & Trans.), *The standard edition of the complete psychological works of Sigmund Freud*, vol. 21. Hogarth Press.

Klein, M. (1946). Notes on some schizoid mechanisms. *International Journal of Psychoanalysis, 27*, 99–110.

Klein, M. (1952). Some theoretical conclusions regarding the emotional life of the infant. In *Developments in Psycho-Analysis* (pp. 198–236).

Lacan, J. (1953–1973). *Écrits and Seminar XI: The four fundamental concepts of psychoanalysis.*

Lacan, J. (1977). *Écrits*: A *selection*. W. W. Norton & Company.

Lacan, J. (1978). *The four fundamental concepts of psychoanalysis* (Seminar XI). W. W. Norton & Company.

Loewald, H. (1978a). Psychoanalysis and the history of the individual. *Psychoanalytic Quarterly, 47*, 327–342.

Loewald, H. (1980). *Papers on psychoanalysis.* Yale University Press.

Lineages and Departures: A Psychoanalytic Genealogy of *Gravitational Psyche*

This book speaks in a voice of rupture, recursion, and paradox—but it does not speak from nowhere. It emerges from a tradition that has always been divided: between the named and the unnamable, the drive and the relation, the cure and the remainder. *Gravitational Psyche* extends this inheritance not by resolving its contradictions, but by intensifying them.

What follows is a symbolic map—**not a full lineage, but a constellation**—tracing how this work emerges from, collides with, and reorients classical and contemporary psychoanalytic thought.

Psychic Topology and the Nonlinear Mind

Thinker	Key Inheritance	Extension/Departure
Freud	Topographic model; primary process	Temporal folding as topological curvature; paradox as foundational
Klein	Part-object relations; splitting	Nonduality of the part-object; splitting as ontological
Loewald	Symbolization; internalization	Symbolic atmosphere as gravitational, not hierarchical
Ogden	Dream space; undreamt dream	Recursive temporality and analyst's gravitational field

Drive, Death, and the Remainder

Thinker	Key Inheritance	Extension/Departure
Freud	Death drive; mystic writing pad	Death drive as recursive return; symbolic trace as Real echo
Lacan	The Real; jouissance; *le reste*	The holographic psyche: remainder as atmosphere

(Continued)

Thinker	Key Inheritance	Extension/Departure
Laplanche	Enigmatic signifier; seduction	Symbolic overflow as gravitational pull toward the unspeakable
Eigen	Ineffable contact; tremble	Recursion and paradox as shapes of psychic survival

Relationality and the Ethics of Presence

Thinker	Key Inheritance	Extension/Departure
Winnicott	True self; holding; play	False self as curator of aesthetic time; performance as defense
Benjamin	Recognition; mutuality; thirdness	Witnessing failure as ethical rupture; non-recognition as depth
Orange	Ethical presence; phenomenology	Attunement to paradox as clinical method
Atwood & Stolorow	Intersubjectivity; contextualism	Psyche as curved field; character as temporality

Paradox, Nonduality, and the Split Mind

Thinker	Key Inheritance	Extension/Departure
Klein	Splitting; depressive position	Holding unresolved splits as ethical stance
Freud	Oceanic feelings; timeless unconscious	Nonduality as structural foundation of psyche
Bion	-K; container-contained dynamics	Symbol collapse as analytic horizon
Heidegger	Language and unnameability	Unsayable as symbolic condensation, not absence
Wittgenstein	Limits of language; negative capabilities	Unformulable as presence, not void

Queer, Postcolonial, and Mystical Currents

Thinker	Key Inheritance	Extension/Departure
Bersani	Erotic shattering; anti-narrative	Submission and dissolution as modes of witness
Sedgwick	Reparative vs. paranoid reading; affect theory	Symbolic shimmer as atmospheric containment
Muñoz	Queer futurity; horizonality	Unformulated experience as utopic horizon, not absence
Fanon	Colonial alienation; symbolic violence	Anti-integration as critique of colonial normativity
Foucault	Care of the self; power/knowledge	Integration as normalization; refusal as freedom

Appendix E

Against the Ideal of Integration: Notes from the Curved Field

Michael Eigen has said, "When I was a little boy I remember seeing a tree. Half of it was withered and dead and the other half was blooming. Then I realized that one could be dead and very much alive, concurrently... We are fractured and whole all at once" (Kara-Ivanov Kaniel, 2013, Tikkun).

Otto Kernberg has given psychoanalysis a lucid and enduring model of structural development. His vision is admirable in its internal coherence: split internal object relations—idealized and persecutory—are brought into relation within the same ego structure, allowing for stable identity, ambivalent affect tolerance, and the capacity for intimacy without collapse.

But the ideal that **integration is the developmental telos**, or worse, that it is synonymous with mental health, must be questioned. This challenge is not theoretical alone. It is existential.

Kernberg's model presumes that the psyche is healthiest when its contradictions are reconciled. But for many, especially those whose psychic lives are shaped by recursive thought, aesthetic containment, and ethical refusal, **unity is not safety—it is violence.** To integrate the internal object world would be to flatten it. To remove its multiplicity, its folds, its conflicting rhythms and nonconforming truths, would be to **colonize psychic life** in the name of coherence.

And that, in the end, is the deeper issue.

The call to integration often functions as a **colonizing gesture**, disguised as care. It emerges from a white, Western, masculinized epistemology that assumes **coherence is desirable** and that dissonance must be metabolized into harmony. It assumes that conflict should be healed, contradiction resolved, unformulated states translated into synthesis. But integration, as it is often deployed, is **the violence of synthesis**—the drive to make the psyche consistent, ordered, and complete, even if doing so **disavows the very excess that makes subjectivity livable**. In this way, integration becomes an **imagined salvation project**—a fantasy of coherence that protects analyst and analysand alike from the terror of the psyche's fundamental unresolvability.

It is worth noting here that Kernberg is a Holocaust survivor.[1] His commitment to the integration of good and bad object relations, and to a vision of internal structure governed by ambivalence and symbolic mediation, may reflect not only theoretical conviction but also an **existential response to the psychic and moral disintegration he witnessed as a young man**. One can read his clinical emphasis on ego strength, reality testing, and the containment of aggression not merely as technical preferences but as an ethical insistence that the psyche *must* be made capable of withstanding its own destructiveness—lest it mirror the horrors of the external world. This context does not weaken the critique. It deepens it. It reminds us that **theories are also defenses**, and that what we elevate as therapeutic may also be a form of mourning.

This is not intended as critique of Kernberg, whose thinking remains one of the most enduring achievements in post-Freudian structural theory. It is a critique of **what we take for granted when we say a psyche has healed**.

Subjectivity does not require coherence to endure. Psychic life is not a sequence of parts awaiting integration, but a curved field of tensions, folds, and recursive currents. Contradictions are not failures of development—they are modes of contact. Structure is not something into which the psyche must be shaped; it is what emerges when paradox is held, not solved.

When the analytic gaze demands integration, it echoes the logic of assimilation. It refuses to tolerate that some forms of psychic life do not seek coherence—they seek company. The refusal to integrate may be not a deficit, but a **mode of ethical persistence**.

This is not a call for chaos. It is a call for **symbolic hospitality to incoherence**. For a psychoanalysis that stops converting everything it touches into a developmental sequence.

This sensibility aligns with a queer theoretical lineage that has long resisted the violence of resolution. **Bersani** taught that the shattering of the self is not necessarily pathological, but erotic. **Sedgwick** warned against reparative reading that forecloses negativity too soon. **José Esteban Muñoz** offered queerness as a field of utopic partiality, not integration. **Fanon** revealed how the psychic effects of colonial violence produce subjectivities that refuse legibility on normative terms. And **Foucault** showed us that power often arrives through the guise of care—that healing, too, can be a regime. In this light, integration is not a cure. It is **an epistemological demand masquerading as care**.

This critique extends a quiet lineage in psychoanalysis that has long refused the ideal of integration, even as it struggled to name the alternative. **Michael Eigen** listens for what cannot be metabolized. He remains in contact with rupture, contradiction, and affective rawness without transforming them into coherent narrative. For Eigen, the psyche's truth is not in resolution, but in **sustained tremble**.

Jessica Benjamin, especially in her later work, approaches the edges of relational failure not as pathology, but as revelation. **Adrienne Harris**, in her theorization of multiplicity and gender, argues for the legitimacy of subjectivities that remain **unresolved, non-unitary, and uncollapsed**. **Donnel Stern** and

Irwin Hoffman each, in different ways, protect the unformulated from premature symbolization, offering a relational ethic of **waiting without knowing**.

And then there is **Lacan**, who names the remainder directly: *le reste*—that which does not submit to symbolization. The Real, for Lacan, is the heart of the psyche that resists all therapeutic effort to bind it. **Laplanche** offers a kindred vision: the **enigmatic signifier** as a wound that forms the subject but cannot be translated without remainder. Both insist: the psyche's core is **not integratable**. It can only be approached, circled, felt—but never cured.

It is here that the critique lands most fully: that **Kernberg's model, in its very elegance, becomes anesthetic**. It transforms unresolvable complexity into developmental sequence. It converts the ache of symbolic life into the appearance of structure. It theorizes away the slippage it cannot bear. The remainder is not integrated—it is denied.

This is not to say his model lacks value. It is to say it lacks nerve for what cannot be metabolized.

To speak of **health** as integration is to reduce it to an aesthetic of internal tidiness. But psychic life is not tidy, and neither is the world. Health, if it exists at all, must be reimagined as the **capacity to live with the unresolvable**—to grieve what cannot be restored, to love without guarantee, to symbolize without final synthesis. Kernberg's vision of integration may itself be a defense—a necessary one, perhaps—against the terrifying complexity of the psyche and its unrelenting contact with a world that offers no stable resolution.

Author's Note

This appendix is not a rejection of integration, nor of psychoanalysis. It is an effort to further the psychoanalytic project by clarifying its limits and re-opening its questions. **Integration remains a meaningful and necessary process in many clinical contexts**—particularly when fragmentation impairs reality testing, or when the psyche requires stabilizing form in order to survive. The capacity to symbolize, metabolize, and relate internal states is essential analytic work.

But when integration becomes a moral endpoint—when it functions as a developmental demand, a normalizing fantasy, or a defense against the psyche's ongoing rupture—it betrays the very spirit of psychoanalysis. This is not a repudiation, but a reclamation. A call to let paradox breathe without insisting it resolve.

I write from within the analytic tradition—with reverence, with resistance, and with a belief that psychoanalysis must remain capable of evolving in response to the lived complexity of the people it serves.

To hold paradox is not to abandon structure. It is to recognize that the structure may already be there, just not in the shape we expected. The psyche does not move toward resolution but bends back on itself—curved, shimmering, unfinished.

Lineage of the Remainder

The following chart traces a lineage of thinkers—analytic, queer, postcolonial, and philosophical—who challenge the integration ideal and offer alternative models of psychic endurance, ethical contact, and symbolic life. Each honors the *remainder* as vital rather than pathological, and helps articulate a psychoanalysis capable of **holding without resolution**.

What follows is a symbolic constellation—not a typology. These figures, past and present, offer clues to the Curved Epistemology explored throughout this book. Some bear its recursive structure in style, others in ethics, some in form, some in failure. Their inclusion is poetic, not diagnostic.

Curved Epistemology: A Symbolic Constellation

Thinker	Core Concept	Form of Resistance to Integration	Symbolic Metaphor	Relevant Texts
Michael Eigen	Contact with raw affect	Refuses symbolization-as-cure	Tremble	The Psychotic Core, Ecstasy
Jessica Benjamin	Moral third, asymmetry, breakdown	Honors failure of mutual recognition	Ethical fracture	Beyond Doer and Done To
Adrienne Harris	Soft assembly, gendered multiplicity	Accepts unintegrated gendered and psychic positions	Assemblage	Gender as Soft Assembly
Donnel Stern	Unformulated experience	Resists premature symbolization	Fog/latency	Partners in Thought
Irwin Hoffman	Hermeneutic field, co-construction	Resists interpretive closure	Echo/ horizon	Ritual and Spontaneity
Lacan	The Real, le reste	Names the unsymbolizable remainder	Rupture/ kernel	Écrits, The Four Fundamental Concepts
Jean Laplanche	Enigmatic signifier	The unconscious as excess beyond integration	Wound/ foreign body	Essays on Otherness
Leo Bersani	Shattering, jouissance	Erotic undoing of the cohesive self	Shatter/ gleam	Is the Rectum a Grave?
Eve Sedgwick	Paranoid vs reparative reading	Opposes premature coherence	Glitter/ residue	Touching Feeling
José Esteban Muñoz	Queerness as horizon, utopia	Sustains partiality, delays closure	Horizon/ shimmer	Cruising Utopia

(Continued)

Thinker	Core Concept	Form of Resistance to Integration	Symbolic Metaphor	Relevant Texts
Frantz Fanon	Colonial alienation and psychic distortion	Reveals integration as racial violence	Mask/ fracture	Black Skin, White Masks
Michel Foucault	Care of the self, disciplinary power	Shows integration as normalizing technique	Apparatus/ frame	Discipline and Punish, History of Sexuality

This is not a system, but a trace—an echo of the field from which this work took shape.

Note

1 Kernberg was born in Vienna in 1928 to a Jewish family and emigrated with his parents to Chile in 1939 to escape the rising threat of Nazism. Though he was not imprisoned in camps, his formative years were shaped by the trauma of state-sponsored annihilation, the destruction of European Jewish life, and the long shadow of ethical collapse in both political and familial structures. This historical trauma likely shaped his clinical emphasis on reality testing, aggression containment, and the moral dimensions of ego integration.

Appendix F
The Curved Structure

Psychoanalytic metapsychology has traditionally described psychic structure along a developmental axis: psychotic, borderline, and neurotic. Each level reflects a mode of organizing reality, symbolizing affect, and relating to others. The higher the structure, the more coherent, reality-oriented, and symbolically integrated the self is presumed to be. Health, in this schema, is understood as a culmination of integration—the synthesis of conflicting internal states into a stable self capable of adaptive functioning.

But this model, while clinically useful, can obscure more than it reveals when it encounters subjectivities shaped not by pathology, but by recursive awareness, paradoxical coherence, and a refusal of premature resolution. A fourth kind of structure—which we call the Curved Structure—emerges not as a deficit but as an ethical stance and structural alternative. It is not an extension of the neurotic structure, nor a refinement of borderline organization. It is an orthogonal orientation: one organized not around coherence but around the symbolic metabolization of contradiction.

Four Levels of Psychic Structure

Structure	Organizing Principle	Primary Defense	Symbolic Mode	Reality Orientation	Clinical Risks
Psychotic	Concrete fusion, intrusion	Denial, projection	Fragmented, literal	Permeable, distorted	Delusion, disorganization
Borderline	Splitting and idealization	Splitting, projective identification	Episodic, vivid, polarized	Divided, unstable	Identity diffusion, relational chaos
Neurotic	Repression and compromise formation	Repression, displacement	Coherent, narrative	Stable, symbolic	Symptom rigidity, repression
Curved	Recursive containment of paradox	Aesthetic-ization, symbolic folding	Curved, layered, atmos-pheric	Reflexive, paradox-embracing	Misrecognition, isolation, ontological instability

Curved Structure Thinkers—Contributions and Examples

Thinker	Signature Contribution	Example Work or Conceptual Moment
Sándor Ferenczi	Trauma dialectics, radical empathy, confusion of tongues	"Confusion of Tongues Between Adults and the Child"
D. W. Winnicott	Holding paradox, transitional space, creative living	*Playing and Reality*— paradox in transitional space
Michael Eigen	Psychic intensity, undreamt dreams, ecstatic suffering	*The Sensitive Self*, *Contact With the Depths*
Judith Butler	Ethics of incoherence, performativity, post-normativity	*Giving an Account of Oneself*
Leo Bersani	Ego-shattering, aesthetic subjectivity, relational undoing	"Is the Rectum a Grave?"
Eve Kosofsky Sedgwick	Reparative reading, queer opacity, affective nuance	*Touching Feeling*—Paranoid vs. Reparative Reading
José Esteban Muñoz	Queer futurity, utopia as method, anticipatory affect	*Cruising Utopia*
Michel Foucault	Dispersed subjectivity, critique of coherence and normativity	*Technologies of the Self*
George Atwood	Reflexive subjectivity, witnessing grief, symbolic atmosphere	*The Abyss of Madness*

The above figures are offered not as "members" of the Curved Structure, nor as endorsers of this formulation, but as individuals whose work, presence, or stylistic sensibility evokes epistemological traits consistent with this curved stance. They appear here as symbolic anchors, gravitational attractors, or resonant inflections—rather than categorical representatives.

Differentiating "Healthy" from the Curved Structure

The classical notion of psychic health presumes increasing integration, symbolic coherence, and adaptability to social norms. But the Curved Structure is not about adaptation—it is about ethical complexity and symbolic truthfulness. It tolerates contradiction without resolving it, maintains awareness of the limits of all meaning systems, and metabolizes affect through recursive aesthetic and philosophical reflection.

Feature	Healthy (Neurotic Ideal)	Curved Structure
Symbolization	Integrative, narrative	Recursive, paradoxical, atmospheric
Conflict	Resolved through synthesis	Held without resolution; metabolized through layered holding
Time	Linear, developmental	Curved, recursive, non-teleological

(Continued)

Feature	Healthy (Neurotic Ideal)	Curved Structure
Reality Testing	External validation, consensual reality	Internal reflexivity; truth as symbolic resonance
Self-Experience	Cohesive, identity-based	Folded, recursive, multi-positional; self as field, not entity
Risk	Rigidity, symptom formation, repression	Misrecognition, ontological doubt, symbolic oversaturation
Ethical Stance	Adaptation, compromise, empathy	Witnessing, principled refusal, symbolic honesty
Goal of Analysis	Greater coherence and flexibility	Greater paradox tolerance and symbolic recursion

Splitting, Identification, and the Curved Structure

While splitting may appear within Curved Structure experience, it is no longer organized around identification or disavowal. The subject does not align with one pole and project out the other, as is common in borderline structure. Instead, the split is held in awareness, sustained as a tension that is neither prematurely resolved nor acted out. This capacity—to remain in relation to paradox without collapsing into either side—is what differentiates the Curved Structure from the borderline level. It is not the absence of division that marks psychic integration, but the non-identification with either side of the divide. What appears as instability from a structural vantage point is, in fact, a higher-order form of reality testing: one that refuses false synthesis and remains ethically attuned to contradiction. This is not fragmentation. It is lucid multiplicity, symbolically held.

Dimension	Psychotic	Borderline	Neurotic	Curved Structure
Identity	Fragmented or fused; reality-boundary breakdown	Diffuse, split between opposing poles	Cohesive but defended; tends toward repression	Multiplicitous but symbolically held; paradoxical identity lived without foreclosure
Defenses	Primitive (denial, delusional projection)	Splitting, idealization/ devaluation, projective identification	Repression, reaction formation, displacement	Recursive awareness, symbolic holding, non-identification with poles
Reality Testing	Severely impaired	Intact but fragile under affective pressure	Stable and intact	Expanded: includes paradox, contradiction, and symbolic ambiguity without collapse
Relation to Splitting	Total collapse or delusional fusion	Identified with one side of the split; disavows the other	Resolves contradiction through symbolic repression	Holds split consciously; does not identify with either pole; paradox becomes ground

On Reality Testing at the Edge of Recognition

There is a paradox at the heart of the Curved Structure: The deeper one's contact with reality becomes, the less likely it is to be recognized.

Traditional psychoanalytic models treat reality testing as the capacity to distinguish internal from external, fantasy from fact, symbol from thing. But what happens when reality itself is paradoxical? When coherence is a defense, and contradiction is what's most true?

At this level, reality testing no longer looks like agreement. It looks like staying in contact with the parts of experience that cannot be confirmed by the other—because the other, too, is defended against what doesn't resolve.

To live inside the Curved Structure is to test not only one's own reality, but the reality of the field itself: its assumptions about wholeness, its hunger for synthesis, its fear of symbolic collapse.

What passes for "healthy" often means believing the right thing at the right time, or not noticing what would disrupt shared meaning. But the one who stays in paradox—who holds the split without identifying with either side—may be closer to the truth of reality than those who appear more integrated.

This is not grandiosity. This is the grief of seeing clearly in a structure that cannot see you back.

Implications

Curved Structure individuals are often misread by traditional models as unintegrated, overly aestheticized, schizoid, or "borderline but organized." In truth, they represent a symbolically saturated, ethically sensitive, and structurally complex position. They live among contradictions not because they cannot resolve them, but because they know resolution is not the task.

Where integration seeks coherence, the Curved Structure curates intensity. Where symptom signals pathology in classical theory, symptom in the Curved Structure may be a gravitational trace of symbolic pressure. Such individuals often appear in analytic work with immense insight, vivid symbolic life, recursive thought patterns, and an uncanny ability to metabolize rupture without foreclosure.

This is not fragmentation. This is curved coherence. It is the structure not of disorder, but of paradox held consciously. It is the psyche metabolizing itself through recursion, witnessing, and refusal.

While the Curved Structure describes a recursive, symbolically saturated stance often misread as fragmentation or excess, it also reflects a structural relation to power and language. Those most fluent in the signifiers of class, education, and cultural dominance may appear "integrated" only because they've learned to foreclose contact with the unknowable. What we often name as psychological normalcy may simply be the ability to perform coherence within dominant symbolic codes—a form of disavowal disguised as stability.

In contrast, those who are structurally marginalized—by race, class, disability, gender, or queerness—may have no choice but to live closer to the limits of symbolization. Without seamless access to the codes that grant legibility, they often navigate experience in ways that are more recursive, more attuned to contradiction, and more honest about the psychic remainder. As Fanon (1952/2008) observed, the colonized subject is required to split between imposed images and lived experience, creating a recursive interiority that the dominant frame misreads as pathology. Glissant (1997) offers a corrective: the right to opacity—the ethical refusal to be made fully knowable or linguistically subdued.

In this light, the Curved Structure is not a disorder of fragmentation, but a structural poetics of survival—an epistemological clarity born of being unable to forget what normative frames are designed to erase.

On the Risk of Not Being Understood

This material is new, unusual, and makes a different demand on the reader; I do not assume comprehension as a precondition for participation. It names something that lives just beyond the reach of most clinical categories: the part of the mind that does not collapse when it splits, the kind of truth that is not rescued by coherence, the form of reality testing that refuses to foreclose contradiction. What I have called the Curved Structure may not appear useful to those who seek clarity, replicability, or diagnostic utility. But some readers may feel an immediate resonance. They will have already stood in this terrain—in the room, in the body, in the trembling space between presence and disappearance—and they will recognize the form before they name it. This structure is not meant to persuade. It is meant to hold what cannot otherwise survive classification.

Figures of the Curved Structure (Selected Lineage)

- Sándor Ferenczi (in his radical sensitivity to trauma and confusion of tongues)
- D. W. Winnicott (late work on paradox and transitional space)
- Michael Eigen (psychic intensity, the undreamt dream, the presence of the infinite)
- Judith Butler (non-coherence and ethical formation)
- Leo Bersani (self-shattering and aesthetic subjectivity)
- Eve Sedgwick (queer performativity and reparative reading)
- José Esteban Muñoz (utopia as anticipatory structure)

- Michel Foucault (dispersed subjectivity and critique of coherence)
- George Atwood (reflexive subjectivity, witnessing grief, symbolic atmosphere)

The inclusion of these names is a gesture of aesthetic and symbolic location, not of ownership or alignment. Some are still living; none were consulted. Their presence here is meant to evoke the multidimensional character of the Curved Structure rather than to claim definitional authority. Like all recursive mappings, this list is partial, porous, and shaped by my own psychic orbit.

Bibliography

Aron, L. (1996). *A meeting of minds: Mutuality in psychoanalysis*. Analytic Press.

Atlas, G. (2015). *The enigma of desire: Sex, longing and belonging in psychoanalysis*. Routledge.

Atlas, G. (2022). *Emotional inheritance: A therapist, her patients, and the legacy of trauma*. Little, Brown Spark.

Atlas, G., & Aron, L. (2017). *Dramatic dialogue*. Routledge.

Atwood, G. (2011). *The abyss of madness*. Routledge.

Atwood, G. E., & Stolorow, R. D. (1984). *Structures of subjectivity: Explorations in psychoanalytic phenomenology and contextualism*. Routledge.

Bakhtin, M. M. (1981). *The dialogic imagination: Four essays* M. Holquist (Ed.) C. Emerson & M. Holquist (Trans.). University of Texas Press.

Barthes, R. (1977). *Image, music, text* S. Heath (Ed.). Fontana Press.

Beck, C. J. (1993). *Nothing special: Living Zen*. Shambhala Publications.

Benjamin, J. (1990a). *The bonds of love: Psychoanalysis, feminism, and the problem of domination*. Pantheon Books.

Benjamin, J. (1990b). An outline of intersubjectivity: The development of recognition. *Psychoanalytic Psychology*, *7*(Suppl.), 33–46.

Benjamin, J. (1995). *Like subjects, love objects: Essays on recognition and sexual difference*. Yale University Press.

Benjamin, J. (1998). *Shadow of the other: Intersubjectivity and gender in psychoanalysis*. Routledge.

Benjamin, J. (2004). Beyond doer and done to: An intersubjective view of thirdness. *The Psychoanalytic Quarterly*, *73*(1), 5–46.

Bersani, L. (2010). *Is the rectum a grave? And other essays*. University of Chicago Press.

Bion, W. R. (1962). *Learning from experience*. Heinemann.

Bion, W. R. (1965). *Transformations*. Heinemann.

Bion, W. R. (1967). *Second thoughts: Selected papers on psychoanalysis*. Karnac.

Bion, W. R. (1970). *Attention and interpretation*. Tavistock Publications.

Bollas, C. (1987). *The shadow of the object: Psychoanalysis of the unthought known*. Columbia University Press.

Bollas, C. (1992). *Being a character: Psychoanalysis and self experience*. Routledge.

Bromberg, P. M. (1998). *Standing in the spaces: Essays on clinical process, trauma, and dissociation*. Analytic Press.

Bromberg, P. M. (2006). *Awakening the dreamer: Clinical journeys*. Analytic Press.

Butler, J. (1997). *The psychic life of power: Theories in subjection.* Stanford University Press.

Butler, J. (2005). *Giving an account of oneself.* Fordham University Press.

Dalai Lama & Varela, F. J. (Eds.). (1997). *Sleeping, dreaming, and dying: An exploration of consciousness.* Wisdom Publications.

Damasio, A. R. (1999). *The feeling of what happens: Body and emotion in the making of consciousness.* Harcourt.

Deleuze, G. (1994). *Difference and repetition* P. Patton (Trans.). Columbia University Press.

Derrida, J. (1976). *Of grammatology* G. C. Spivak (Trans.). Johns Hopkins University Press.

Derrida, J. (1978). *Writing and difference* A. Bass (Trans.). University of Chicago Press.

Derrida, J. (1982). *Margins of philosophy* A. Bass (Trans.). University of Chicago Press.

Donnellan, A. M., Hill, D. A., & Leary, M. R. (2012). Rethinking autism: Implications of sensory and movement differences for understanding and support. *Frontiers in Integrative Neuroscience, 6,* Article 124.

Eigen, M. (1986). *The psychotic core.* Aronson.

Eigen, M. (1993a). *The electrified tightrope.* SUNY Press.

Eigen, M. (1993b). *The psychotic core.* Jason Aronson.

Eigen, M. (1998). *The psychoanalytic mystic.* Free Association Books.

Eigen, M. (2001). *Ecstasy: A way of knowing.* Wesleyan University Press.

Eigen, M. (2004). *The sensitive self.* Wesleyan University Press.

Eigen, M. (2005). *The psychotic core.* Karnac.

Engler, J. (2003). Being somebody and being nobody: A re-examination of the understanding of self in psychoanalysis and Buddhism. In J. D. Safran (Ed.), *Psychoanalysis and Buddhism: An unfolding dialogue* (pp. 35–79). Wisdom Publications.

Epstein, M. (1995). *Thoughts without a thinker: Psychotherapy from a Buddhist perspective.* Basic Books.

Epstein, M. (1998). *Going to pieces without falling apart: A Buddhist perspective on wholeness.* Broadway Books.

Epstein, M. (2007). *Psychotherapy without the self: A Buddhist perspective.* Yale University Press.

Fanon, F. (2008). *Black skin, white masks* R. Philcox (Trans.). Grove Press (Original work published 1952).

Ferenczi, S. (1988). Confusion of tongues between the adults and the child. In J. Dupont (Ed.) M. Balint & N. Z. Jackson (Trans.), *The clinical diary of Sándor Ferenczi* (pp. 156–167). Harvard University Press (Original work written 1932).

Ferenczi, S. (2018). *Final contributions to the problems and methods of psychoanalysis.* Routledge.

Ferro, A. (2006). *Avoiding emotions, living emotions.* Routledge.

Fink, B. (1997). *A clinical introduction to Lacanian psychoanalysis: Theory and technique.* Harvard University Press.

Foucault, M. (1966/1970). *The order of things: An archaeology of the human sciences* A. Sheridan (Trans.). Pantheon Books (Original work published 1966).

Foucault, M. (1977a). *Language, counter-memory, practice: Selected essays and interviews* D. F. Bouchard (Ed.). Cornell University Press.

Foucault, M. (1977b). *Discipline and punish: The birth of the prison* A. Sheridan (Trans.). Pantheon Books

Foucault, M. (1978). *The history of sexuality: Volume 1: An Introduction* R. Hurley (Trans.). Pantheon Books.

Foucault, M. (1988). *Technologies of the self* L. Martin, H. Gutman, & P. Hutton (Eds.). University of Massachusetts Press.

Freud, S. (1900). The interpretation of dreams. In J. Strachey (Ed. & Trans.), *The standard edition of the complete psychological works of Sigmund Freud*, vols 4–5. Hogarth Press.

Freud, S. (1912). Recommendations to physicians practicing psycho-analysis. In J. Strachey (Ed. & Trans.), *The standard edition of the complete psychological works of Sigmund Freud*, vol. 12. Hogarth Press.

Freud, S. (1914a). On narcissism: An introduction. In J. Strachey (Ed. & Trans.), *The standard edition of the complete psychological works of Sigmund Freud*, vol. 14. Hogarth Press.

Freud, S. (1914b). Remembering, repeating and working-through. In J. Strachey (Ed. & Trans.), *The standard edition of the complete psychological works of Sigmund Freud*, vol. 12. Hogarth Press.

Freud, S. (1915). The unconscious. In J. Strachey (Ed. & Trans.), *The standard edition of the complete psychological works of Sigmund Freud*, vol. 14. Hogarth Press.

Freud, S. (1920). Beyond the pleasure principle. In J. Strachey (Ed. & Trans.), *The standard edition of the complete psychological works of Sigmund Freud*, vol. 18. Hogarth Press.

Freud, S. (1923). The ego and the id. In J. Strachey (Ed. & Trans.), *The standard edition of the complete psychological works of Sigmund Freud*, vol. 19. Hogarth Press.

Freud, S. (1925). A note upon the mystic writing-pad. In J. Strachey (Ed. & Trans.), *The standard edition of the complete psychological works of Sigmund Freud*, vol. 19. Hogarth Press.

Freud, S. (1930). Civilization and its discontents. In J. Strachey (Ed. & Trans.), *The standard edition of the complete psychological works of Sigmund Freud*, vol. 21. Hogarth Press.

Freud, S. (1937). Constructions in analysis. In J. Strachey (Ed. & Trans.), *The standard edition of the complete psychological works of Sigmund Freud*, vol. 23. Hogarth Press.

Freud, S. (1953–1974). *The standard edition of the complete psychological works of Sigmund Freud* J. Strachey et al. (Eds.), vols. 1–24. Hogarth Press.

Gallese, V. (2007). The "shared manifold" hypothesis: From mirror neurons to empathy. *Journal of Consciousness Studies*, 8(5–7), 33–50.

Ghent, E. (1990). Masochism, submission, surrender: Masochism as a perversion of surrender. *Contemporary Psychoanalysis*, 26(1), 108–136.

Glissant, E. (1997). *Poetics of relation* B. Wing (Trans.). University of Michigan Press.

Goldman, A. (2012). *Clinical practice at the edge of caring: Affect, action, and analytic process*. Routledge.

Green, A. (1993). *The dead mother: The work of André Green* A. Sheridan (Trans.). Routledge. (Note: Original French 1983; English translation 1993).

Green, A. (1999). *The chains of eros: The sexual in psychoanalysis* A. Weller (Trans.). Karnac Books.

Grotstein, J. S. (2000). *Who is the dreamer who dreams the dream? A study of psychic presences*. Routledge.

Hacking, I. (1995). *Rewriting the soul: Multiple personality and the sciences of memory.* Princeton University Press.

Harris, A. (2005). Gender as soft assembly. *Studies in Gender and Sexuality*, 6(1), 87–120.

Harris, A. (2009). *Gender as soft assembly*. Routledge.

Heidegger, M. (1962). *Being and time* J. Macquarrie & E. Robinson (Trans.). Harper & Row (Original work published 1927).

Heidegger, M. (1977). *Poetry, language, thought* A. Hofstadter (Trans.). Harper & Row (Original work published 1971).

Herman, J. L. (1992). *Trauma and recovery.* Basic Books

Hoffman, I. Z. (1998). *Ritual and spontaneity in the psychoanalytic process: A dialectical-constructivist view.* Routledge.

Kapp, S. K., Gillespie-Lynch, K., Sherman, L. E., & Hutman, T. (2013). Deficit, difference, or both? Autism and neurodiversity. *Developmental Psychology*, 49(1), 59–71.

Kara-Ivanov Kaniel, R. (2013, May 21). Therapist from the depths: A conversation with Michael Eigen. Tikkun. https://www.tikkun.org/therapist-from-the-depths-a-conversation-with-michael-eigen/

Kernberg, O. F. (1975). *Borderline conditions and pathological narcissism.* Jason Aronson.

Kernberg, O. F. (1984). *Severe personality disorders: Psychotherapeutic strategies.* Yale University Press.

Klein, M. (1946). Notes on some schizoid mechanisms. *International Journal of Psychoanalysis*, 27(3–4), 99–110.

Klein, M. (1952). Some theoretical conclusions regarding the emotional life of the infant. In M. Klein, P. Heimann, S. Isaacs, & J. Rivière (Eds.), *Developments in psycho-analysis* (pp. 198–236). Hogarth Press.

Klein, M. (1957). On the development of mental functioning. *International Journal of Psychoanalysis*, 38, 284–293.

Klein, M. (1975). *Love, guilt, and reparation and other works 1921–1945.* Free Press.

Kristeva, J. (1989). *Black sun: Depression and melancholia* L. S. Roudiez (Trans.). Columbia University Press.

Lacan, J. (1953–1973). *Écrits and Seminar XI: The four fundamental concepts of psychoanalysis.*

Lacan, J. (1977). *Écrits: A selection.* W. W. Norton & Company.

Lacan, J. (1978). *The four fundamental concepts of psychoanalysis (Seminar XI).* W. W. Norton & Company.

Lacan, J. (1991). *The seminar of Jacques Lacan: Book II, The ego in Freud's theory and in the technique of psychoanalysis, 1954–1955* (J.-A. Miller, Ed.; S. Tomaselli, Trans.). W. W. Norton & Company.

Lacan, J. (1998a). *The four fundamental concepts of psychoanalysis* J.-A. Miller (Ed.) A. Sheridan (Trans.). W. W. Norton & Company (Original work published 1973).

Lacan, J. (1998b). *Écrits* (1st complete ed.) B. Fink (Trans.). W. W. Norton & Company (Original work published 1966).

Laplanche, J. (1999). *Essays on otherness* J. Fletcher (Trans.). Routledge.

Levinas, E. (1969). *Totality and infinity: An essay on exteriority* A. Lingis (Trans.). Duquesne University Press.

Loewald, H. W. (1960). On the therapeutic action of psycho-analysis. *International Journal of Psycho-Analysis*, 41, 16–33.

Loewald, H. W. (1975). Psychoanalysis as an art and the fantasy character of the psychoanalytic situation. *Journal of the American Psychoanalytic Association*, 23(2), 277–299.

Loewald, H. W. (1978a). Psychoanalysis and the history of the individual. *Psychoanalytic Quarterly*, *47*(2), 236–255.

Loewald, H. W. (1978b). Psychoanalysis as a process. *Psychoanalytic Quarterly*, *47*(3), 431–449.

Loewald, H. W. (1978c). Primary process, secondary process, and reality. *Psychoanalytic Quarterly*, *47*, 43–64.

Loewald, H. W. (1978d). Primary process, secondary process, and language. *Psychoanalytic Quarterly*, *47*(1), 28–54.

Loewald, H. W. (1978e). *Psychoanalysis and the history of the individual*. International Universities Press.

Loewald, H. W. (1980). *Papers on psychoanalysis*. Yale University Press.

Magid, B. (2002). *Ordinary mind: Exploring the common ground of Zen and psychotherapy*. Wisdom Publications.

McWilliams, N. (2011). *Psychoanalytic diagnosis: Understanding personality structure in the clinical process* (2nd ed.). Guilford Press.

Merleau-Ponty, M. (1962). *Phenomenology of perception* C. Smith (Trans.). Routledge and Kegan Paul.

Merleau-Ponty, M. (1968). *The visible and the invisible* A. Lingis (Trans.). Northwestern University Press.

Mitchell, S. A. (1993). *Hope and dread in psychoanalysis*. Basic Books.

Mottron, L. (2021). A radical change in our autism research strategy is needed: Back to prototypes. *Autism Research*, *14*(10), 2213–2220.

Mottron, L., Dawson, M., Soulières, I., Hubert, B., & Burack, J. (2006). Enhanced perceptual functioning in autism: An update, and eight principles of autistic perception. *Journal of Autism and Developmental Disorders*, *36*(1), 27–43.

Muñoz, J. E. (2009). *Cruising utopia: The then and there of queer futurity*. NYU Press.

Ogden, T. H. (1992a). *The primitive edge of experience*. Jason Aronson.

Ogden, T. H. (1992b). *The matrix of the mind: Object relations and the psychoanalytic dialogue*. Jason Aronson.

Ogden, T. H. (1994). The analytic third: Working with intersubjective clinical facts. *International Journal of Psychoanalysis*, *75*(1), 3–19.

Ogden, T. H. (1997a). Reverie and interpretation. *The Psychoanalytic Quarterly*, *66*(4), 567–595.

Ogden, T. H. (1997b). Reverie and metaphor: Some thoughts on how I work as a psychoanalyst. *International Journal of Psychoanalysis*, *78*(3), 719–732.

Ogden, T. H. (2004). *This art of psychoanalysis: Dreaming undreamt dreams and interrupted cries*. Routledge.

Ogden, T. H. (2005). *This art of psychoanalysis: Dreaming undreamt dreams and interrupted cries.* Routledge.

Orange, D. M. (1995). *Emotional understanding: Studies in psychoanalytic epistemology*. Guilford Press.

Orange, D. M. (2009). *Thinking for clinicians: Philosophical resources for contemporary psychoanalysis and the humanistic psychotherapies*. Routledge.

Panksepp, J. (1998). *Affective neuroscience: The foundations of human and animal emotions*. Oxford University Press.

Panksepp, J., & Biven, L. (2012). *The archaeology of mind: Neuroevolutionary origins of human emotions*. W. W. Norton & Company.

Phillips, A. (1993). *On kissing, tickling, and being bored*. Harvard University Press.

Phillips, A. (2012). *Missing out: In praise of the unlived life*. Farrar, Straus & Giroux.

Rubin, J. B. (1996). *Psychotherapy and Buddhism: Toward an integration*. Issues in the Practice of Psychology series. Springer.

Sacks, O. (1995). *An anthropologist on Mars: Seven paradoxical tales*. Alfred A. Knopf.

Safran, J. D. (2003). *Psychoanalysis and Buddhism: An unfolding dialogue*. Wisdom Publications.

Safran, J. D., & Muran, J. C. (2000). *Negotiating the therapeutic alliance: A relational treatment guide*. Guilford Press.

Sedgwick, E. K. (2003). *Touching feeling: Affect, pedagogy, performativity*. Duke University Press.

Siegel, D. J. (1999). *The developing mind: How relationships and the brain interact to shape who we are*. Guilford Press.

Stern, D. B. (1997). *Unformulated experience: From dissociation to imagination in psychoanalysis*. Analytic Press.

Stern, D. B. (2010). *Partners in thought: Working with unformulated experience, dissociation, and enactment*. Routledge.

Stern, D. B. (2015). *Relational freedom: Emergent properties of the interpersonal field*. Routledge.

Stern, D. N. (1985). *The interpersonal world of the infant: A view from psychoanalysis and developmental psychology*. Basic Books.

Stern, D. N. (2004). *The present moment in psychotherapy and everyday life*. W. W. Norton &Company.

Stolorow, R. D., & Atwood, G. E. (1992). *Contexts of being: The intersubjective foundations of psychological life*. Analytic Press.

Trungpa, C. (1973). *Cutting through spiritual materialism*. Shambhala Publications.

Tulku Urgyen Rinpoche. (1999). *As it is: The instructions of Dzogchen master Tulku Urgyen* E. Pema Kunsang (Trans.). Rangjung Yeshe Publications.

Van der Kolk, B. A. (2014). *The body keeps the score: Brain, mind, and body in the healing of trauma*. Viking Press.

Williams, D. L., Goldstein, G., & Minshew, N. J. (2006). Neuropsychologic functioning in children with autism: Further evidence for disordered complex information-processing. *Child Neuropsychology: A Journal on Normal and Abnormal Development in Childhood and Adolescence, 12*(4–5), 279–298.

Winnicott, D. W. (1958). The capacity to be alone. In D. W. Winnicott (Ed.), *The maturational processes and the facilitating environment* (pp. 29–36). Karnac.

Winnicott, D. W. (1960a). Ego distortion in terms of true and false self. In D. W. Winnicott (Ed.), *The maturational processes and the facilitating environment* (pp. 140–152). International Universities Press.

Winnicott, D. W. (1960b). The theory of the parent–infant relationship. *The International Journal of Psycho-Analysis, 41*, 585–595.

Winnicott, D. W. (1965). *The maturational processes and the facilitating environment: Studies in the theory of emotional development*. International Universities Press.

Winnicott, D. W. (1967). The location of cultural experience. *International Journal of Psychoanalysis, 48*(3), 368–372.

Winnicott, D. W. (1971). *Playing and reality*. Tavistock Publications.

Wittgenstein, L. (1953). *Philosophical investigations* G. E. M. Anscombe (Trans.). Basil Blackwell.

Index

For Product Safety Concerns and Information please contact our EU
representative GPSR@taylorandfrancis.com
Taylor & Francis Verlag GmbH, Kaufingerstraße 24, 80331 München, Germany